# Praise for *Aches and Gains*

"When you're in pain and you are desperate for an expert, Dr. Christo is just that. He's also filled with compassion and a wonderful bedside manner. Pain is inevitable but Dr. Christo helps relieve your suffering."

**—Naomi Judd, singer, author, and humanitarian**

"There's no other book like it—eye-opening, motivational, and powerful. Dr. Paul Christo responds to this tremendous problem with new insights and reliable options. His care and good will for all of us in pain shines brightly, and his desire to bring forth the best and highest in everybody permeates his work."

**—Clay Walker, multi-platinum country music artist**

"*Aches and Gains* offers far-reaching therapeutic options for pain relief. Dr. Christo, and his interesting patients and prominent personalities from all walks of life, carefully guide anybody dealing with this multidimensional disease through its complexities in a remarkably understandable and compelling manner. Pain can strike us at any time in life. We are now fortunate to have a book that both serves as a beacon of hope and as a source of many evidence-based and emerging treatments that can really help."

**—Rollin M. Gallagher, MD, MPH, editor-in-chief, Pain Medicine; past president, American Academy of Pain Medicine**

"This book is a terrific resource that everybody should pay attention to. It's cutting-edge, easy to read, and inspirational. Dr. Paul Christo gives you the tools to move beyond your pain and into the realm of healthy living. Believe me, he is talking to YOU! I am honored to be a part of this movement!"

**—Gunnar Peterson, Beverly Hills–based personal trainer**

"Dr. Christo has created a brilliant, comprehensive guide into the world of pain packed with research-based information while also dispensing his wise, compassionate guidance. Every person will need to navigate the realm of pain in some capacity at sometime in their lives. This stellar work gives them an invaluable roadmap."

**—Kathleen Hall, PhD, CEO, The Stress Institute**

"If you suffer from pain, know somebody who does, or want to limit your chances of de it, *Aches and Gains* is a must read. Dr. Christo covers this universal problem with great and compassion."

**—Coach Lou Holtz, 2008 College Football Hall of Fame Coach, r ESPN analyst, motivational speaker, New York Times best-selli author**

"Dr. Paul Christo's insightful book *Aches and Gains* is a breath of fresh air, particularly at a time when we, as a nation, are experiencing an opioid-addiction catastrophe. This book offers true healing and 'another therapeutic option' without the dangerous effects of harsh drugs. Human beings will do anything to take away pain. It is refreshing to read a book that offers another path. If you are experiencing pain, I highly suggest you read Dr. Christo's book before you consider any treatments."

***—Suzanne Somers, actress and best-selling author***

"*Aches and Gains* is a great resource for patients suffering with chronic pain. Dr. Christo shares his clinical and scientific expertise in a way that is engaging, informative, and empathetic, and doesn't focus only on pills or surgery. The stories of famous individuals with pain are unique and informative, and demonstrate that pain can impact anyone. I think anyone reading this book will have a greater understanding of the causes of pain and strategies for managing it—giving them the tools to ultimately get back their lives."

***—Roger Chou, MD, professor of medicine, division of General Internal Medicine and Geriatrics, Oregon Health & Science University***

"Dr. Christo's *Aches and Gains* provides an incredibly comprehensive overview of the many forms that pain can take, how it impacts the lives of its sufferers, and, most inspiringly, the multiple treatment options that are available for the tens of millions who suffer from chronic pain. Importantly, Dr. Christo strikes an impressive balance between conveying information that will be helpful to people experiencing pain while staying true to the current state of pain science. He artfully intertwines stories from real people with evidence-based information to both inspire and educate the reader. This book will help arm people in pain with knowledge and hope, empowering them to take control over their pain and their lives."

***—Roger B. Fillingim, PhD, distinguished professor and director of the University of Florida's Pain Research & Intervention Center of Excellence***

"Dr. Christo gives a truly unique and balanced overview of all potentially valid possibilities for those who suffer and have the desire to take back their function and quality of life. I would recommend this book for anyone who suffers from pain, who has loved ones in this condition, or would like to know things we can do to help this terrible problem for our society."

***—Timothy R. Deer, MD, president, International Neuromodulation Society***

"In the area of pain management, Dr. Paul Christo has devoted his career to helping those in need, and making a difference to improve their lives. His new book *Aches and Gains* is a wonderful culmination of his vast experience and knowledge. I recommend it as a helpful tool in pain management."

***—Tim Janis, renowned composer***

# Aches and Gains

## A Comprehensive Guide to Overcoming Your Pain

### Paul J. Christo, MD

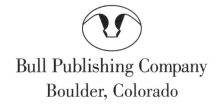

Bull Publishing Company
Boulder, Colorado

Bull Publishing Company

P.O. Box 1377

Boulder, CO  USA  80306

www.bullpub.com

**Library of Congress Cataloging-in-Publication Data**

Christo, Paul J.

ISBN 978-1-945188-09-1 (paperback)

Interior design and production by Dovetail Publishing Services

Cover design and production by Shannon Bodie, Bookwise Design

*For those yearning to make their lives greater, richer, and healthier.*

*For my family—Dana, Ashton, and Francesca; and my parents.*

# Contents

# Part I
# Understanding and Treating Your Pain

# Part II
# Medical Therapies for Pain: Traditional and Innovative

# Part III
# Integrative Therapies for Pain

# Featured Celebrity Stories
## (listed in order of appearance in the book)

**Jennifer Grey**    Star of *Dirty Dancing* and *Ferris Bueller's Day Off.* Jennifer takes us down her path of overcoming the neck pain that almost paralyzed her.

**Ty Warner**    The creator of the Beanie Baby. Ty shares his triumphs over Tech Neck and the creation of a simple toy called the "Peek-A-Boo."

**Gunnar Peterson**    Fitness trainer to the stars. Gunnar highlights effective exercise strategies for pain relief.

**Joe Montana**    Legendary quarterback. Joe describes how he successfully treated his arthritic knee pain.

**Jerry Mathers**    Star of *Leave It to Beaver.* Jerry shares the lifestyle changes he made to combat painful diabetic neuropathy.

**Clay Walker**    Country music star. Clay reveals his strategies for getting past the pain of multiple sclerosis.

**Peggy Fleming**    Figure skater and Olympic gold medalist. Peggy talks about moving beyond sports pain.

**Michael McCreary**    Former Baltimore Ravens defensive end. Michael discusses how managing pain is a team sport.

**Mark Peel**    Executive chef and owner of Bombo. Mark shares how carpal tunnel syndrome, thoracic outlet syndrome, and low back pain have not prevented him from thriving in his career.

**Prodigy**    Rapper and author. Prodigy describes how he overcame the pain of sickle cell anemia.

**Ally Hilfiger**    Daughter of fashion designer, Tommy Hilfiger. Ally chronicles her unbelievable journey through a decade of pain and confusion from undiagnosed Lyme disease.

**Lisa Swayze**    Wife of the late actor Patrick Swayze. Lisa provides a moving account of caring for Patrick during the last 22 months of his life with pancreatic cancer.

# Foreword

Four months before I graduated from the United States Naval Academy, I suffered my first bout of multiple sclerosis (MS), losing 80% vision in my left eye. One of the many topics that Dr. Christo's book covers so well is that feeling of embarrassment when pain creeps into your life. I was 22 years old at the time, in the best shape of my life, lifting weights and looking good. I didn't want to admit to anyone—including myself—that something was wrong with me.

If I'd caught the problem back then, maybe I could have nipped it in the bud, or at least started on a treatment regimen to mitigate its symptoms. Instead, I let it fester. It wasn't until 1999, after I felt a sharp and chronic pain in my feet, that I finally took action, consulting with various doctors, one of whom delivered the shocking news: He said that I had MS I'd be in a wheelchair in four years, and dead by age 57.

Another feeling that Dr. Christo writes about so eloquently is the feeling of hopelessness that goes hand in hand with chronic pain. Lying awake every night in tears from the pain, as I counted down to 57, wondering if I should expedite the inevitable—it felt like that moment when you get to the top of a hill, look up, and see this impossible mountain. I realized I had a choice to make: I could spend the rest of my life feeling sorry for myself, or I could look at my illness as a call to action and start climbing.

Dr. Christo outlines all the tools you need for the climb, beginning with seeking help from loved ones. "The emotional distress and helplessness that often accompany pain," he writes, "can be just as destructive as the physical aspects of the pain."

He also writes about taking your health into your own hands, which, for me, has been essential. After my diagnosis, I made dramatic changes to my diet and exercise routine. I poured myself into an intense treatment regimen and sought out experimental therapies. I appreciate Dr. Christo's thoroughly researched section on cannabis, including various ingestion methods, its complex structure, and its therapeutic effects. After doctors prescribed opioids for my pain, triggering a severe addiction and irreversible damage to my body, I was told to try cannabis as part of my treatment. For me, cannabis has been more than a treatment for the pain. It's become a lifesaver.

Finally, as Dr. Christo advises, you can never lose hope. That's easier said than done, especially when the pain keeps coming back, again and again; but it's necessary. Personally, I found hope—and purpose—in sharing my experience with others by writing books, promoting healthy living, and starting an MS Foundation. Helping others, I've found, gets me "out of my head" and gives me a reason to wake up in the morning, to keep battling the pain, and to continue climbing that mountain.

*Montel Williams*

# Preface

## The Cost of Pain

Throughout the world, pain is poorly controlled—80% of the world population has little or no access to treatment for moderate or severe pain. In fact, the World Health Organization estimates that pain threatens to condemn one out of every 10 people alive today to die a painful death. It's that serious. Pain touches all of us during our lives and has become a pressing humanitarian crisis.

Chronic pain affects 116 million U.S. adults, and 40% of people living in developing countries. It doesn't spare the more vulnerable members of society, affecting 20% of all children and increasing in prevalence in senior adults. Chronic pain is growing in magnitude as well. Those surviving HIV, cancer, and cardiovascular disease are now able to live longer lives, but find themselves living a poorer quality of life due to continual pain from their disease or from interventions needed to treat the disease, such as chemotherapy, radiation therapy, or surgery.

Sadly, not everybody makes it. Compared to those without chronic pain, people living in pain are twice as likely to commit suicide. Pain not only takes lives and debilitates individuals and families, but it costs the U.S. economy more than half a trillion dollars annually. And despite these alarming facts, research funding is lower for the study of pain in the United States than it is for any other chronic health problem. The quest for relief continues, however.

Pain relief is a multi-billion dollar industry. Each year, millions of Americans empty their wallets for pain medications, surgery, and various other therapies in a desperate attempt to alleviate their symptoms. Many turn to alternative medicine—from acupuncture and yoga to dietary supplements and aromatherapy. Still others use illegal substances or become entangled in other addictive behaviors, searching in vain for relief from suffering they do not understand. Sometimes the quest to ease pain can become more frustrating than the pain itself.

But it doesn't have to be this way. Recent advancements in both medicine and technology have revolutionized the way we understand and treat pain. Pain may be part of life, but chronic pain and the frustration it brings with it do not have to be part of your daily experience.

## The Experience of Pain

An individual's experience with pain is as unique as his or her fingerprints. As a pain medicine specialist at the Johns Hopkins Hospital in Baltimore, Maryland, I have seen firsthand that pain can manifest so differently—sharp or dull, severe or muted, pounding or burning. It can occur intermittently or all the time, touching one part of the body or every part. None of us experience pain in quite the same way, but no matter who you are, when you experience pain, it is almost always impossible to ignore.

Pain is *supposed* to get our attention and often serves a vital function in our survival. After all, if the nerves in your fingers didn't immediately alert you that the stove was hot, you could get some serious burns before you pulled your hand away. The memory of the pain also reminds you not to get too close next time. Pain plays a role in helping us assess illness as well as injury. That sharp pain in your chest tells you that your cold has progressed to the point where you need to see your doctor.

But pain can take on a life of its own. Think of a home security system: The alarm goes off to alert you that your home and possessions may be in danger. But what would happen if the alarm malfunctioned and couldn't be disarmed? Its constant blaring could make your home uninhabitable. Chronic pain behaves the same way—a siren that persists long past the point of doing any good, interfering with every aspect of life. It becomes a *disease itself*, rather than just a symptom of another condition.

Chronic pain is a special kind of pain. It is a complex process of changes in and reorganization of the central nervous system (brain and spinal cord). It's typically defined as pain lasting for three months or more. We're realizing that the environment, genes, and imbalances in neurotransmitters can all contribute to the origin of chronic pain. In some ways, chronic pain is like Parkinson's disease or Alzheimer's disease. The progression of all of these disorders leads to substantial changes to nerves in the brain and spinal cord. Chronic pain is unlike these conditions as well though; we're learning that we may be able to restore normal or near normal nerve function once chronic pain has developed by implementing effective treatments.

As the pain-relief industry has grown, it has become more and more challenging to distinguish the real solutions from the snake oil. Some "experts" market potions and techniques that have absolutely no science behind them. And at the same time, far too many authentic medical doctors are completely unaware of the wide range of tools and techniques scientifically proven to help patients combat and defeat pain. I know, because I was one of those doctors: I knew everything medical school taught me about how to treat my patients, but I knew very little about how to help them with their pain.

## Why I Wrote This Book

Although I knew I wanted to go into medicine from a young age, my journey took some interesting detours along the way. I grew up in Moraga, California, a suburb of San Francisco. Soon after entering high school, I organized a squad of Boy Scouts to feed the hungry at a soup kitchen in Oakland. Organizing this event was the last step in meeting all of the requirements for the rank of Eagle Scout. I felt confident in my ability to pull it off until I learned that the shelter was expecting 300 people that day!

With a lot of organizing and delegating, I was able to purchase, prepare, and distribute food to all of those people and earn the rank of Eagle Scout. It was a tremendously moving experience for many reasons, but my heart was particularly affected by meeting the many homeless people who walked with a limp or had visible wounds on their bodies. Some had dried blood on their faces or limbs. Others winced as they sat down. Most were middle-aged and alone, but some brought their family members—young children or parents—all of whom suffered from the pain of hunger. This was more than a day of service for me. It was a window into a world of suffering that I never knew existed.

I often wonder whether that one day as a young Scout led me to choose a life of easing pain—pain resulting from visible wounds as well as unseen sources. During the promotion ceremony, my scoutmaster said something that has stuck with me since, "Scouting is far more than fun in the outdoors. Scouting is a way of life. Scouting is growing into responsible manhood, learning to be of service to others." My scoutmaster modeled this service as a leader and a professional. He was a cardiologist and the example he set strengthened my own personal desire to become a physician. I wanted to continue serving others, but I wanted to be able to offer those in need more than just a ladle of soup.

My college years gave me the chance to volunteer on the suicide prevention hotline for the city of South Bend, Indiana, and later serve as a summer intern-scholar on two adolescent mental health units in Green Bay, Wisconsin. Though I had set my sights on medical school, I elected to spend one year working as a chemist for a medical diagnostics company called Microgenics Corporation. The company was filled with ambitious college graduates eagerly pursuing careers in science. This time greatly enhanced my teamwork, negotiation, and organizational skills, which have served me very well as a doctor and especially as a pain specialist.

Medical school offered me the opportunity to work as a research fellow at the National Institutes of Health (NIH) in Washington, D. C. While working in the Clinical Brain Disorders Branch, I helped develop a novel approach for analyzing the magnetic resonance imaging (MRI) brain images of schizophrenic twins. I was poised to become a neuropsychiatrist, like my mentor at the NIH. But like all medical students, I was required to rotate through various medical specialties, and my time with anesthesiologists during my fourth year of medical school changed the course of my career forever.

I was intrigued with the procedures I saw used in the operating room, such as nerve blocks, spinals, epidurals, applied physiology and pharmacology. I was amazed by the powerful pain-relieving effects of morphine given to patients intravenously during surgery. I could watch patients' heart rates and blood pressure drop and their breathing become slower and deeper as they drifted peacefully into a state of calm. By the end of my rotation in the operating room, my focus had shifted to anesthesiology and analgesia.

My interest in pain medicine intensified during my internship. I treated many patients in the clinic for chronic obstructive pulmonary disease (COPD), pneumonia, and hypertension with reasonable success. However, I often felt helpless when treating patients suffering from chronic back pain, arthritic pain, or neuropathic pain. Few of the nonsteroidal anti-inflammatory drugs (NSAIDs), such as ibuprofen (Motrin) or naproxen (Aleve), that I recommended during this period were able to bring true relief to these painful conditions. I knew opioids would alleviate the pain more effectively, but I never felt comfortable prescribing them, even short-acting ones such as oxycodone (Percocet) or hydrocodone (Vicodin). Like doctors today, many physicians back then wanted to avoid opioids but really didn't know what else to use when the usual drugs failed.

As a physician, nothing is more frustrating than watching your patients suffer and feeling like you can't do anything about it. As I gained more clinical experience, some patients would tell me how opioids were "life-saving," while others wanted nothing to do with them and feared addiction. Pain was everywhere and on everyone's mind. Yet, as a new doctor, I received no formal education on pain care. Furthermore, I had no knowledge of pain-relieving injection treatments, implantable devices, neuropathic medications, cognitive behavioral therapies, or the physical restoration methods that can be so critical to alleviating chronic pain.

In short, even after I became a doctor, I felt ill-prepared to care for people in pain. Unfortunately, I have found that this is the norm and not the exception among healthcare professionals. Very few doctors understand the basics of pain diagnosis and treatment any better than I

did as an intern. This lack of knowledge and experience on the part of physicians results in unnecessary and prolonged suffering for many patients.

Today, I treat patients who are experiencing all kinds of pain, and I educate healthcare professionals and pain sufferers all over the country about the vast array of methods available for pain control. While raising awareness about the under-treatment of pain, I have had the opportunity to lead many educational programs during regional and national pain conferences, to speak at national and international medical meetings, and to be a an investigator in research projects published in peer-reviewed journals. I've also served on advisory committees for national pain organizations; chaired annual pain medicine conferences for pain specialists and primary care physicians; consulted for the development and expansion of a pain center in the Middle East; and mentored students interested in pain medicine and research. I've even served as the pain expert for the Web Chat Series on Pain Management for the Tribune newspapers and made guest appearances on various radio and television programs. In short, I've not only been able to help my own patients conquer their pain, I've been able to reach out to other healthcare professionals and the general public.

## Educating the Healers

My life's work is focused on improving the lives of people in pain through clinical care, education, and clinical investigation. The education component is multifaceted, and it begins with the physician population. Despite considerable gains in diagnostic and therapeutic approaches to pain, for many people, that chronic pain alarm system just keeps blaring day and night. Until our doctors are better educated about these new advancements, countless patients will continue to suffer from treatable pain across the country and throughout the world. We always need to do more research, but we also need to make sure that clinicians can easily access the results of the research we've already conducted. We must continually improve clinicians' overall knowledge of pain diagnosis and treatment to alleviate unnecessary suffering. A critical step toward this goal is empowering physicians to partner with patients along the way, to listen to them and advocate for them.

Although there is still tremendous work to do, I have seen many encouraging developments over the past several years. My position as a speaker and educator has enabled me to train physicians from a variety of medical backgrounds—such as physiatry (rehabilitation physicians), anesthesiology, neurology and rheumatology—in state-of-the-art and evidence-based diagnostic and therapeutic approaches to managing pain. Many of my trainees have expanded pain programs in other academic settings or private practice settings, and some have even created new pain centers.

Medical residents who rotate through our pain treatment center are empowered to make informed decisions for pain patients in the operating room, hospital setting, or in outpatient clinics. As greater numbers of trainees complete our program, more physicians will have the skills to improve treatment for patients with pain and serve as compassionate advocates for pain education.

## Educating the Public

As gratifying as it is to educate fellow doctors and healthcare workers in cutting-edge pain management techniques,

I have also learned that there is a tremendous need to educate the public. Patients who learn about the options available to them can work much more effectively with their healthcare providers to control and eliminate pain. Both policymakers and the public need to be aware that chronic pain is a *legitimate medical condition*. The recognition of this fact fosters greater access to pain care, reduces the stigma associated with chronic pain, and promotes effective research. When pain is treated as a legitimate concern, chronic pain patients are better able to become active participants in their own care, chronicle the effects of pain-relieving medications and procedures, and participate in multidisciplinary treatment options such as mind-body therapies and various methods of physical restoration.

The more I began to share information about pain relief and management with general audiences, the more I learned how crucial it is to dispel some extremely popular myths surrounding pain and its treatment. These include:

- Myth: Pain is not a valid medical condition.
- Myth: Pain medications like morphine always lead to addiction.
- Myth: Pain builds character and is simply a "part of life."
- Myth: Healthcare professionals can easily identify and quantify a patient's pain experience.

In addition to multiple media and public speaking appearances, I began a weekly radio talk show in 2011 that is now nationally syndicated on Sirius XM Radio. The program, called *Aches and Gains*, highlights compelling stories of people who have found relief, shares information about cutting-edge treatments from contributing experts, and suggests ways that people in pain can improve their daily lives. Several celebrities with pain, including Joe Montana, Naomi Judd, Montel Williams, the late Maya Angelou, and Jennifer Grey, have brought their own stories of success to the show. Their stories make us realize that nobody is immune to pain, but together we can overcome it.

I wrote this book as an extension of my work to ensure that everyone has an opportunity to learn about the newest and best methods for diagnosing and relieving pain. My goal is to make all the relevant medical information comprehensible for the general public so that you can understand what is going on in your body and what to do about it.

If you or a loved one suffers from poorly controlled pain, this book is about learning to live either pain free or with effective, practical pain management. This book is for anyone who currently suffers from pain and it is also for anyone who is concerned about developing pain in the future. Since pain can strike us at any stage of life, I cover ways to treat pain from infancy to old age.

While no book can properly diagnose your condition or replace your primary care doctor or local pain specialist, I have done my best to address the pain you're feeling, explain it, and offer possibilities for relief, so that you can live the life you were meant to live.

# Acknowledgments

I'd like to acknowledge the perpetual encouragement of my friend and mentor, Mark Hubbard. As an entrepreneur and media-savvy individual, Mark has listened, provided guidance, and then shared his connections. He has been an invaluable resource for creating the radio show from which this book was conceived. It is also important to thank my many radio show guests who have shared their stories of overcoming hardships so that others may benefit. I'm also appreciative of the creative force of Ty Ford, friend and producer. Special thanks to my editor, Erin Mulligan for her critical review and suggestions on the manuscript. I wish to extend my appreciation to my colleagues, past and present at the Johns Hopkins Blaustein Pain Treatment Center for their training and collegiality. Finally, I'm indebted to my wife, Dana for her generosity and self-sacrifice. She made this book possible.

# Introduction

## Why This Book?

This book is designed to provide a down-to-earth understanding of painful conditions that many of us will experience in life. It can serve as your guide to learning about your pain, how to prevent your pain from continuing, and what to do if your pain becomes chronic. It provides options for supporting a loved one in pain and how to cope if you have pain yourself.

I've distilled important evidence from research findings, added recommendations from my expertise as a pain specialist, and combined these with insightful suggestions from contributing experts and success stories from guests on my radio show, *Aches and Gains*. These guests include celebrities, well-respected experts, and everyday people—all have valid experiences and make worthwhile suggestions about overcoming pain.

A special feature of this book includes links to specific radio shows that correspond to the topics covered in each chapter. Listening to the shows will supplement your understanding and expand your learning about a particular condition. They all aired live on Sirius XM Radio and were subsequently made into podcasts. Each show is easily downloaded to your smartphone or computer.

Interspersed throughout the book are real stories of celebrity guests from my radio show who have overcome their pain: sports figures such as Joe Montana; actors such as Jennifer Grey and Jerry Mathers, The Beaver; music stars such as Naomi Judd, Clay Walker, and Prodigy; Ally Hilfiger, producer, artist, and daughter of fashion designer Tommy Hilfiger; executive chef Mark Peel; composer Tim Janis; talk show host Montel Williams; and Lisa Swayze, wife of the late actor Patrick Swayze. There are also revealing accounts of Elvis Presley and President John F. Kennedy. Each of their stories reminds us that pain touches everybody, and like them, we can overcome pain too.

## Organization of the Book

The book is organized into three parts. The first part, Understanding and Treating Your Pain, delves into common pain conditions and how best to treat them. The second part, Medical Therapies for Pain: Traditional and Innovative, concentrates on conventional as well as less known medications used to ease pain and then launches into the exciting world of pain-relieving devices and the "brave new world" of regenerative therapies such as stem cells. Finally, the third part, Integrative Therapies for Pain, examines the benefits of modifying everyday activities such as diet and sleep in order to control pain, and also introduces the reader to the realm of mind-body and spiritual practices, which can be surprisingly effective as pain managing strategies.

## General Strategies for Overcoming Pain

Many patients want a road map for overcoming pain. There is no single path, but there are some steps and strategies that can help you get your life back from chronic pain.

- *Step 1:* A good practical first step in gaining control of any type of pain is keeping a pain journal. In this journal, note the triggers, the quality of the pain, the pain's duration, and any associated physiological responses, such as sweating or memory problems. Keep note of how your mood changes and whether you find yourself missing out on activities. Also keep track of anything that makes the pain better.

- *Step 2:* Bring your pain journal to your doctor or healthcare professional. Share how your pain began and how it has influenced your life, and mention all previous treatments whether they have helped or not.

- *Step 3:* While you work with your healthcare team to address your pain, make sure you are also doing all you can at home to stay as healthy as possible. This step involves implementing the everyday suggestions from this book about eating healthy, anti-inflammatory foods, exercising, managing your stress, and optimizing your sleep. Most doctors don't discuss the value of these strategies in appointments, so I have described them in the book for you to incorporate yourself. Even if they reduce your pain by just 25%, they are moving you closer to your goal of feeling more in charge of your life and making a healthy change.

- *Step 4:* Possess the personal force and belief that you can improve. This will advance your upward progress. I have seen optimistic patients gain from cultivating a positive attitude when others without it out lag behind. See yourself feeling better and doing things you want to do. Have this image in your mind continually. This stabilizes your path to wellness. Without a positive attitude, the disappointments tend to crush your spirit. It's like a badly built house with walls that are not strong enough to sustain the roof. If the walls are unstable, the roof crumbles down and the house falls into ruins. Strengthen the walls with a never-ending belief in creating a new self, of being more than you are now.

- *Step 5:* Ask for help and be open to treatments. Don't eliminate recommendations based on what you have heard from friends or the Internet. Inform yourself of the facts and don't stop learning about your condition and your pain until you find the relief you need. Relief may come from cutting-edge treatments or holistic methods of pain relief. Or a combination of techniques may achieve the most striking result. If you are not looking, you won't find help or relief.

## An Important Message about Caregiving

Take care of yourself if you are taking care of someone else in pain. Many people care for a family member or friend in chronic pain. They take them to medical appointments, help them get dressed and bathe, prepare meals, clean the house, and maintain a job. Dealing with anger, depression and suicidal thoughts, anxiety, and withdrawal from life on the part of the patient in pain is taxing for any caregiver. The entire process exacts a substantial emotional and physical toll. Make sure you carve out time for yourself by taking breaks, participating in support groups, or getting somebody else to step in from time to time.

## No One Is Immune to Pain, but Together We Can Overcome It

Pain can strike at any time, from infancy to older age. Chronic pain can gradually chip away at our capacity to enjoy even the most basic pleasures in life and dissolve our ability to accomplish our dreams. The key to overcoming pain rests in taking ownership of your own health, not giving up, and reaching out to experts for guidance. I hope this book will draw back some of the many veils that can cover new opportunities for feeling better, opportunities that will make a difference in your life and allow you to see what is possible.

## What about the Opioid Epidemic?

No doubt you are familiar with the opioid epidemic. This phrase is prevalent in all forms of media—print, radio, television. There is definite cause for concern over the non-medical use of opioids and the 2016 Centers for Disease Control and Prevention (CDC) guideline is curbing opioid prescriptions to help control the problem. There are countering opinions on the value of this strategy and its impact on legitimate chronic non-cancer pain patients using opioids for relief. In my experience, most patients on chronic opioid therapy take their medications responsibly. The non-medical use and abuse occurs more often in those obtaining opioids from family members and friends or by other means. That is not to say that patients using opioids are immune to risk. On the contrary, they require close monitoring, education, and discontinuation if they lose control over opioid use or don't improve their function or quality of life. Only a minority of patients should be considered for opioid therapy after careful assessment of risks, benefits, and medical necessity. As you will see from reading this book, there are an array of non-opioid pain-relieving options for patients—and that is good news. Pain specialists are able to offer many of these strategies and alternative practitioners provide access to the others. This book is full of information about these options. My hope is that you will read it and explore these options and find something that works for you.

# PART

# I

# Understanding and Treating Your Pain

# CHAPTER

# 1

# Headache Pain

When Priya first walked into my office, she had come to the end of her rope. A young mother of two who had once led an extremely active life, she had been battling debilitating migraines since becoming pregnant with her first child. The pain would appear without warning, beginning in her eyes and the back of her neck. It moved up through the base of her skull, blurring her vision and causing her eyes to water. Finally, her entire head would be so crushed with pressure and pain that over-the-counter medications, such as aspirin or acetaminophen (Tylenol), did nothing.

Headaches are not unusual. It's estimated that 46% of adults across the world have an active headache disorder. But the pain Priya experienced went far beyond the typical tension headache. It caused nausea and vomiting, condemning her to lie in bed in a dark room for days at a time. Her husband would beg the children to stay quiet so Mommy could rest. In addition to interfering with their daily routine, the family found themselves canceling vacations and social engagements when Priya's migraines mercilessly incapacitated her for days.

Priya's doctors prescribed increasingly strong prescription pain pills, suppositories, and patches to try to manage these episodes. And while the medications enabled her to "sleep off" the migraine if she caught it early enough, they did little to nothing if she didn't catch it in time. Her days were haunted by the anxiety that a headache could appear at any time. Finally, her doctors resorted to injectable opioid painkillers and, in time, sent her to me.

The key to Priya's long-term relief came from an unlikely ally: Botox injections. Known primarily for its cosmetic abilities to minimize wrinkles, botulinum toxin (Botox) is actually a neurotoxin produced by the same bacteria that causes serious food poisoning. In small doses, Botox blocks the signals sent from nerves to muscles, preventing the muscles from contracting. New research now suggests that Botox may also reduce pain and inflammation by inhibiting neurotransmitters, which are the chemical messengers that transmit pain signals and sensitize the spinal cord to pain. Its utility for treating migraines was discovered when a number of the patients who were getting cosmetic treatments reported experiencing migraine relief as well.

I treated Priya by inserting a tiny needle into the muscles of her forehead, scalp, and along the back and sides of her head. I also gave her injections in the back of her neck and even above her shoulder blades. Research supports the efficacy of precise needle insertion sites, which target the muscles and trigger zones that are the sources of pain. Unlike muscle relaxants or injectable pain relievers, which focus on relieving pain after a headache has begun, Botox injections are used to prevent headaches. After regular treatment, Priya's headaches became less frequent and less intense. Although not yet medication free, Priya has regained a significant level of control over her migraines and, as a result, is living a richer, fuller life.

## Understanding Headache Pain

Headaches can range from garden-variety tension type headaches to full-blown migraines. As I noted in Priya's story, an estimated 46% of adults across the world have an active headache disorder, and 99% of women and 93% of men experience headache pain in their lives.

### Causes of Tension Type Headache (TTH) Pain

Everyday headaches known as tension type headaches (TTH) can be triggered by any number of common causes including, allergies, stress, fatigue, injury, illness, sun exposure, dehydration, or caffeine withdrawal, to name just a few. The pain from TTH is typically mild-to-moderate in intensity, on both sides of the head, and doesn't throb. Patients of mine who are experiencing TTH will say that they feel like a tight cap is on their heads or a tight band constricts their heads. Some even have nausea. Diagnostic testing (magnetic resonance imaging (MRI) or computed tomography (CT scan) is usually not needed for TTH.

Physicians currently believe that sensitization of pain receptors in the muscle or fascia around the head lead to these types of headaches. Pain receptors around blood vessels and tendons may also be sources of pain. If these pain receptors continue to send signals to the central nervous system, then chronic TTH develops. Similar to brain imaging studies in patients with chronic low back pain, one study in patients with chronic TTH showed a decrease in a certain type of brain tissue called gray matter in those areas of the brain involved with pain processing. This highlights the importance of treating TTH so that it doesn't become chronic.

Tension type headaches are often the normal reactions of the body to problems that the pain should prompt us to correct. A dehydration headache reminds you to drink more water. A person suffering from a cold or the flu will hopefully be driven by a mild headache to get much needed rest. Often, mild headaches can be remedied or prevented by getting adequate rest, drinking more liquids, and taking steps to reduce stress, tension, and anxiety in your life.

## Causes of Migraine Headache Pain

Unlike everyday tension headaches, migraine and cluster headaches arise from spontaneous pain signals that serve no health-related purpose. People who suffer from these types of headaches on a regular basis are often born with sensitivity to certain stimuli. When present, those stimuli, such as light, sound, certain foods or food additives, can spark unbearable, throbbing, and usually one-sided pain.

Twelve percent of the U.S. population suffers from migraine headaches. An attack usually unfolds gradually over the course of hours to days, and most migraine sufferers (including myself) don't experience an aura, a strange sensation such as dizziness, ear-ringing, or flashes of light experienced before the headache. If left untreated, an attack will continue for several hours or even days. I suffer from episodic migraine headaches, which happen occasionally, whereas others experience chronic migraines, attacks occurring 15 days or more monthly for at least three months with headaches lasting four hours or more.

Migraines appear to be connected to hormones, since three times as many women experience them as men, most often during their childbearing years. Fortunately, women suffer less frequently after menopause, and migraines are relatively uncommon in children. We also believe that there is a genetic basis to migraines, but gene studies have not yet clarified which ones are actually linked to the disorder.

Migraine headaches begin at the "headache center" of the brain, a small area in the brainstem. This bundle of nerves is like a busy central traffic intersection between the brain and the body; nearly every neural signal from the brain to the body or from the body to the brain passes through it. When this part of the brainstem becomes overstimulated, it amplifies the effect of normal environmental stimuli. Sufferers suddenly feel as if someone turned up their hearing aids too high or forced them to wear night vision goggles in broad daylight, resulting in tremendous pain and nausea. Along with nausea and light sensitivity, many patients experience sound sensitivity.

Physicians used to believe that dilatation of blood vessels caused migraine headaches, but current research supports a process known as cortical spreading depression, a wave of electrical activity spreading across the brain, and specifically the cerebral cortex. This is thought to cause the aura of migraine, trigger a nerve of the face called the trigeminal nerve, and disrupt the natural barrier between brain tissue and blood. It's a complex process that leads to inflammation of the membranes enclosing the brain that are known as the meninges. This inflammation ultimately generates the headache. Nerve inflammation may intensify and prolong the migraine and may also sensitize nerves in a way that they "turn on" more easily, with greater force, and spontaneously. It's this sensitization in the brain that may explain why migraines worsen with coughing, bending, or quick head movements and may account for the throbbing quality of the pain.

Although not necessarily a source of migraine headaches, a condition known as occipital neuralgia can lead patients to feel one-sided head pain that's burning, deep, throbbing, and shooting, along with scalp tenderness to light touch. Patients can have symptoms that begin in the back of the head and travel to the top of the head (greater occipital nerve), or travel to the side of the head near the ear (lesser occipital nerve). There can be tenderness over the nerves, but not always. We believe that irritation or entrapment of the nerves may be the reason for occipital neuralgia, and many cases are related to whiplash injuries and head trauma. Certain patients report radiating pain up to the forehead or discomfort behind the eyes along with features of migraines. There certainly can be an overlap between this headache type and migraines. Occipital nerve blocks are shown to help patients with migraines as well as patients with the other primary headache disorders discussed in this chapter, TTH and cluster. I've had several referrals from neurologists to evaluate patients for nerve blocks with migraine-like headaches associated with occipital neuralgia. When nerve blocks are used for pain treatment and management, a local anesthetic medication is injected around a specific nerve in the body.

It is important to note that sinus headaches are often misdiagnosed. Many patients actually meet the diagnostic criteria for migraine. Sinus pain headache usually presents as a pressure-like sensation located on both sides of the head and behind the eyes. In addition, patients often have nasal congestion or obstruction with sinus headaches.

## Causes of Cluster Headache Pain

Cluster headaches—so-called because of the group of headaches that attack closely together that most sufferers experience—involve similar areas of the brainstem as migraines, but cluster headaches also affect the nose, sinuses, and eyes. It's not clear what happens during the cluster attack, but it's thought that the hypothalamus, trigeminal nerve area, and nerve inflammation of a sinus deep inside the head may all contribute. Cluster headaches cause substantial disability and impair quality of life.

This headache type is classified among a group of headaches called the trigeminal autonomic cephalgias. The one-sided attacks can be vicious, making patients rock back and forth or pace relentlessly. The pain is on one side of the face—around or above the eye, or in the temporal region. The attacks can strike up to eight times per day, and usually last between 15 minutes to three hours. Compared to migraine headaches, this is short, but the excruciating nature of the cluster headache attack makes it seem like an eternity. Many times, cluster attacks continue every day for weeks before a period of remission. Patients may awaken in the middle of the night with severe pain, red and watery eyes and inflamed sinuses. This is due to the changes in the autonomic nervous system and specifically, the activation of the parasympathetic system and the blunting of the sympathetic system. Patients experience a droopy eyelid, small pupil size, tearing, and nasal congestion during the attacks. Cluster headache pain is not connected to any other medical problem: It's as if that burglar alarm has been triggered for no reason.

Thankfully, cluster headaches occur rarely, in less than 1% of the population. They affect men more than four times as often as women. There is some evidence that these headaches are inherited, and that cigarette smoking may be a risk factor for development.

No special testing is needed for diagnosis of cluster headaches (which is true for migraines as well). However, most doctors will order an MRI or CT scan of the brain when the diagnosis of cluster headache is first made. This excludes brain abnormalities that might be the source of the headache pain (tumors or aneurisms, for example). This is based on reports of patients thought to have cluster headaches, but who ended up having brain abnormalities instead. In contrast, an MRI is usually not needed for patients with classic migraine headaches or TTH.

## Headache Pain and Triggers

Although it is unclear why some people experience migraines and cluster headaches and others do not, some factors have been shown to trigger symptoms in multiple patients. Stress, skipping meals, weather, sleep disturbances, perfumes, smoke, exercise, and even sexual activity can trigger headaches in some individuals. Alcohol consumption has been shown to increase the frequency and severity of migraine and cluster headaches: the darker the alcohol, the greater the chance of a problem. For instance, dark rum can trigger my own migraines (as will sleep loss, red wine, and sometimes stress). Caffeine, another common trigger, is a double-edged sword. A cup of coffee or large glass of soda can actually help get rid of a headache, but if you regularly drink more than one or two cups of coffee, tea or soda per day, you are at a higher risk of migraine, tension, or even chronic daily tension type headaches.

Stress is one of the most frequent triggers of both migraine and tension headaches, so managing stress is an important part of controlling headaches. If you suffer from headache pain, it makes sense to invest time in getting to know your triggers. Keeping track of other possible headache triggers in a journal and avoiding them can be a huge step toward conquering your headache pain.

## When to Call Your Doctor about Headache Pain

Most headaches are very common and usually no cause for alarm. For example, I've had some patients worry that their headache may be caused by a brain tumor. Even though brain tumors can cause headaches, only a very small number of patients with headaches actually have brain tumors. However, there are some headaches that may require medical attention and serve as warning signs of possible serious disease:

- A "thunderclap" headache in which the pain comes suddenly and intensifies rapidly. This may reflect a bleed inside the brain called a subarachnoid hemorrhage.

- A "first headache," or a particular kind of headache experienced for the first time, particularly if you're over 40 years old. New headaches can

suggest metastasis in a patient with cancer, encephalitis in a patient with Lyme disease, or an infection in a patient with HIV, for example.

- A headache that is unusually intense in comparison to the kind you usually get.

- A change in headache patterns (for example, awakening with a headache in the morning when you normally only get them at night).

These red flag symptoms do not necessarily indicate a severe health threat, but they should be checked out by your doctor and usually require a brain MRI or CT.

## Treating and Preventing Headache Pain

If you suffer from headache pain, it is important to determine what kind of headaches you are experiencing and identify your triggers. Being able to discuss this with your physician will help your medical team find the right treatment for your headache pain. Depending on the type or severity of your headache, there are a variety of simple, effective treatments available.

### Treating Tension Type Headache Pain

The typical tension type headache (TTH), can be treated with nonsteroidal anti-inflammatory drugs (NSAIDs) such as aspirin, acetaminophen (Tylenol), ibuprofen (Motrin), or even a cup of coffee. Ibuprofen (Motrin) leads to fewer side effects than other NSAIDs according to several studies. Some patients of mine have benefited from naproxen (Aleve) or diclofenac (Voltaren) as well. If these medicines don't help enough, then combining caffeine with acetaminophen or aspirin may be even more effective than taking a single drug alone. Adding caffeine can cause more side effects, though. These mainly consist of gastrointestinal upset.

A specific tricyclic antidepressant medication, amitriptyline (Elavil) can reduce the number and intensity of tension type headaches, and it even decreases tenderness of the muscles surrounding the head. Reducing this tenderness is important because it can prevent pain amplification from occurring in the spinal cord and brain. Other drugs in that family, nortriptyline (Pamelor) or protriptyline (Vivactil) are alternatives, but amitriptyline has the best evidence of efficacy. There are also many over-the-counter medications, such as decongestants or antihistamines that target sinus or allergy-related headaches.

Trigger point injections, injections of small amounts of local anesthetic into specific "tight" muscles in the scalp, jaw, and neck, can decrease tension type headache frequency as well as the need for medications.

Integrative therapies can help with TTH too. For example, consider biofeedback, cognitive behavioral therapy, and relaxation techniques including hypnosis (which are discussed in detail in Chapter 19, Mind-Body Techniques for Pain Relief). These treatments can reduce the triggers of TTH and thereby their frequency. These treatment options also emphasize self-care and focus on achieving a better awareness and control of stress-inducing events. I've had a few patients tell me that acupuncture has eased their TTH and others have mentioned that physical therapy incorporating cranio-cervical exercises has reduced their headache frequency.

Make sure you don't overuse medications used to treat episodic TTH or migraines. Overmedicating can actually *cause* headaches known as medication overuse headaches (MOH) or "rebound headaches." When this happens, patients say that they experience headaches when they wake up in the morning every day (or almost every day). The risk of MOH is greatest for patients taking opioids, combination analgesics, such as aspirin/acetaminophen/caffeine (Excedrin), and butalbital-containing medications (Fioricet). Make sure that you limit use to around nine days a month and two doses per day if you have TTH. Fortunately, MOH usually stops once the overuse has stopped.

### *Treating Migraine Headache Pain*

A migraine often requires more individualized medication than a TTH. A large, single dose of medicine typically treats acute migraines better than small doses spread out during the day. For less intense attacks, NSAIDs or combination analgesics similar to those used for TTH are effective. When these aren't sufficient, the triptans, a series of seven drugs, or a combination triptan-NSAID are specifically designed to treat migraines and are currently "the gold standard" for aborting acute migraine attacks. The most recent evidence indicates that a triptan-NSAID combination seems be even better at controlling acute migraine attacks than either drug alone. If this combination brand drug called Treximet (sumatriptan-naproxen sodium) is too expensive, you can take each drug separately.

Many studies have found the triptans to be beneficial for acute migraines. Triptans work by binding to the serotonin receptors (the channels which regulate the "traffic" of chemical messengers to the brain). This causes the blood vessels feeding the brain to constrict, preventing neurotransmitter release and blocking pain pathways in the brainstem. This in turn relieves swelling and makes the neurons (the nerve cells) in the spinal cord and brain less sensitive.

There is some evidence that triptans probably also lower levels of the neurotransmitter called calcitonin gene related peptide (CGRP), a strong dilator of blood vessels located in the brain and in the outermost membrane covering the brain. The role of serotonin and CGRP in migraine development is unclear, but current and future drug therapy alters levels of these molecules in ways that help control symptoms.

All triptans are available orally; two can be injected into the nose and one can be given by injection into the thigh. If one triptan doesn't alleviate your pain, then try another. Both patient experience and the research indicate that failure of one drug does not predict the same failure of another drug in the same family. There are instances when people should avoid using triptans. These instances are related to the type of migraine, to uncontrolled hypertension, and to pregnancy, for example. You need to discuss the risks and benefits of specific triptans with your doctor. Remember that triptans are most effective when taken as early as possible during an acute attack.

Dihydroergotamine (DHE 45) is a different class of medicine that patients use for acute migraine relief, and the evidence shows DHE 45 to be effective for relieving migraine symptoms. It constricts blood vessels and binds to the serotonin receptors like the triptans do. DHE 45 is available in many forms:

intravenous, intramuscular, subcutaneous, and intranasal. An anti-nausea medicine is often given along with DHE 45. Patients with hypertension, a certain type of heart disease, or who are older adults aren't candidates for this medicine because of the risks, though.

While some patients do feel that opioids or barbiturates (butalbital) treat their migraines, most doctors administer these only as a last resort. Neither of these medicines is as effective as the migraine-specific drugs (the triptans and DHE 45) just discussed.

Transcutaneous magnetic stimulation (TMS), an innovative therapy for depression, may be able to help control acute migraine attacks with aura. The evidence for TMS is growing. Its application is supported in spinal cord injury pain, trigeminal neuralgia, post-stroke pain, and fibromyalgia too. TMS is noninvasive, targets the cerebral cortex (outer layer of the brain) with magnetic fields, and may help heal areas inside the brain that have been altered due to chronic pain.

When TMS is applied, either a helmet is placed on the head or a metallic arm hovers over the head during the 20-minute treatment sessions, typically performed in a hospital setting. There is also a portable TMS device available in certain centers in the United States (Spring

TMS) and in England that is much more practical to use. One particular study had patients place the handheld device against the backs of their heads as soon as the aura began and found that it substantially reduced headache pain two hours afterwards. These patients were pain-free up to 48 hours after treatment as well. You may want to look into this therapy if you need to avoid medications or don't respond to them. However, it's not widely available yet. Patients with epilepsy should not use a TMS device due to the risk of seizure.

The success of triptans led many researchers to believe that a drug had to affect the blood vessels to provide migraine relief. Physicians still refer to migraines as "blood vessel" headaches. More recent theory, however, holds that not just blood vessels but primarily nerves and nerve inflammation contribute to migraines. A new series of drugs called calcitonin gene related peptide antagonists (CGRP antagonists) address the neurological component of migraine pain. CGRP, like serotonin, is thought to play a key role in migraine development. CGRP antagonists have been tested in clinical trials and some have proven as effective as the triptans. Unlike triptans, CGRP antagonists don't work by simply constricting the blood vessels;

rather, they block the dilation of vessels and reduce nerve transmission in the central nervous system. These antagonist drugs, along with an exciting group of biological drugs called "monoclonal antibody drugs" that also target CGRP or its receptor, show promise for treating migraine pain The monoclonal antibody drugs may offer even more beneficial effects by offering relief for weeks, or even months, after each dose.

## Preventing Migraines

If chronic migraines are affecting your life, the best thing is to prevent them. Options for preventing chronic migraine attacks include lifestyle modifications, drug therapy, botulinum toxin (Botox), specific herbals, integrative therapies, and transcutaneous electrical nerve stimulation.

In terms of your lifestyle, make sure you optimize your sleep hygiene, eat meals routinely, and identify and manage your migraine triggers. A headache diary helps patients keep track of the number and severity of monthly headaches and increases awareness of headache triggers. Patients of mine use both avoidance of triggers and coping techniques such as cognitive behavioral therapy (CBT). (CBT is discussed in detail in Chapter 19, Mind-Body Techniques for Pain Relief.)

Avoiding triggers can be tough, so a newer behavioral strategy called "learning to cope" may be something to try. It teaches patients how to desensitize themselves to headache triggers by exposure to these triggers in a stepwise fashion. Early work in this area seems promising based on a small study showing significant reduction in headaches and need for medication.

In addition to using drugs to address acute migraine headaches, some patients turn to medicines to prevent migraines. For example, drugs used for hypertension (high blood pressure) have also been prescribed to prevent headaches. The best evidence of antihypertensive drug therapy for migraine prevention exists for the beta blockers, especially propranolol (Inderal), motoprolol (Toprol), and timolol (Betimol). The results don't happen immediately. It may require several weeks of therapy before they make a difference, and three months or so before it can be determined if the drugs are effective. Some patients are not candidates for these medications, so consult with your doctor about your specific needs. The literature suggests that other types of antihypertensives might be effective and each needs to be tailored to your specific condition.

Like the type of antidepressant drug mentioned for treatment of tension type headaches, tricyclic antidepressants (TCAs) can be useful for migraine prevention too. For instance, amitriptyline (Elavil) is often the first medicine used at lower doses and at bedtime, but the other TCAs (such as nortriptyline [Pamelor] or desipramine [Norpramin]) can help as well. I often prescribe the TCAs (which are discussed more fully in Chapter 14, Pharmacological Therapies) for headache pain with good results. As a matter of fact, I've have patients with untreated chronic migraines surprised to discover their benefits when using a TCA for a different pain condition.

Anticonvulsants (also covered in Chapter 14, Pharmacological Therapies) such as topiramate (Topamax) and valproate (Depakene) are recommended by the American Academy of Neurology as beneficial for migraine prevention. One study looking at topiramate found that patients reported relief for up to six months after stopping the drug. Valproate can cause several side effects and shouldn't be used by women of childbearing age.

I've had many patients like Priya tell me that botulinum toxin (Botox) has made a difference in the frequency and intensity of their chronic migraines. It's a quick procedure performed in the office that requires many small needle insertions into the face, head, neck, and upper back. The needles cause mild pain, but rarely do patients refuse to repeat the injections because of this temporary pain. The effects generally last for three months, but the length of symptom relief varies by patient. I treat certain patients every eight to 10 weeks, and others every five months, for example. It's an FDA-approved treatment for chronic rather than episodic migraine prevention.

One NSAID in particular, naproxen (Naprosyn), offers some benefit in migraine prevention, and others, such as ibuprofen, may also help. NSAIDs typically offer better relief for acute migraine headaches, though. Early investigations into vitamin B2 (riboflavin) at 400 mg per day has shown quite a bit of improvement in headache intensity, frequency, and number of attacks.

There are options for prevention beyond traditional medical therapies as well. For example, studies show that biofeedback can be quite effective for treating migraine headaches in adults and children. (You can learn more about biofeedback in Chapter 19, Mind-Body Techniques for Pain Relief). Even though an herbal supplement called butterbur has shown benefit in studies and has been used for prevention, there are concerns about liver toxicity and cancer if the product contains molecules called pyrrolizidine. Research also suggests that aromatherapy can be effective in migraine prevention. Herbals and aromatherapy are discussed more in depth in Chapter 20, Alternative Medicine and Pain Relief, and Chapter 21, Aromas, Music, and Pain Relief.

Acupuncture may help to decrease the number of migraine days per month according to a couple of research trials. Transcutaneous electrical nerve stimulation (TENS) positioned in the supraorbital region (above the eye) and used for 20 minutes a day might also reduce the frequency of migraines. Both of these treatments are quite safe. Review Chapter 20, Alternative Medicine and Pain Relief, and Chapter 15, Pain-Relieving Devices, for more details about these techniques.

### Treating Occipital Neuralgia Pain

Injections of local anesthetic or steroid around the greater occipital nerves located along the back of head have been shown to be effective in patients with occipital neuralgia as well as certain patients with cluster and migraine headaches. These injections are quick, safe, and performed in the clinic. Interestingly, occipital nerve blocks may influence the activity of many nerves associated with primary headache disorders (TTH, migraine, and cluster) because their positive effect lasts longer than the duration of local anesthetic used for the block. This may account for why TTH, cluster headaches, and migraine headaches respond to these nerve blocks. (Recall that when nerve blocks are used for pain treatment and management, a local anesthetic medication is injected around a specific nerve in the body).

Although the benefits of the injection can be short, a promising treatment option called pulsed radiofrequency (PRF) can extend the duration of relief for several months. In a PRF procedure, doctors place a needle near the nerve. The needle is attached to a wire that is plugged into a machine. Once activated, the needle transmits a low intensity electrical field around the nerve to reduce the firing of pain signals in that nerve. Other mechanisms may play a role too. Research studies suggest benefit for patients with occipital neuralgia, and new research shows improvement in migraines. I've performed this procedure on select patients with migraines and occipital neuralgia and seen good results.

Another option for relieving occipital neuralgia is occipital nerve stimulation, or more generally referred to as peripheral nerve stimulation. This is in contrast to spinal cord stimulation (discussed in Chapter 15, Pain-Relieving Devices), which affects nerves in the spinal cord rather than peripheral nerves such as the occipital nerves in the back of the head. (Peripheral nerves are part of the peripheral nervous system, the large network of nerves that connect the brain and spinal cord—the central nervous system—to the body.)

Occipital nerve stimulation requires the pain specialist or neurosurgeon to place a thin wire (lead) into the back of the scalp near the occipital nerves. Patients control the delivery of current through the wire and around the nerves during a trial or "test drive." If relief is significant, the wire and a pacemaker-like battery are implanted under the skin. This therapy is often reserved for those not getting enough relief from other pain treatments. The literature shows extended pain control and lower use of pain medications with occipital nerve stimulation. As with any surgical procedure, complications can occur such as migration of the wire or even erosion of the wire through the skin.

## Treating Cluster Headache Pain

To treat cluster headaches specifically, inhaling 100% oxygen with a face mask for 15 minutes or a taking a triptan can help. These treatments are viewed as the first steps. Of the triptans, sumatriptan (Imitrex) and zolmitriptan (Zomig) have shown to be most effective in treating cluster headaches in studies. A third option is injecting lidocaine, a local anesthetic, into the nose, or taking a drug called ergotamine orally. In the hospital, intravenous dihydroergotamine (DHE 45) can be effective in treating cluster headache pain (like it is in treating acute migraine pain).

Exciting neurostimulation procedures for treating cluster headaches are both on the horizon and currently available. Currently available, one procedure involves electrically stimulating the *sphenopalatine ganglion*, a clump of nerves positioned behind the base of the nose to treat cluster headache. A small lead (wire) is surgically implanted through the upper gum. Using a handheld remote control, patients operate the device. It's called the Pulsante SPF Microstimulator System and the evidence is favorable for producing pain relief in 15 minutes, reducing attack frequency, and maintaining benefit for up to two years.

Vagus nerve stimulation (VNS) represents another technique being studied and used for cluster headaches. European researchers have developed transcutaneous (placed over the skin instead of implanted) VNS devices. One of these, GammaCore has been shown to reduce the symptoms of acute headache attacks and to perhaps decrease the frequency of future attacks. It's approved in Europe for both migraine and cluster headaches and recently FDA approved for episodic cluster headaches. This transcutaneous stimulator device is pocket sized and portable. A patient places it against the side of the neck to stimulate the vagus nerve, reducing the number of attacks per week. Finally, deep brain stimulation (DBS) may come to the aid of those completely resistant to all other treatments. Imagine having tiny electrodes surgically placed deep inside the brain, connected to a wire that travels under the skin, down the side of the neck, and then to a pacemaker-like battery implanted under the collar bone. That's DBS. Although it sounds frightening, this therapy can be a lifesaver for pain and the tremors due to Parkinson's disease. Promising studies of DBS for cluster headaches may convert this treatment from investigational to a more standard one for a select group of people. More information about these neurostimulation techniques is included in Chapter 15, Pain-Relieving Devices.

## Preventing Cluster Headaches

The key to cluster headaches is prevention, just as it is for migraines. The acute therapies mentioned in the previous paragraphs don't reduce the number of cluster attacks, but they can abort an attack. An antihypertensive drug, verapamil, is the drug of choice for cluster headache prevention. Because the doses may be high, patients may be asked to get an electrocardiogram (ECG or EKG). Verapamil is usually well tolerated and can take two to three weeks to take effect. Steroids are another option—either oral prednisone or intravenous steroid if necessary.

To help lessen her dependency on medication, Priya plans to experiment with several alternative treatments that have helped many of my other patients, including yoga, meditation, and acupuncture. (More information on these and other cutting-edge headache therapies can be found in Part 3, Integrative Therapies for Pain.) Although she still has some good and bad days, she is eager to continue participating in her own recovery. Thanks to her perseverance and willingness to try new treatments, Priya is more in control than ever and has tremendous hope for the future.

## Hope for Headache Pain Relief

Headache is a practically universal human experience and among the most common conditions known to humankind. It can be disabling but is very treatable with medications, alternative therapy, and innovative neurostimulation techniques.

To learn more about various self-care and pain treatment options and therapies, read the chapters in Part 2, Medical Therapies for Pain: Traditional and Innovative, and Part 3, Integrative Therapies for Pain. There you will find more information and ideas for working with your physician and other healthcare providers to find ways to prevent, manage, and address your pain.

You can also learn more about headache pain by listening to the headache episode of my weekly radio talk show that is nationally syndicated on Sirius XM Radio. The program, called *Aches and Gains*, highlights compelling stories of people who have found relief, shares information about cutting-edge treatments from contributing experts, and suggests ways that people in pain can improve their daily lives. You can find the broadcast on headache pain at the following URL.

**Headache**

http://paulchristomd.com/headaches

## Suggested Further Reading

Abeles, Frederick. *Break Away: The New Method for Treating Chronic Headaches, Migraines, and TMJ without Medication*. Cluster One Media, 2015. This book focuses on treatments without medication.

Bernstein, Carolyn. *The Migraine Brain: Your Breakthrough Guide to Fewer Headaches, Better Health*. Simon & Schuster, 2008. Popular book for people suffering from migraines.

Buchholz, David. *Heal Your Headache*. Workman Publishing, 2002. Originally published in 2002, this remains the best-selling book on the market for headache sufferers.

## Other Resources to Explore

The Daily Headache: Blogger Kerrie Smyres writes about the issues migraineurs want to know about, including research, opinions and forum.

MAGNUM: The National Migraine Association: Their mission is to raise public awareness about migraines as a debilitating neurological illness. Find out how you can help.

The National Headache Foundation: The world's largest non-profit voluntary organization for finding migraine treatment clinics, resources and local community programs.

WebMD—Migraines: WebMD is a comprehensive website which provides health tips, information, slideshows and support for medical issues from A to Z; their migraine page is particularly helpful.

CHAPTER

# 2

# Joint and Soft Tissue Pain

Actress Jennifer Grey—known for her roles in wildly successful eighties films such as *Dirty Dancing* and *Ferris Bueller's Day Off*—recaptured America's heart when she won the TV dance competition *Dancing with the Stars* in 2010 at the age of 50. Not only was Jennifer able to keep up with her partner, Derek Hough (a professional dancer half her age), but week after week, she also amazed the judges with routines that were both artistically expressive and technically flawless.

Just a few years earlier, however, Jennifer had been suffering from neck pain so severe it nearly paralyzed her. The chronic pain made it challenging for her to fulfill the physical demands of acting. After a while, just tilting her head to have makeup applied was enough to bring her to tears. Just a short period of time after being nominated for a Golden Globe Award in 1988, Jennifer's entire career was in jeopardy because of her suffering.

On a typical workday, Ty Warner, creator of the Beanie Baby, toy manufacturer, and philanthropist, spent about six to seven hours a day looking down at his computer. "I could almost spend a full working day texting and looking at a monitor," he said. But then he started feeling pins and needles from his shoulder to his fingertips, severe neck tightness, and headaches. It became hard to concentrate and tougher to endure every day. The pins and needles made him wonder whether he was having a heart attack, so he consulted his primary care doctor who reassured him that he wasn't. While there, his doctor examined his neck and upper back, eliciting Ty's symptoms, and observed his posture, noting a forward roll to his shoulders. He then learned how much Ty was flexing his neck to text or email. The doctor told Ty he was not alone and told him how frequently he was seeing the "Tech Neck" problem that had been making Ty uncomfortable for the past six months.

## Understanding Joint Pain

Pain in joints—such as the vertebrae in the neck—is very common. In this chapter, we look at common joint pain that is not necessarily related to arthritis or athletic injury. (We cover arthritis and athletic injury specifically in Chapter 3 and Chapter 7, respectively.) In this chapter, we also discuss an emerging problem: chronic pain in the soft tissues (muscles, tendons, ligaments, nerves, for example)—of the neck. This problem is sometimes referred to as "Tech Neck."

## Understanding Neck Pain

About 75% of the adult population in the United States face some type of neck pain during their lives. It can have a negative effect on our productivity and quality of life. For 90% of sufferers, the pain goes away in three months or less. The remaining 10% may develop chronic neck pain. Neck pain ranks as the fourth leading cause of years lost to disability, and many patients with neck pain also experience headaches, joint pain, back pain, and depression. Although neck pain can be excruciating, there are a variety of remedies, primarily non-surgical, that can be very helpful.

Jennifer Grey's 20-year battle with neck pain began with a car accident. X-rays after the head-on collision revealed no broken bones, so doctors assumed she just had a bad case of whiplash that would eventually go away. When the pain didn't subside, she tried chiropractic treatment and a few other alternative methods, but the pain only seemed to get worse. As time passed, Jennifer began experiencing severe cervicogenic headaches—one-sided head pain that radiated from the back of her head to the front. This type of headache can cause head pain from the muscles, nerves, bones, or joints in the neck. The pain is often caused by neck movement or awkward head positions. Whenever Jennifer felt anxious or tense, her neck pain would travel to her shoulders, tightening her muscles. This isn't unusual. Patients often describe one-sided shoulder, neck, or arm pain too. For Jennifer, often this led to a headache, which made it almost impossible to concentrate and to work.

Soon Jennifer was planning every aspect of her life around her pain. She began to cut out many of her favorite pastimes, such as yoga, weight lifting, and other physical activities, fearing a flare-up. She no longer had her full range of motion, and she had to worry about a crippling headache interfering with her performances. Day after day, she asked herself why the pain wouldn't go away.

At the end of her rope, Jennifer consulted a spinal surgeon and finally learned the truth: She didn't have whiplash at all. Instead, she was suffering from a severe disc herniation, which was compressing her spinal cord. "My head was basically falling off my neck," she explained on my radio program. Fortunately, neck surgery was successful, and today, Jennifer manages her neck pain with exercise, occasional medicines, and nerve blocks.

## Causes of Neck Pain

Neck pain has a multitude of common causes, including whiplash injury, facet joint disease, illness, arthritis (which we cover in Chapter 3, Arthritis Pain), compression fractures (often due to osteoporosis), and herniated discs. As we age, both the bones and the soft tissues that make up the spine begin to wear out, including the discs between the vertebrae, which act as shock-absorbers. Discs that become herniated—damaged or "slipped" out of place—like Jennifer's can irritate the spinal nerves or spinal cord itself, creating pain that can radiate down the arms or to parts of the body depending on the location of the herniation. Discs that don't herniate but do degenerate can cause neck pain only. The term for this neck pain is cervical discogenic pain. The neck can feel painful with range of motion, and pain can lead to restricted range of motion.

Cervical discogenic pain may be the most common cause of neck pain, especially in those younger than 50 years. The symptoms are often worse in situations when the neck doesn't move (for example, driving, doing computer work, or reading). Neck muscles frequently contract causing spasms and tightness. The pain results from degenerative changes to the disc structure that cause pressure to be unevenly distributed between the disc, vertebral bodies, and facet joints. The facet joints are joints formed by the overlap of two segments of the vertebra. They allow us to bend and twist our necks. Small nerves supply sensation to these joints, which can be targeted for pain relief.

If you've experienced whiplash and suffer from neck pain, then the facet joints are probably the reason. Whiplash injury is common and often happens after motor vehicle accidents. Patients with whiplash may experience bad neck pain, spasm, headaches in the back of the head, and limited range of motion. The cause of the pain probably is injury to multiple parts of the neck, such as the spinal nerves, discs, ligaments, or especially the facet joints. Whiplash pulls the joints of the neck apart and then snaps them back together, often causing muscle strain, ligament damage around the back of the neck and shoulders, and occasionally even damage to the discs of the neck and spinal column itself. Such injuries often lead to what is known as "diffuse neck pain," which radiates to other parts of the body such as the back, limbs, and head. Neck stiffness, headaches, dizziness, and even memory problems can accompany whiplash injury and shouldn't be ignored. Some patients, like Jennifer, also experience headaches, or pain in their shoulders or upper back. Unfortunately, imaging the neck with magnetic resonance imaging (MRI) or computed tomography (CT) doesn't usually identify the source of pain, and a high percentage (50%) of patients continue to have symptoms a year after the injury.

If you experience neck pain, you may have had your doctor diagnose you with cervical strain. This is a general term that implies muscle spasms in the neck or upper back from injury or even from "Tech Neck" like Ty Warner experienced. I've seen more and more patients with acute strain from poor posture or poor sleeping habits, so try to pay attention to how you position your body while sitting in front of a computer, texting, or lying in bed.

In today's high tech world, using a smartphone or other handheld device is the norm. We use them at work, take them on trips, bring them to bed, and use them in the bathroom. They are everywhere. People use them excessively in both developed and developing nations. The length of time we are looking down to type or read messages is escalating, leading to strain and stress on the neck muscles, misalignment, and potential disc degeneration.

More than likely, you're reading this book with your head bent, shoulders forward, and eyes focused in front of you. If you have a mobile device (smartphone, iPad, laptop computer), you're tilting your head even more forward and for greater periods of time—probably two to four hours per day on average. That's a long time. The advent of these mobile devices has led to a new "diagnosis": Tech or Text Neck. Tech Neck is essentially repetitive strain injury from constantly looking down to type or read text messages, answer emails, or check social media sites. It's also become especially worrisome in teenagers and younger children who spend hours playing video games or surfing on hand-held devices. When you bend your head to use your smart devices, it's often at a 60-degree angle. That's equivalent to 60 pounds of pressure on your neck, or it's like carrying an eight-year-old on your neck for hours each day.

Cervical spondylosis is another common cause of neck pain. Cervical spondylosis—the "wear and tear" caused by age-related changes to the neck—can produce osteophytes (bone spurs), which narrow the space around spinal nerves or the spinal cord, called stenosis, causing

pain. Injury to soft tissues of the neck such as the fascia (layers of fibrous tissues), ligaments, tendons, and muscles are also common sources of pain. Degenerative changes in the discs, facet joints, and vertebral bodies begin showing up on an MRI over the age of 30, but that doesn't correlate to the presence of pain. Tumors and infections can also lead to neck discomfort, although these are less common.

### When to Call Your Doctor about Neck Pain

Although most neck pain is not dangerous, you should be aware of some danger signs. These include progressive weakness or rapid sensory changes in the arms, fever, or even a change in bowel or bladder function. Sensory changes might manifest as numbness or pins and needles in the arm. If a person has neck pain along with fever, chills, or weight loss, for instance, we wonder about a tumor or an infection. On the other hand, bowel or bladder dysfunction, problems walking, and arm clumsiness may lead to a diagnosis of cervical myelopathy, disease of the spinal cord. Pain shooting down one or both arms can indicate disc herniation or stenosis (the narrowing around the spinal nerves or spinal cord), or other neurologic conditions that should be examined by a physician.

## Diagnosing Neck Pain

Unfortunately, all x-rays can tell your doctor about your neck is whether or not you have fractured your vertebrae; they reveal nothing about the muscles, ligaments, or other soft tissues. Still, in some cases, x-rays are sufficient. MRIs provide a much more complete picture of the discs, spinal cord, and spinal nerves of the neck. There are specific reasons for imaging the neck; these reasons depend on your age, the length of time you've had the symptoms, and whether you're having progressive neurologic problems. Blood tests are not routinely needed for neck pain, and neither is electrodiagnostic testing—EMG/NCT (electromyography/nerve conduction testing)—unless there is a suspicion of nerve problems in the arm.

A discogram is a much more invasive procedure with questionable utility. During a discogram, the doctor inserts a thin needle into the small discs of the neck and injects a special dye, which fills part of the disc as well as any cracks, and makes the cracks visible on an x-ray or CT scan. Most of the time, the pain specialist performs this test for the spine surgeon in order to determine whether a cervical fusion will benefit the patient. Unfortunately, the discogram injection process itself may temporarily worsen neck pain symptoms, especially when the needle is inserted into the disc in the neck that is generating the pain.

## Treating Neck Pain

It is usually best to start treating neck pain as noninvasively as possible. Acetaminophen is a good first medicine to try and it can help with mild-to-moderate intensity pain. Anti-inflammatories such as meloxicam (Mobic) or over-the-counter nonsteroidal anti-inflammatory drugs (NSAIDs) such as ibuprofen are also a good start, along with physical therapy (PT) and small range of motion exercises. On occasion, tramadol (Ultram), a mild opioid, may be needed for short periods of time. Primary care doctors can manage initial symptoms and then refer the patient to a pain specialist if necessary.

PT is directed at providing therapeutic exercises using heat, ice, electrical stimulation, traction, and myofascial release. Several studies suggest that stretching the neck and shoulder blade area along with strengthening provide relief. We don't know the optimal number of sessions for benefit and, frankly, insurance companies typically limit the duration. I often suggest two to three PT sessions per week for two months and then reassess the patient.

Patients wonder whether neck collars are important and the answer is no according to the literature. Sometimes collars can even delay improvement of acute neck pain. That said, I've had some patients wear a soft collar at night to help them sleep, but I limit use to three hours a day for a couple of weeks so that the neck muscles don't atrophy.

Chapter 23, Pain Relief through Movement, highlights several original methods of postural correction that can be applied to easing neck pain. For the growing numbers of patients with Tech Neck, re-structuring neck posture is key. For example, make sure that your head is up and not tilted down, ears area aligned with your shoulders, and the shoulder blades are retracted (shoulders rolled back) when you're sitting in front of a computer, standing, or walking. Just having an awareness of good neck posture will help remedy the problem.

Patients of mine get massages and take hot showers before bedtime. I personally do both and have found they help to break up the tense, tight muscles in my neck and upper back. Some patients perform home exercises in the shower

while the hot water pours over the neck. At work, take frequent breaks; every 20 minutes, try to stand up, move your neck, take note of your posture, and walk around. There are smartphone applications that track safe viewing and alert us if we are at risk for Text Neck. When possible, consider making phone calls or engaging voice recognition on your smartphone to avoid texting.

Some easy at-home or in-office exercises include the following:

- *Neck rotation:* Turning the head to the right, holding it for five to 10 seconds, returning it to center, and then turning it to the left.

- *Neck tilting:* Tilting the head toward the right ear, holding, returning to center, and then tilting it to the left

- *Neck bending:* Touching your chin close to your chest, holding, and then returning your head upright again

- *Shoulder rolls:* Pulling your arms backwards while trying to pinch your shoulder blades together, then returning the arms forward

Repeat each exercise about 10 times and hold each position five seconds or so. Heating your neck with warm water from the shower, bath, or moist towels from the microwave facilitates the stretches. Doing these exercises two to three times per week maintains neck flexibility too.

If these methods don't bring sufficient relief, particularly if you've tried them for two to three months, it may be time to try a more aggressive approach such as the following options:

- Trigger point injections—inserting a small needle into specific neck muscles that are tense, tight, or in spasm—can bring welcome relief. These can be performed with or without local anesthetic such as lidocaine. I usually don't inject steroid into the muscles because it can cause injury or isolated muscle cell death (necrosis). Studies have revealed benefit from these injections and clinically, patients report less muscle tightness.

- Physicians can also perform medial branch nerve blocks (facet blocks) of the neck joints under fluoroscopic (x-ray) guidance. These tiny nerves provide sensation to the joints of the neck and blocking them with local anesthetic temporarily interrupts their ability to transmit impulses which can ease neck pain. If the diagnostic nerve blocks provide approximately 50% relief, the nerves are then treated with radiofrequency denervation, which can reduce pain for several months. Radiofrequency denervation (also called radiofrequency ablation or rhizotomy) is the standard of care for facet-mediated pain. During a radiofrequency denervation, electrical current produces a small, controlled lesion in the nerve to safely block pain signals for extended periods of time. A small insulated electrode (needle) is placed near the nerve, and then high frequency current produced by a generator heats up the tissue. In contrast, pulsed radiofrequency procedures avoid tissue destruction by applying an electrical field to the nerve without a substantial rise in temperature.

- Epidural steroid injections offer relief if patients have cervical radicular pain (shooting pain down the arm from a herniated disc), stenosis around the spinal cord or spinal nerves (narrowing around the nerve), or neck surgery. This is supported by several studies. However, the injections often need to be repeated intermittently for continued benefit.

◆ Muscle relaxants such as cyclobenzaprine (Flexeril), tizanidine (Zanaflex), and carisoprodol (Soma) offer relief for acute neck pain by working on the areas of the brain that cause the neck muscles to contract. They are not as effective for chronic neck pain as they are for acute injuries. Because these medicines can cause sleepiness, I start with low doses and at night. While Soma can help certain patients control their chronic neck pain, some physicians avoid it because it contains a sedative-hypnotic agent with anti-anxiety properties similar to Valium. This means it carries greater risk and should be monitored.

There are other treatment options as well. A group of medicines called the tricyclic antidepressants (TCAs), which we discussed in Chapter 1, Headache Pain, and discuss in more detail in Chapter 14, Pharmacological Therapies, have proven helpful to treat neuropathic neck pain. Neuropathic means that nerves are injured or dysfunctional, sending the wrong signals to the spinal cord or brain. Neuropathic neck pain can manifest as burning pain, shooting pain down the arm, pain from even the lightest touch, and/or areas of tingling or numbness. (We cover neuropathic pain in much more detail in Chapter 4, Neuropathic Pain.) The two most commonly used TCAs are nortriptyline (Pamelor) and amitriptyline (Elavil). I've found them helpful in certain patients with neck pain alone or neck and arm pain combined.

Duloxetine (Cymbalta) can provide relief too, and it is FDA approved for musculoskeletal pain, a common source of neck pain. Anticonvulsants are important treatments for neuropathic pain, including pregabalin (Lyrica) and gabapentin (Neurontin). I frequently use gabapentin for neck pain as well.

Some patients dealing with muscular pain in the neck find a topical NSAID patch (Flector) containing diclofenac helpful. Although I don't routinely prescribe it for neck pain, I've had patients tell me that the topical lidocaine patch seems to decrease their symptoms.

Traction—the act of stretching the spine using a traction table or similar device—was once thought to be beneficial to neck and back pain, but multiple studies now cast its benefit in doubt. However, spinal manipulation, often performed by chiropractors using high velocity thrusts at the neck joints can offer benefit particularly for younger patients with acute mechanical neck pain—pain due to the muscles, ligaments, and joints, for instance. It's probably less useful for chronic neck pain.

Transcutaneous electrical nerve stimulation (TENS), along with exercise for chronic neck pain, has been found to improve both pain and disability while enhancing strength. The TENS device delivers low voltage electricity through electrodes (similar to EKG pads) placed over the painful area and is generally safe and well tolerated. You can learn more about TENS in Chapter 15, Pain-Relieving Devices.

Some pain doctors have also had success with spinal cord stimulation (which is also discussed in Chapter 15), a technique that delivers small electrical impulses to the region of the spinal cord in the neck to reduce pain that shoots down the arm or stays in the neck. It's similar to a heart pacemaker but "paces" the spinal cord instead of the heart. For those with low back and shooting leg pain (failed back surgery syndrome), complex regional pain syndrome (see Chapter 4, Neuropathic Pain), and other neuropathic pain conditions, spinal cord stimulation (SCS) has made a favorable, long-term difference in their lives. Reports have also demonstrated significant long-term economic value. We have emerging evidence that SCS can improve pain symptoms and quality of life in those with persistent neck pain after surgery or from degenerative disc disease in the neck. In my experience, SCS can likewise alleviate discomfort in the arm from neuropathic pain conditions resulting from complex regional pain syndrome or neck surgery, and that's consistent with some of the research findings.

Acupuncture, covered in Chapter 20, Alternative Medicine and Pain Relief, can be an option for neck pain sufferers given that we do have some evidence that it relieves neck pain and disability. Qigong (pronounced chee gung), a Chinese practice involving slow movements, meditation, and breathing exercises, compares favorably to exercise therapy in lowering chronic neck pain and disability for many months. Cognitive behavioral therapy (CBT), a mind-body technique discussed in Chapter 19, Mind-Body Techniques for Pain Relief, is worth the investment. It relaxes the body, reduces stress, and furnishes practical self-management strategies. There is evidence that aromatherapy (massage) can be effective for neck pain too; it's covered in Chapter 21, Aromas, Music, and Pain Relief.

Sometimes surgery is necessary to stabilize the neck and prevent nerve or spinal cord damage. But barring a traumatic injury to the neck or significant compromise of the spinal cord or spinal nerve roots exhibiting worrisome symptoms, surgery should be a last resort. For chronic neck pain alone (compared to neck pain with shooting arm symptoms) make sure the surgeon clearly outlines the potential for benefit. Most of the time, a customized approach that incorporates nerve blocks, medications, neurostimulation, and complementary therapies helps patients regain control of their lives without resorting to surgery.

## Understanding Low Back Pain

After headaches, low back pain (LBP) is the most frequent complaint of chronic pain sufferers, affecting between 70% and 80% of the adult population. It's a major cause of disability across the world with a lifetime risk reaching as high as 84%. In addition, the socioeconomic costs have surged to an estimated $100–$200 billion per year due to direct or indirect medical costs associated with missed work days and decreased workplace productivity. Every component of the spine—the facet joints, intervertebral discs, nerves, and muscles—can contribute to pain and discomfort. The most common kind of low back pain is axial back pain, also known as lumbosacral pain; it occurs around or just below the waist and is often aggravated by particular activities and relieved by rest. Think of it as being located just in the low back region. In contrast, radicular pain—commonly known as sciatica—shoots down into the leg with or without low back pain, signaling that a nerve is being irritated.

New diagnostic techniques are revealing that the damage to the body from chronic low back pain may be far more extensive than previously imagined. Advances in brain imaging using functional MRI show areas of the brain (prefrontal cortex) that are degenerating because of chronic low back pain. Nobody would have imagined that chronic pain sufferers could actually lose brain tissue, but they can. Researchers have observed a loss in gray matter—the brain tissue that stores memories and processes information—among patients with chronic low back pain. Fortunately, treating low back pain can reverse this loss and restore healthy brain activity. It's noteworthy to mention that this gray matter loss isn't specific to LBP either. It also has been found by researchers studying patients with fibromyalgia, chronic tension type headaches, and irritable bowel syndrome, for instance.

## Causes of Low Back Pain

Herniated discs are the most common cause of sciatica, but most episodes resolve on their own in six to eight weeks and don't require surgery. Still up to 40% of people experience frequent recurrences of symptoms. Unlike acute disc herniation, the changes causing axial back pain do not typically improve on their own. Discogenic pain (pain coming from the disc itself) is the problem in many cases of chronic low back pain.

The disc acts as a shock absorber or weight bearer that lies in between the vertebral bodies, allowing movement between them. The outer part of the disc is made of dense collagen fibers, while the inner part is gelatinous and contains water. When we talk about disc degeneration or herniation, we mean that tears develop in the outer fibers and dehydration occurs in the inner part. Axial or radicular back pain can result from this degenerative process—the disc height decreases, the facet joints become arthritic and overly stressed, compression of the spinal nerves can occur from stenosis (narrowing around the nerve), and inflammatory molecules are released from the disc that sensitize nerves.

Recall from our previous discussion on neck pain that the facet joints along the spine are designed to assist with spinal movement, but they are present to limit twisting movement and prevent the vertebral body from moving too far forward.

Overall, the vast majority of patients seen in the primary care setting have nonspecific LBP, which means it's not possible to reliably identify a specific source of pain. In my experience, a good deal of both acute and chronic low back pain is due to strain of the muscles and ligaments of the low back, which physicians refer to as musculo-ligamentous strain. Multiple muscle groups help to control movement of the lumbar spine, and their density has been found to be reduced in patients with LBP. Further, this muscular "atrophy" is linked to conditions that precipitate pain such as disc space narrowing, facet joint arthritis, and slippage of the vertebral body forward or backward known as spondylolisthesis. This is why exercising these muscles becomes critical in stabilizing the lumbar spine and alleviating pain.

Although the disc accounts for a large proportion of pain in patients with axial back pain, the lumbar facet joints are estimated to be the cause in 15%–30% of patients. We see this facet joint pain condition more often in older adults—greater than 65 years of age—and it happens progressively. In contrast, disc pain more frequency appears in those younger than 45 years old, and disc pain patients report that they can't endure sitting whereas lying down makes the pain better. Facet pain is worse with standing and reduced when sitting or lying down, taking the weight off the joints.

Another principal cause of low back pain is radicular. Radicular pain, which is commonly referred to as sciatica, causes shooting pain down the leg and occurs mostly from a herniated lumbar disc at either L4-5 or L5-1. When we talk about radicular pain in the low back or other parts of the body, we classify it as neuropathic (See Chapter 4, Neuropathic Pain). This means that there is some type of problem with the nerves or sensory pathways in the body. Neuropathic pain can be a characteristic of chronic back pain.

Along with disc herniation, radicular pain (sciatica) can be due to lumbar spinal stenosis. Stenosis is a narrowing in the size of the spinal canal, the passageway for the spinal cord or the spinal nerves. As you might imagine, when the spinal canal volume gets tighter, pressure on the spinal cord or spinal nerves develops, leading to pain or neurological impairment. Lumbar spinal stenosis causes a special symptom that physicians call neurogenic claudication—radicular pain (sciatica) that is initiated or worsened by standing or walking and quickly improves with sitting down. Patients will say that their symptoms ease when they lean forward as if pushing a shopping cart at the store. This makes sense anatomically because the area inside the spinal canal and around the spinal nerves widens when we lean forward and narrows when we stand.

Low back pain can also be the result of an inherited spine abnormality. Scoliosis—the sideways curvature of the spine—often appears in the preteen and early teenage years when children experience a growth spurt. It is important that scoliosis be diagnosed promptly and monitored carefully to ensure it does not progress to the point where it causes significant pain.

Many women experience low back pain during pregnancy. Back muscles and ligaments may be strained by the changes in their bodies. Certain professions which involve heavy lifting or extensive exposure to strong vibrations—such as driving a truck or flying a jet—also put people at risk for low back pain. You can read more about workplace injuries in Chapter 9, Workplace Injury and Pain.

Low back pain can also occur for no obvious reason, but often the modern office is a contributor. Sitting for long periods in an uncomfortable chair, hunching over a desk, staring at a computer monitor, or using a computer mouse can all trigger pain. A study of office workers concluded that 40% did not get out of their chairs to talk to colleagues, while 70% spent five or more hours sitting at a desk each day. It is not surprising that sedentary work (along with smoking, obesity, and depression) is a risk factor for experiencing LBP.

The sacroiliac joint is often involved in chronic low back pain; up to 30% of sufferers may find it to be the cause. Its role in low back pain is probably underestimated by primary care doctors and surgeons. The sacroiliac joint represents the fusion of the sacrum—the large, triangular bone at the base of the spine—and the ilium, the largest bone of the pelvis. It causes pain in younger athletes and older adults, the majority of the time in the low back and buttock. Arthritis, as well as injuries to the ligaments and muscles that support the joint, tend to produce the painful symptoms. Risk factors for sacroiliac pain include constant strain or trauma on the joint from jogging or falls, abnormal body postures and movements (biomechanical abnormalities),

or pregnancy. In 40%–50% of patients, some event triggers the pain; motor vehicle accidents and falls represent the two most common events.

Spine surgery is a less well known but frequent cause of sacroiliac joint pain, especially for patients who have had fusions extending to the sacrum. In these cases, steroid injections in or around the joint can provide temporary relief, but radiofrequency ablation of the nerves supplying the joint has been found to give patients more lasting relief. A new technique called *cooled radiofrequency ablation* provides a greater chance of successfully controlling pain by more effectively targeting the nerves that provide sensation to the joint. The evidence suggests anywhere from three months to one year of benefit.

## When to Call Your Doctor about Low Back Pain

As with neck pain, the overwhelming majority of acute incidents of low back pain will get better on their own. Rest, over-the-counter pain relievers, and a gradual return to regular activity resolve a large percentage of cases. There is no need to go to the emergency room unless you experience sudden leg weakness, loss of feeling in your lower extremities, or a loss of bowel or bladder control.

Obviously, if you have accompanying symptoms like a high fever or you have a personal history of cancer, infection, or other illness, you will also want to see your physician.

Although patients often expect doctors to order an image (x-ray, MRI, CT) to establish a diagnosis, the research tells us that earlier imaging does not change pain or functional outcomes in the short term or long term for those with LBP lasting up to three months or for radicular pain (sciatica). Imaging becomes more important if the LBP or radicular pain doesn't improve, significant spinal cord compression is suspected, or if there are progressive neurological problems.

## Treating Low Back Pain

While bed rest was a standard recommendation for acute low back pain (LBP) for decades, several studies have now demonstrated that patients can recover just as quickly and completely without bed rest. Randomized, controlled, clinical trials—a type of medical experiment considered to be the gold standard—have failed to demonstrate beneficial effects of bed rest for patients, and one systematic review (a literature review that critically analyzes many research studies) reported that bed rest may even lead to slightly more pain and less functional recovery than a program of gentle, regular movement. Bed rest can even cause several complications that may delay or prevent recovery, including muscle atrophy and joint contractures (deformity due to disuse).

When low back pain doesn't get better on its own, there are a variety of approaches that can be very helpful. Heat therapy and physical therapy exercises that strengthen the abdominal muscles can help many patients. This is especially true of pregnant women and new mothers. The focus on stretching and strengthening the low back and core can relieve the strain caused by the growing fetus on the muscles and ligaments of the lumbar spine.

Because low back pain is highly individual, you will want to work closely with your healthcare providers to ensure that you are exploring every non-surgical option for your pain. Sometimes low back pain is caused or exacerbated by our habits: how we sit, stand, run or lift things. Physical therapy and chiropractic interventions can help improve body mechanics if the pain is caused by posture problems or overuse injuries. If your lower back pain is due to muscular strain, then ergonomically correct chairs at the workplace can be very helpful. Office workers should also be sure to stand up every hour and walk for three minutes. Make sure your computer monitor is at the right height and find wrist supports for using the mouse.

## Low Back Pain and Pharmacological Therapies

Muscle relaxants, also known as antispasmodics, can help make the pain manageable while the area heals and seem to be more effective for acute rather than chronic pain. I rarely prescribe these medications, however, because they cause so much sedation. That said, they can help with sleep at night and sometimes are effective in small doses during the day. Nonsteroidal anti-inflammatory drugs (NSAIDs) can be useful medicines for chronic low back pain, but they need to be used judiciously given their effects on the stomach, kidney, and clotting system.

I've had some success with tricyclic antidepressants (TCAs; see Chapter 14, Pharmacological Therapies), such as amitriptyline and nortriptyline, for easing chronic low back and neck pain. While they are most helpful for neuropathic pain conditions such as migraines, painful diabetic neuropathy, and chronic

shingles pain (postherpetic neuralgia), patients with back pain do report relief. Another drug called duloxetine (Cymbalta) may also help musculoskeletal back pain. It's approved by the FDA for musculoskeletal pain along with fibromyalgia and painful diabetic neuropathy.

Although falling into disfavor (due to the concern about abuse and overdose), opioid medications such as tapentadol (Nucynta) and tramadol (Ultram) have shown effectiveness for acute and chronic LBP. Long-term benefits of opioids, however, are unproven and use needs to be determined based on careful review of the risks and potential benefits for individual patients.

For radicular pain (sciatica), pain specialists and other doctors often use anticonvulsant medications or antidepressant medications alone or together. Gabapentin (Neurontin) and pregabalin (Lyrica) are first line treatment options in clinical practice. The research findings about the effectiveness of this treatment are not conclusive, though. TCAs, mentioned earlier in this section, show positive effects in other neuropathic pain conditions and are therefore applied to treat radicular pain conditions. I've seen patients improve with each group of these medicines and have needed to prescribe both of them together if the relief isn't adequate.

Injection therapies can help too. In the spine, there are multiple pain generators—facet joints, discs, nerves, and muscles—that we can target. Frankly, many pain syndromes can present with several possible sources, and anesthetic blocks can help establish the basis for the pain. Therapeutic injections can provide durable relief, although they often need to be repeated. Pain specialists perform epidural steroid injections (ESIs) for radicular pain (sciatica). ESIs contain local anesthetic and/or steroid and are injected into the epidural space surrounding the spinal cord to alleviate the discomfort of shooting leg pain and to reduce any inflammation. There are different approaches to the ESI: transforaminal (targeting the spinal nerve specifically), interlaminar (targeting the spinal cord), and caudal (targeting spinal cord from the tailbone area). Each has certain benefits and risks that you should discuss with your pain doctor.

Although steroids are not opioid "painkillers," they interrupt the body's inflammatory response, disrupting the pain transmission by nerves. Injections have been found to provide substantial benefit for six weeks or longer. In practice, I treat patients who get several months of relief, but the duration varies according to their history. Interestingly,

a recent study suggested that ESIs may even possibly reduce the need for spine surgery in the short term.

## Low Back Pain and Other Therapies

Radiofrequency denervation (also called radiofrequency neurotomy) is another minimally invasive technique that can bring good relief to low back pain caused by the facet joints due to arthritis, degeneration, or traumatic injury, for example. This technique uses radiofrequency energy (heat) to disrupt the pain signals in the nerves and limit their ability to communicate those signals to the spinal cord and ultimately to the brain. The targeted nerves are primarily involved with sensation and do not control muscles in the arms or legs, and the procedure is very safe.

Typically, a physician will perform diagnostic blocks before radiofrequency denervation. If patients report meaningful relief of their pain—typically an improvement greater than 50%—then the physician will offer the radiofrequency denervation procedure for extended relief. Both the diagnostic block and the radiofrequency procedures are performed under fluoroscopic (x-ray) guidance. You may encounter some doctors using ultrasound instead. Appropriately selected patients who undergo lumbar radiofrequency facet denervation (applying heat to the nerves supplying the facet joints in the low back) and sacroiliac joint denervation (applying heat to the nerves supplying the sacroiliac joint) can experience sustained pain relief.

Pain-relieving devices are discussed in Chapter 15, but one device that can be invaluable for refractory radicular pain (sciatica) and sometimes axial back pain is spinal cord stimulation (SCS). It's similar to a cardiac pacemaker, but it's directed to the spinal cord, spinal nerves, or brain. Neurostimulation is the general term for this type of therapy and it refers to the process of applying electrical current to the nervous system for pain relief. Many physicians reserve SCS for patients who continue to suffer from back and shooting leg pain despite other treatments and whose quality of life is impaired. Much of the supportive evidence for SCS is associated with radicular pain from failed back surgery syndrome. Many patients have axial back pain alone and, traditionally, SCS has been limited in achieving meaningful benefit in this area. New programming capability and higher frequency stimulation, however, is honing in on axial back pain in ways that weren't possible in the past. Personally, it's been exciting to see more patients with back pain alone respond to this therapy.

Pain pumps, also known as intrathecal pumps or intrathecal drug delivery systems (IDDS), can supply very small doses of medication such as morphine or bupivacaine (a local anesthetic) directly to the spinal fluid to control back pain. More often used for cancer pain, these pumps are occasionally provided to patients with refractory LBP from failed back surgery syndrome or spinal stenosis. You can find a comprehensive discussion of pain pumps in Chapter 15, Pain-Relieving Devices.

Trigger point injections are helpful if select muscles are identified as tense or tight and they are generating pain. In my experience, botulinum toxin (Botox) also provides relief, but only for those muscles in spasm or that exhibit substantial tension.

Many patients have successfully treated their low back pain with alternative therapies including cognitive behavioral therapy (CBT), biofeedback, hypnosis, acupuncture, massage therapy, and exercise. We explain more about these kinds of treatments in Part 3, Integrative Therapies for Pain, specifically in Chapters 19 and 20. Interestingly, aromatherapy massage can also be effective for low back pain, discussed more fully in Chapter 21, Aromas, Music, and Pain Relief.

## Low Back Pain and Exercise

Exercise such as walking, pool exercise, or strength training with light weights can be beneficial to people experiencing low back pain. Yoga and other group methods of postural correction, such as Feldenkrais, can provide benefits at the same time they foster new friendships and a sense of community. Patients of mine have enjoyed the dual advantages of these strategies and you can learn more about them in Chapter 23, Pain Relief through Movement.

Gunnar Peterson, a guest on my radio show and well-known trainer for professional athletes, celebrities, and everyday people, emphasizes functional training—training the body for activities performed in daily life. This technique is especially applicable for those with chronic pain by modifying exercises that allow people to perform everyday activities more easily and without injuries. Gunnar has seen firsthand how clients lower their risk of injury by gaining strength and applying new information about how to lift, bend, and move.

Remember that it's important to maintain an exercise program for sustained benefit. Of course, maintainance is critical for many of the pain therapies discussed in this book (injections, medications, acupuncture, behavioral therapy, and diet, for example). It can be a struggle to exercise and keep doing it regularly, even if you're not in pain. Gunnar has some useful advice for us, though, on how to make exercise an ongoing part of our lives: "Schedule it and treat it like a doctor's appointment or job interview or a first date. Make it [as] unthinkable to cancel as any of those events would be. Prioritize it."

Many patients are afraid that exercise will make their pain worse or lead to further damage. This rarely happens. The general term related to a fear of movement is called kinesiophobia. The scientific research tells us that this fear and avoidance can worsen LBP outcomes by delaying recovery and heightening disability. In contrast, exercise can improve LBP and function even as we get older.

## Low Back Pain and Spine Surgery

Back surgery is sometimes indicated for severe scoliosis, cancer, severely herniated discs that compromise the spinal cord or spinal nerves, stenosis (narrowing) around the spinal cord or spinal nerves, or for fractures to the vertebrae. In these situations, discectomy, laminectomy, or fusion surgery may be undertaken to ensure that the spine is stabilized and to protect the spinal cord from damage.

In cases where fusion surgery may be appropriate, patients may report pain in their backs, legs, or both. If the spinal cord or nerves are significantly impaired, people may begin noticing weakness in their legs, or even lose bowel or bladder function. Spine surgery is more useful for pain that radiates or shoots down the legs than for low back pain alone. I remind my patients to ask spine surgeons how much relief they are likely to get from a procedure such as a discectomy, laminectomy, or fusion if pain is the only reason the procedure is undertaken. This is because the role of surgery in addressing non-specific low back pain is highly questionable. As a matter of fact, the authors of one study comparing decompression and fusion question the usefulness of a variety of surgical treatments.

Prosthetic disc replacements are offered for low back pain and degenerative disks (discogenic pain). Disc prostheses serve as an alternative to fusion surgery. But while joint replacement surgery has improved tremendously over the past several years, artificial discs have not enjoyed the same level of success as newer hip and knee replacement surgeries have. Disc replacement surgery for low back pain is expensive, the recovery takes time, and the results have been mixed at best. In short, science simply hasn't yet developed an artificial disc that works as well as the real thing. Interestingly, a recent study comparing disc replacement

to rehabilitation alone found that by two years after the surgery, the benefit to the surgical group was clinically insignificant. However, if patients have herniated discs or spinal narrowing that compresses nerves or the spinal cord and causes worrisome symptoms, then surgical intervention may indeed be warranted.

## New and Innovative Treatments for Low Back Pain

There are many exciting developments in treating low back pain that we can look forward to in the future. In addition to improved artificial discs, surgeons are working to develop less invasive surgical techniques with lower risks and faster recovery times. Surgical techniques are constantly improving, and we are also seeing advances in minimally invasive procedures to widen the spinal canal as a treatment for various problems putting pressure on the spinal cord.

One such procedure is called the *mild* procedure (minimally invasive lumbar decompression). This technique helps reduce leg pain (sciatica) caused by lumbar spinal stenosis. Although the pain often referred to as sciatica can have several causes, a thickened ligament in the back of the spinal canal is one that can lead to compression of the spinal cord or spinal nerves.

This often leads to buttock pain, leg pain, and sometimes back pain. The condition is known as neurogenic claudication and was described earlier in this chapter.

The *mild* procedure uses a special instrument under fluoroscopic guidance to remove excess ligament from the spinal canal in order to decompress and expand the narrowed part of the spinal canal. Although higher quality studies need to be performed, it appears that the procedure is safe in experienced hands and can provide improvement in pain over time. Compared to the most common surgical option—laminectomy—the *mild* procedure may offer similar relief and less risk.

Another promising and recently developed minimally invasive therapy is called *intradiscal biacuplasty*. As I noted earlier, pain arising from the discs (discogenic pain) accounts for a considerable amount of chronic low back pain. With injury or aging, the disc can degenerate, leading to cracks or tears in the outer layer. Further, inflammatory molecules called cytokines are released that sensitize nerves, and nerves can also sprout into other parts of the disc causing pain. Biacuplasty uses radiofrequency waves to heat or coagulate the nerves located in the lumbar discs to reduce low back pain. Under fluoroscopic guidance,

two electrodes are placed through the patient's back and then into the rear portion of the disc for about 25 minutes.

In general, patients have reported good relief and improved function from biacuplasty with just minor aches in the muscles of the low back from the procedure. The results of several studies on this intervention strongly support its ability to reduce pain and increase physical activity up to year in patients who are candidates. This therapy may offer patients an alternative to spinal fusion or artificial disc replacements in the future. This is particularly relevant as we see more criticism of disappointing outcomes related to spinal surgery and routine conservative care for LBP.

Exciting biologic therapies for treating low back pain are also on the horizon. These include stem cell therapy that may help regenerate and realign the fibers in the disc and platelet-rich plasma therapy, which may stop the progression of disc degeneration. Early and encouraging investigations on transplanting genetically engineered stem cells into damaged spinal nerves of animals may help patients with sciatica in the future. You can read more about promising regenerative therapies in Chapter 16, Regenerative Biomedicine.

# Understanding Knee Pain

The knee is the largest joint in the body. Our knees bear five times our weight when we walk, run, and climb. The knee is made up of the thigh bone, shin bone and knee cap, lubricated and supported by cartilage and a cartilaginous structure called the meniscus, and held together by the quadriceps muscle and several ligaments. The synovial fluid found inside the knee joint produces hyaluronic acid, which aids in lubricating the joint.

When any of these components of the knee become damaged, intense pain can result. Up to 19% of adults experience knee pain due to injury or disease like arthritis, covered in the next chapter. The pain can often be debilitating, but the good news is that there are many steps we can take to prevent knee pain and the treatments are constantly improving.

## Causes of Knee Pain

Knee injuries are caused by overuse or trauma. The soft tissues (ligaments, meniscus, tendons) are a common source of knee pain, but problems with the hard tissues (bone, articular cartilage) can lead to pain as well. Each year, at least one million people tear their meniscus—the cartilage that acts as a shock absorber in the knee. (This is different from the articular cartilage, which covers the ends of the long bones and makes the joint movements smooth.) Meniscus injuries happen most often when a person falls, pivots, or twists the knee incorrectly while putting weight on it, or takes a blow to the knee in a sport or accident. Osteoarthritis (OA), covered in Chapter 3, Arthritis Pain, degrades and thins the articular cartilage of the knee. OA of the knee is a leading cause of pain and disability worldwide.

## Excess Weight and Knee Pain

Besides avoiding dangerous sports and activities, the most important step individuals can take to prevent knee pain is to maintain a healthy weight. The average person takes two to three million steps per year. Minimizing the load on the knees can go a long way toward reducing the wear and tear. Optimizing your weight can extend the life and health of the joint. Building overall strength and flexibility also helps maintain good body mechanics, which greatly reduces the chances of twisting the joint incorrectly and damaging the meniscus.

# Treating Knee Pain

Along with a full examination of the knee, diagnostic imaging using MRI gives us a clear view of the structures of the knee. Obtaining images earlier after the onset of knee pain provides a more accurate diagnosis and can spare patients from incorrect therapies and even unnecessary arthroscopy. Although MRI imaging is expensive, it may be more cost-effective long term.

## Knee Pain and Pharmacological Therapies

The initial course of pharmacological treatment for knee pain is acetaminophen (not to exceed 4000 mg per day). One brand-name acetaminophen manufacturer recommends 3000 mg per day. The rule of thumb is to use the lowest dose for the shortest period of time. If there is an inflammatory element to the pain or acetaminophen is too weak, then oral nonsteroidal anti-inflammatory drugs (NSAIDs; ibuprofen, naproxen) are more effective. There's no compelling evidence that one NSAID is superior for the knee. The choice relates to patient factors and side effects of the individual NSAIDs. In large analyses of clinical trials, NSAIDs reduce pain more effectively than acetaminophen, and that's what I see in my practice.

Topical NSAIDs such as diclofenac (Voltaren Gel or Pennsaid) are FDA-approved for osteoarthritis (OA) and can ease painful joints. They can be used instead of oral NSAIDs but need to be applied three to four times daily. Diclofenac comes in a topical patch too, and I've found it effective for knee OA in my patients. Even topical local anesthetics, such as lidocaine, may be effective for short-term relief of knee pain. I've had more success with topical NSAIDs applied to the knee, though.

Another medication called capsaicin, which is derived from the active ingredient in hot chili peppers, can ease knee arthritic knee pain. It works by depleting a pain neurotransmitter known as substance P so that transmission of pain signals from the knee to the spinal cord and brain is dampened. This drug is typically offered when oral or topical NSAIDs are insufficient. It's supposed to be applied three to four times daily but may be just as effective once or twice daily based on clinical experience. The limiting factor to this treatment is local skin irritation—redness, stinging, or burning. One study reported these side effects in 40% of patients. The irritation goes away, but some of my patients just can't tolerate even brief periods of worsening pain. Once you have touched the medicine, you must avoid touching your eyes, lips, and genitals until you cleanse your hands.

Several studies involving many patients support the benefit of steroid knee joint injections for OA. I repeat injections every three months if they are effective. They can be performed at the bedside using anatomical landmarks or ultrasound, or done using fluoroscopy. Side effects are infrequent and there was no evidence of adverse effects on the knee structures in a two-year evaluation of patients whose knees were injected with triamcinolone (a specific steroid that is commonly injected) every three months.

In addition to the anti-inflammatory effects, steroids can benefit the knee joint by increasing the concentration of hyaluronic acid (HA), a naturally occurring molecule present in the synovial fluid, which acts as a lubricant and shock absorber during joint movement. HA is decreased in osteoarthritic joints. If steroid injections produce little response, then I offer injections of hyaluronic acid (Synvisc). HA can accomplish several desirable actions in the joint: reduce synovial inflammation, restore the effect of the synovial fluid, and protect the cartilage from eroding. The research has shown that knee pain and function improve while side effects in general are minimal. HA injections can last up to six months. I typically inject the knee with HA once a week for three weeks.

## Knee Pain and Other Therapies

More recently, I've provided genicular nerve blocks followed by cooled radiofrequency treatment (CRF) for chronic, intolerable knee pain due to OA, pain due to knee replacement surgery, or for knee pain in patients who are not candidates for knee surgery. When nerve blocks are used for pain treatment and management, a local anesthetic medication is injected around a specific nerve in the body. This technique targets three nerves which are involved with knee joint sensation. To predict who will have a good response to the treatment, fluoroscopic or ultrasound-guided diagnostic local anesthetic blocks are administered first. CRF is then offered to patients who report 50% or more relief of pain from the local anesthetic blocks. The CRF procedure uses fairly large electrodes that are placed along the three nerves, so I offer light sedation for most patients.

Some physicians use conventional radiofrequency denervation or even pulsed radiofrequency treatment instead of CRF for the same purpose. All three procedures use thermal energy to interrupt pain signals traveling from the knee joint to the spinal cord, but CRF produces a larger effect on the nerve tissue, thereby increasing the chances for an effective outcome—longer term relief and maybe more significant relief. CRF is a safe, minimally invasive therapeutic option for knee pain that is supported by the literature. As up to 7% of patients experience debilitating knee pain after total knee replacement, it's fortunate that genicular nerve denervation is available.

Have you heard about leeches for knee pain? Throughout history, they have been used to treat pain. Medicinal leeches (*Hirudo medicinalis*) are still part of some medical systems. Leech saliva contains anti-inflammatory substances as well as other substances that are thought to reduce pain. A couple of preliminary studies in patients with knee OA have shown that putting four to six medicinal leeches on the knee for about 70 minutes improved pain, stiffness, and functional ability. Leeches even compared favorably when tested against topical diclofenac.

Cutting-edge regenerative techniques such as prolotherapy, platelet rich plasma, and stem cell therapy may all contribute to easing pain and restoring knee function. These therapies are discussed in Chapter 16, Regenerative Biomedicine.

## Knee Pain and Surgery

When the meniscus is damaged, orthopedists usually remove the torn tissue. However, there is a growing bias toward saving the tissue rather than replacing it, if possible. The theory is that the more tissue that can be retained, the lower the chance of developing arthritis. Because of this, certain treatment centers are re-growing and then replacing a damaged meniscus with human tissue rather than removing it surgically. If the joint isn't completely collapsed from arthritis, partial replacements of the worn-out portion of the knee can be performed robotically using a combination of metal and plastic components. The incision is small, patients can go home the same day, and they can walk very soon if not immediately following the surgery.

When all other options have been exhausted and there is "bone on bone" contact, a total knee replacement can help. It's reserved as a last procedure, especially since some studies show that as many as 50% of patients report continued knee pain following surgery. Aggressive rehabilitation before and after the joint replacement is critical to establishing and maintaining range of motion.

Hall-of-Fame quarterback Joe Montana always understood that a certain amount of pain was part of his job. Although Montana started playing football in the Pop Warner League at the age of eight, it wasn't until his career with the San Francisco 49ers that he began to experience pain in his knee. That pain—caused by repeatedly planting and twisting his left leg in order to throw the football, coupled with the repeated hits he sustained over the years—eventually led to at least seven arthroscopic surgeries on his knee.

While playing in the National Football League, Montana had access to excellent doctors and physical therapists who used a combination of anti-inflammatory medicines, ice, and other treatments to keep him on the field. Unfortunately, when he retired, Joe did not leave the knee pain behind. He has received hyaluronic acid (Synvisc) injections into his knee—supplementing the existing fluid to help lubricate and cushion the joint—to manage the pain.

Joe has also found relief from drinking Joint Juice, a liquid supplement made up of glucosamine and chondroitin. Glucosamine is a naturally occurring chemical found in the body, especially in the synovial fluid surrounding joints. Chondroitin is also found in the body and specifically in the joint cartilage. Both glucosamine and chondroitin have anti-inflammatory effects and stimulate the production of hyaluronic acid in the joint. Chondroitin even promotes collagen synthesis (the formation of an important structural protein in cartilage or bone, for example). The primary reason to take both together is the synergistic benefit they exert on the destructive processes underlying osteoarthritis. Though not formally designated as such, we may realize their potential as disease-modifying drugs. It took about 20 to 30 days before Joe's knee felt noticeably different from the supplement, so patience is required if this route is pursued. These substances help to stimulate lubrication of the joint so patients feel less stiff. Aromatherapy massage can help with knee pain too. This treatment is discussed in Chapter 21, Aromas, Music, and Pain Relief.

Joe Montana's two Super Bowl wins and eight Pro Bowl appearances came at a cost, but he has not allowed the residual pain to prevent him from enjoying his life. He still throws the football around with his two sons and travels across the country to watch them play. He also maintains a healthy weight and stretches and exercises regularly. Montana encourages individuals coping with knee pain to follow their doctors' advice, stay as active as they can, strengthen the muscles supporting the knee, and keep working to improve their condition. It takes real effort.

# Understanding Shoulder Pain

Shoulder pain is yet another form of joint pain that is extremely common and it too can have a variety of causes. Because of its complex anatomy, the shoulder joint is more mobile than any other joint in the body. Impingement, tendonitis, and rotator cuff tears are among the most widespread conditions that lead to shoulder pain.

## *Causes of Shoulder Pain*

Typically, shoulder pain can be classified either as rotator cuff syndrome, which can result from performing a new or strenuous activity for the first time or over an extended period of time, or "frozen shoulder," a numbness or stiffness in the shoulder causing pain and limited motion. "Weekend Warriors," those of us in sedentary jobs who are active on the weekends, are particularly at risk for acute rotator cuff injuries. If you must pitch that softball game on Saturday, be sure to warm up first!

The rotator cuff consists of four muscles and their tendons, which stabilize the glenohumeral joint (shoulder joint) and help move the arm. Each tendon inserts into the humerus (upper arm bone). A fall or accident can tear one or more of these tendons away from the humerus, requiring surgery to reattach it. Rotator cuff injury is a common cause of shoulder pain, especially among the middle and older adult populations. The tendons can weaken through long-term wear and tear. Over time, tiny tears in these tendons show up as weakness, soreness, stiffness, or outright pain. Reaching overhead often aggravates shoulder pain if the rotator cuff is involved. Some studies indicate that as many as half of all adults over 50 will have partial or full tearing of the rotator cuff tendons. These tears are very rare in people under 30 with the exception of athletes who use their shoulders more aggressively.

Conditions such as osteoarthritis (OA) or trauma can cause pain in the acromio-clavicular joint, the joint on the top outer part of the shoulder between the clavicle (collar bone) and the acromion. Patients who have this problem typically use a finger to identify the end of the collar bone as the area of pain. Sometimes shoulder pain can come from spinal nerve compression in the neck and radiate to the back of the shoulder area and arm. Other times, medical problems related to the heart, liver, or abdomen (diaphragm irritation) can "refer" pain to the shoulder.

Frozen shoulder is a general diagnosis; adhesive capsulitis is the medical term. It refers to stiffening of the shoulder joint itself (glenohumeral joint). Some patients wake up with stiffness in their shoulder that inhibits or prevents arm movement. Many patients complain of achiness at night, difficulty putting on a coat, or washing their hair. Many times, there is no apparent cause for this condition.

Diabetes is a major risk factor for frozen shoulder as are as other diseases, such as stroke. Make sure you follow up with any exercise programs for immobilization of the shoulder joint (sling placement for a shoulder or elbow injury, for example) because immobilization can also lead to frozen shoulder.

## Treating Shoulder Pain

Outside of medication, the best treatment for frozen shoulder focuses on increasing mobility by doing exercises to strengthen the muscles and loosen the stiffness. If the stiffness persists, check with your doctor about getting into a physical therapy program with guided stretching or using a "pulley unit" that attaches to a door.

As with other kinds of joint pain, over-the-counter pain relievers can help address shoulder pain. Since pain often limits movement in cases of frozen shoulder, medicines such as acetaminophen, anti-inflammatories, and short-acting opioids like oxycodone can help, but for a limited duration. Sometimes, a five-day course of oral steroids is a great option too. An injection of steroid into the joint (glenohumeral joint injection) has been found to be as effective as oral steroids, but as with other kinds of pain, it's best to try the less invasive option first. If they are injected too frequently, steroids can harm the collagen framework of cartilage, tendons, and ligaments.

In some cases of rotator cuff tears or shoulder bursitis (the inflammation of the fluid-filled bursa sac, which cushions most joints), a procedure called a subacromial bursa injection with local anesthetic and steroid can offer relief. These injections are generally low risk and can facilitate physical therapy by increasing range of motion. They are performed at the bedside using surface landmarks or under ultrasound imaging guidance.

For those with painful arthritis of the shoulder who wish to avoid surgery, injections of hyaluronic acid (HA) into the shoulder joint can provide benefit. As mentioned in the discussion of knee pain in this chapter, hyaluronic acid exists in the synovial fluid of joints and act as a lubricant and shock absorber. Treatment typically involves one injection each week for three weeks. This may be a good option for the aging population who may not be candidates for other treatments such as nonsteroidal anti-inflammatory drugs (NSAIDs), aggressive physical therapy, or surgery.

Prolotherapy, the injection of high-concentration dextrose (a sugar) that is one of the cutting-edge therapies examined in Chapter 16, Regenerative Biomedicine, may be an option for rotator cuff tendon problems too.

## Shoulder Pain and Surgery

The two major surgeries performed to treat shoulder pain are rotator cuff surgery and full shoulder replacement. By the time people hit retirement age, they might have multiple tears along an entire tendon in the shoulder. The decision to operate is made by weighing the level of discomfort against the risk of surgery. MRIs are usually ordered when the doctor is concerned about a complete tear. Other factors doctors consider when contemplating surgery include:

♦ Age of the patient

♦ Source of the tear (trauma or wear and tear)

♦ Severity or size of the tear

♦ Location of the tear (dominant arm: left-handed /right-handed)

♦ The patient's overall health

♦ The patient's overall activity level and the tear's effect on lifestyle

Shoulder replacement, when indicated, can almost universally eliminate pain and free the patient to be more active. However, patients with shoulder replacements must be careful; playing tennis, heavy weightlifting, or participating in other activities that are hard on the shoulders after the replacement can jeopardize the life span of the joint. That doesn't mean you can't be active, though. Many patients can play golf, ride a bike, jog, and even swim. Fortunately, shoulder replacements last a long time if cared for properly. Studies indicate that 17 years after replacement, only 5% of patients require additional surgery.

## New and Innovative Treatments for Shoulder Pain

The future of shoulder relief includes a new procedure called a "reverse prosthesis." This is a unique shoulder replacement designed for people who have bad arthritis or significant rotator cuff injuries, which prevent traditional shoulder replacements. Reverse prostheses offer good pain relief but haven't been sufficiently studied in the United States to determine how long they last.

# Understanding Temporomandibular Joint Disorder (TMJ)

According to the American Academy of Orofacial Pain, about 75% of Americans experience symptoms of temporomandibular joint disorder (TMJ) during their lifetimes. TMJ contributes to almost 18 million lost work days per year in the United States alone. In recent years, the condition is more often being referred to as temporomandibular disorder because more than the joint is believed to cause the symptoms. TMJ is not one particular ailment, but rather a constellation of symptoms involving the facial muscles and the jaw in particular. Jaw muscle dysfunction, problems with the temporomandibular joint, and spinal problems in the neck all occur together in this condition.

The temporomandibular joint is the "hinge" between the base of the skull and the jaw, and consists of two moving joints in series with a disc between them. When healthy, this "joint and disc" combination provides a wide range of motion for the lower jaw to move up and down, as well as side to side. TMJ symptoms include facial and jaw pain, soreness, stiffness and even the inability to open the mouth. Sometimes early symptoms feel very similar to a headache, but on bad days, TMJ can completely restrict the ability to use the jaw. After pain, ear discomfort or dysfunction is a frequent symptom reported by patients—tinnitus (ringing in the ears), stuffiness, or pain. Many times, patients go for an evaluation of TMJ after the ear, nose, and throat (ENT) specialist rules out a primary ear problem. The headache is typically different from those we talked about in Chapter 1, Headache Pain. TMJ headaches are located around an ear and radiate to the temple, jaw, or neck, usually described as dull and continuous, and worse in the morning.

Freelance writer Yumiko began experiencing significant facial pain after a regular dentist visit. Instead of lessening, within two weeks an unbearable throbbing had enveloped her head, radiating to her neck and shoulders. Soon, she couldn't yawn, chew, swallow, or even speak without pain. Her diet became limited to soups, yogurt, and heavily steamed vegetables that required little chewing.

Even after she was correctly diagnosed with temporomandibular joint disorder (TMJ), Yumiko's quest for treatment proved long and frustrating. First, a dentist attempted to realign her jaw with a plastic mouthpiece, which resulted in more pain. She was prescribed a variety of muscle relaxants and other medications that left her feeling groggy and unable to engage in her normal daily activities. Her next doctor prescribed physical therapy, which did begin relieving her discomfort and giving her hope. But her recovery only began in earnest when she found a compassionate family doctor who focused on her pain first and her teeth and jaw second.

At her doctor's advice, Yumiko tried ultrasound massage on her neck and face and thermal treatments, such as icing down her facial muscles and applying heating pads to her neck. Yumiko also purchased a transcutaneous electrical nerve stimulation (TENS) unit. The TENS device delivers low voltage electricity through electrodes (similar to EKG pads) placed over the painful area and is generally safe and well tolerated, which she used along her temples and her jaw. After three long years of suffering, Yumiko was finally on her way back to a normal life.

Risk factors for TMJ include being young and female. Women are one and a half times as likely to develop TMJ as men. TMJ occurs in women mostly during their reproductive years. TMJ does not result from wear and tear or overuse. If you haven't experienced TMJ during your reproductive years, you most likely will not develop it later in life. If you have rheumatoid arthritis, you are more likely to develop TMJ pain, and if you like to chew gum or bite a pencil along with other repetitive jaw movements, you may develop TMJ pain. Some research points to an association between chronic TMJ and post-traumatic stress disorder (PTSD), depression, and anxiety, illustrating a behavioral aspect of this condition. Contrary to popular belief, a clicking noise in the jaw is not indicative of TMJ unless it is associated with pain. Noise in joints is frequent in healthy people and isn't necessarily a sign of disease.

Untreated TMJ can result not only in pain but also in excessive weight loss, low energy, and malnutrition. The psychological effects, as with any untreated pain, can also be devastating. Doctors have noted a link between TMJ and fibromyalgia, as many patients with one condition tend to have the other. (We discuss fibromyalgia in more detail in Chapter 4, Neuropathic Pain.)

---

## Treating Temporomandibular Joint Disorder (TMJ)

Conservative treatments for temporomandibular joint disorder (TMJ) include cold or heat packs, massage therapy, vibration therapy, nutritional therapy, and even acupuncture. Teaching patients to alter their head posture and sleeping position, or to avoid repetitive oral behavior, such as chewing pens or biting nails, can help. Mouth splints are useful more in the context of reducing tooth grinding.

Pharmacologic therapies, such as tricyclic antidepressants, are quite safe and allow pain control over longer periods of time. These are often the drugs of choice for persistent musculoskeletal pain associated with TMJ. Brief courses of nonsteroidal anti-inflammatory drugs (NSAIDs) may help or in combination with other medications. Muscle relaxants, such as cyclobenzaprine (Flexeril), can also help with muscle spasm and pain. Flexeril is structurally related to the tricyclic antidepressants, and once metabolized, works similarly. Anti-epileptic medicines, such as gabapentin (Neurontin), can be very beneficial for patients who have had surgery and report sharp, shooting pain afterwards. We don't have good evidence that long-term opioid or benzodiazepine therapy (diazepam [valium], clonazepam [klonopin]) is effective in controlling TMJ pain.

Other treatments include trigger point injections (inserting a needle into tense, taught, painful muscles usually with local anesthetic or steroid), although multiple injections can create muscle scarring and inflammation. One of the most invasive therapeutic measures is arthrocentesis, or joint aspiration. This involves actually draining synovial fluid from the joint in question, removing inflammatory molecules called cytokines. Patients who undergo such a procedure may experience relief for five to six months before the pain typically returns and the procedure may have to be repeated.

Surgically replacing the temporomandibular joint, while tempting in an era when such procedures seem to work miracles, can be a disaster. Thus far, artificial joints don't seem to be able to bear the load required for the jaw to function normally. As a result, surgically replaced joints tend to wear out far too quickly to justify the procedure unless there is severe functional disability or degeneration of the joint, often due to trauma or disease. Still, patients with persistent pain or substantial joint limitations may need surgical intervention if they have loose bone fragments in the joint, for example. Oral and maxillofacial surgeons can offer advice on specific procedures.

Current research is focusing on understanding the overlap of TMJ disorder with other pain conditions in the body. The good news is that, even with conservative, noninvasive treatment, studies indicate that 60%–70% of sufferers from TMJ will fully recover. The resources of the TMJ advocacy group (www.tmj.org) provide valuable guidance, featuring patient stories and information from expert clinicians and scientists.

The options for people with TMJ are varied. Early investigations into stem cell therapy for TMJ are discussed in Chapter 16, Regenerative Biomedicine; hypnosis and biofeedback are discussed in Chapter 19, Mind-Body Techniques for Pain Relief; and acupuncture is discussed in Chapter 20, Alternative Medicine and Pain Relief. All these discussions include strategies for improving daily life for those with TMJ. Fortunately, many patients respond to treatment and just a small number develop chronic pain.

## Hope for Joint and Soft Tissue Pain Relief

Yumiko's recovery took several months of physical therapy, a soft food diet, and ultrasound treatment combined with home remedies including ice packs and heating pads. She was later able to return to a nearly normal diet, and she even trained for and ran a marathon.

Jennifer Grey's surgeon performed a fusion and foraminotomy. This connected the vertebrae in her spine to prevent them from moving (fusion) and widened the opening where the nerves exit the spinal canal (foraminotomy). The procedure was a success and greatly reduced her pain while stabilizing her spine. After recovering from her neck pain, Jennifer became a spokesperson for Partners Against Pain, where she helped others with chronic pain learn their options and how to advocate for themselves.

Massage, warm baths, and Epsom salts alleviated Ty Warner's neck pain. He first noticed that his headaches were gone followed by improvement in his neck pain and pins and needles sensation. Not only did Ty also adopt a better posture, but he created a new toy to help prevent "Tech Neck." It's called the "Peek-A-Boo," so named because its big, sparkly eyes peek over the phone. It's designed to hold a smartphone hands-free. You can place the "Peek-A-Boo" on your desk, a table, or an airplane tray while it supports the device for texting, playing games, or watching TV. "It's a cradle for the smartphone, and kids really like them," Ty told us. They cost $5 to $6, but they are not just for children. Ty has noticed that lawyers and accountants are using them on their desks in professional settings. Personally, I've found that I don't flex my neck nearly as much when I use the "Peek-A-Boo" as I do when I put the phone in my lap.

Joint and soft tissue pain, while sometimes excruciating, does not have to last forever. By working with your healthcare providers, getting the correct diagnosis, and trying conservative, noninvasive treatments first, you can conquer your joint and soft tissue pain.

You can learn more about joint pain by listening to the joint and soft tissue pain episodes of my weekly radio program, *Aches and Gains*. You can find the broadcasts on joint pain at the following URLs.

**Neck Pain**

http://paulchristomd.com/neck-pain

**Text Neck**

http://paulchristomd.com/text-neck

http://paulchristomd.com/text-neck-2

**Knee Pain**

http://paulchristomd.com/knee-pain

**Low Back pain**

http://paulchristomd.com/low-back-pain

**Shoulder Pain**

http://paulchristomd.com/shoulder-pain

**Tempomandibular Disorder**

http://paulchristomd.com/temporomandibular-disorder

# Suggested Further Reading

Diana, Richard. *Healthy Joints for Life: An Orthopedic Surgeon's Proven Plan to Reduce Pain and Inflammation, Avoid Surgery and Get Moving Again.* (n.p.): Harlequin, 2014. Orthopedic surgeon and former NFL player Richard Diana applies his unique experience and training to relieve joint pain by reducing inflammation. http://tinyurl.com/y926pnff

• For more details visit the author's website: http://www.richdiana.com

Esmonde-White, Miranda. *Forever Painless: End Chronic Pain and Reclaim Your Life in 30 Minutes a Day.* (n.p.): Harper Wave, 2016. This book provides detailed instructions for gentle exercise designed to ease discomfort in the feet and ankles, knees, hips, back, and neck. http://tinyurl.com/ya4mek6j

Fernandez de las Penas, Cesar. *Neck and Arm Pain Syndromes: Evidence-informed Screening, Diagnosis and Management.* (n.p.): Churchill Livingstone, 2011. This book discusses the management of neuromusculoskeletal pathologies and dysfunctions of the upper quadrant, including joint, muscle, myofascial and neural tissue approaches. http://tinyurl.com/ydhr6s6u

Gokhale, Esther. *8 Steps to a Pain-Free Back: Natural Posture Solutions for Pain in the Back, Neck, Shoulder, Hip, Knee, and Foot.* (n.p.): Pendro Press, 2008. A step-by-step guide to help those suffering from back pain to re-educate their bodies and regain good posture. http://tinyurl.com/ya5fhc4w

Goodman, Eric. *True to Form: How to Use Foundation Training for Sustained Pain Relief and Everyday Fitness.* (n.p.): Harper Wave, 2016. Dr. Eric Goodman discusses how to integrate mindful movement into daily activities to make readers fit, healthy and pain free. http://www.harpercollins.ca/9780062315311/true-to-form

Jakobson Ramin, Cathryn. *Crooked: Outwitting the Back Pain Industry and Getting on the Road to Recovery.* (n.p.): Harper, 2017. An essential examination of the back pain industry, exploring what works, what doesn't, what may cause harm and how to get on the road to recovery. https://www.harpercollins.com/9780062641809/crooked

Kubey, Craig, and McKenzie, Robin. *7 Steps to a Pain-Free Life: How to Rapidly Relieve Back, Neck, and Shoulder Pain.* (n.p.): Plume, 2014. This book teaches readers about common causes of lower back, neck pain and shoulder pain, the vital role discs play in back and neck health, and easy exercises that alleviate pain. http://tinyurl.com/yc6nrj7y

Olderman, Rick. *Fixing You: Hip & Knee Pain: Self-treatment for IT Band Friction, Arthritis, Groin Pain, Bursitis, Knee Pain, PFS, AKPS, and Other Diagnoses.* (n.p.): Boone Publishing, 2011. With illustrations and patient stories, this book teaches readers about how poor pelvic muscle performance and walking habits result in hip and knee pain. http://tinyurl.com/ya5csrgt
   • Additional video clips of all exercises: www.FixingYou.net

Phillips, Edward M. *The Joint Pain Relief Workout: Healing Exercises for Your Shoulders, Hips, Knees, and Ankles.* (n.p.): Harvard Health Publications, 2014. This book is a special health report from Harvard Medical School that covers exercises that can help relieve ankle, knee, hip, or shoulder pain. http://tinyurl.com/y876buo9

Sarno, John E. *Healing Back Pain: The Mind-Body Connection Mass Market.* (n.p.): Grand Central Life & Style, 2010. Dr. John E. Sarno uses research into Tension Mytostis Syndrome to identify how stress and other psychological factors attribute to back pain. http://tinyurl.com/y853dy3u

## Other Resources to Explore

SpineUniverse offers patient education on conditions related to the spine in a clear accessible format. The content is developed by a team of experts. Also featured on the site is a video directory with exercises to relieve back pain: https://www.spineuniverse.com/videos/all

# 3

# Arthritis Pain

Kiki was just a teenager when she first felt the strange pain in her chest. After a few days, she was barely able to take a breath or bend over. In the weeks after a barrage of tests confirmed that her heart was healthy, the pain began to spread to her hands, knees, and even her toes. Her joints soon became hot to the touch.

After a litany of further tests, Kiki learned she had arthritis. Within six years, the pain would confine her to wheelchair and prevent her from even lifting a fork to her mouth to eat.

## Understanding Arthritis Pain

Arthritis—the general inflammation of the joints—affects millions of Americans. Although we often talk about arthritis as if it were a single disease, there are actually more than 100 different kinds of arthritis. The symptoms for the various types can be quite similar, but they have very different causes. In this chapter we'll examine three of the most common kinds of arthritis: osteoarthritis, rheumatoid arthritis, and gout. As you'll see, correctly pinpointing the cause of arthritis pain can be crucial to treating it effectively.

## Understanding Osteoarthritis

Patients with moderate to severe osteoarthritis (OA) typically wake up each morning with throbbing pain in their large joints, such as the hips and knees. The pain makes it extremely tempting to resist movement, but as we'll see, staying in bed all day is one of the worst things you can do when battling osteoarthritis.

Osteoarthritis is by far the most common form of arthritis, and one of the most common disabling diseases in developed countries. Fifteen percent of adults over the age of 60—45 million people in the United States and many more worldwide—suffer from this progressive disease. Eighty percent of patients with osteoarthritis experience restrictions in movement, and 25% of those patients cannot perform the basic activities of daily living. Risk for OA increases greatly with age. Given our current long life expectancies, experts anticipate that OA will rank as the fourth leading cause of disability by the year 2020. OA generally occurs more often in women than men, with the exception of patients under 40 years old, in whom cases are equally distributed between the genders.

What actually happens in the progression of osteoarthritis? The ends of our bones are covered with cartilage, which lubricates our joints and makes their movements smooth. The joint itself is joined by a capsule, which is lined by a layer called the synovial membrane. Osteoarthritis occurs as the cartilage (which should have a slick surface) wears down with age and use. The surface of the cartilage first becomes irregular; then, over time, it begins to thin in various spots. Finally, it begins to develop ulcers and holes, eventually exposing the bone.

Bone, once exposed, also undergoes changes similar to the weakening and small fractures associated with osteoporosis. This can cause the synovial membrane to become inflamed, releasing fluid and causing the joint to swell. The membrane also releases chemical messengers called mediators, which bind to the receptors in the nerve endings, causing pain. When the joint doesn't move properly, patients may feel weak and off balance too.

All the tissues in the joint can be involved in osteoarthritis. Sufferers experience mild to moderate pain that is often worse when they stand or are active and improves when they sit and rest. Thirty minutes or less of morning stiffness is a characteristic symptom. Most osteoarthritis pain can be categorized as either a constant dull aching or an intermittent sharp pain. The latter type of pain can be severe enough to stop people in their tracks.

OA can affect just one or multiple joints, or manifest throughout the body. When it involves particular joints, it typically attacks the knees, hips, hands or feet, or the facet joints of the low back and neck (discussed in Chapter 2, Joint and Soft Tissue Pain). In the more generalized form, OA causes pain in the hands, thumb joint, low back and neck, knees, and hips—a lot of locations. OA develops in both hands and both knees, but more frequently in just one hip.

A diagnosis of OA is made based on history and examination. No laboratory studies are needed, assuming a typical presentation. If the diagnosis is unclear, then x-rays of the joint are ordered to look for features of OA (joint space narrowing and osteophytes [overgrowth of bone], for example). Just as images of the low back don't clearly "show" pain, changes detected on x-ray don't correlate well with symptoms of OA.

## Causes of Osteoarthritis

Our joints are constantly working; many support body weight while allowing us to lift, bend, and move. Osteoarthritis is caused by the daily mechanical wear and tear on these hardworking joints. Despite appropriate treatment, many people continue to experience osteoarthritic pain that interferes with both their physical function and psychological well-being.

Besides age, other risk factors for OA include being overweight or obese and having previous fractures or other injuries to the joints. Injuries often lead to the buildup of scar tissue, which can then become easily inflamed. There can be a strong genetic component as well; family history of osteoarthritis is an independent risk factor, as well as inherited abnormalities in the shape of the bones that make up the joint.

Certain occupations put people at greater risk for osteoarthritis. Repetitive use of the hands at work or activities that strain the elbows or knees also set people up for developing osteoarthritis later in life. For example, frequent kneeling, bending, heavy lifting, and moving up and down stairs multiple times a day increases the risk of developing osteoarthritis of the knee. Certain kinds of athletes are also more prone to osteoarthritis; we cover this in more detail in Chapter 7, Sports Injury and Pain.

On the opposite end of the spectrum, sedentary lifestyles also contribute greatly to the development of osteoarthritis. Not only does lack of movement contribute to obesity (a leading risk factor for OA), but it also stiffens joints and leads to muscle loss. Weaker muscles encourage joints to become unstable, putting them at further risk of injury. The right kind of movement increases blood circulation, helping joints stay properly nourished.

We do not yet understand exactly why women are more likely than men to develop osteoarthritis. The current hypothesis is that sex hormones have a protective effect on the cartilage and women become more vulnerable to cartilage damage after menopause when estrogen levels sink dramatically. Men do not experience a comparable drop in testosterone. Unfortunately, estrogen supplementation for women after menopause doesn't help treat the symptoms or underlying disease.

### Preventing Osteoarthritis

The Arthritis Foundation has three major recommendations to prevent osteoarthritis. The first is to prevent or reverse obesity through diet and exercise; the second is to improve or maintain a healthy level of physical activity; and the third is to avoid joint injury.

To increase your activity level, many physicians recommend starting with aquatic exercise or supervised physical therapy. The water provides a buoyant force that decreases joint compression and allows movement without the constraints of body weight. Aerobic and weight training can both have a positive impact on pain, so consider incorporating each into your workout. Exercises such as walking, swimming, bicycling, or tai chi protect the joints while enhancing muscular strength. Remember to wear protective equipment when playing sports, so that you can safeguard your joints from injury.

Maintaining a healthy weight, building muscle strength while concentrating on balance and proprioception (body positioning awareness), and drinking plenty of water are some practical steps to take to maintain healthy joints.

## Treating Osteoarthritis Pain

Once you've been diagnosed with osteoarthritis (OA), there are many effective ways to control it. Unfortunately, no pharmacologic therapies halt the progression of joint damage, but they certainly can ease pain, limit disability, and reduce suffering. As with other joint pain, the first step is to try acetaminophen (Tylenol) and over-the-counter nonsteroidal anti-inflammatory drugs (NSAIDs).

If you're going to take oral medicines, try acetaminophen first. In my experience, patients use doses that are too low for a good effect, so consider using up to 3000 mg per day. That's considered a safe dose and some physicians recommend up to 4000 mg per day. If you use acetaminophen daily and over the long term, your doctor may regularly test your blood to monitor liver function, particularly related to underlying liver disease or heavy alcohol use. If you don't get sufficient relief from acetaminophen, turn to the NSAIDs, especially if there is evidence of inflammation, such as a swollen knee or finger. Although acetaminophen has weak anti-inflammatory properties, it isn't as effective for inflammatory pain or overall pain as the NSAIDs.

No single NSAID is superior to another for OA based on the literature. I give my patients a trial for one to two weeks on each before switching to another. NSAIDs that are typically prescribed include naproxen, ibuprofen, and celecoxib. Celecoxib does not inhibit the clotting process and has a decreased risk of gastrointestinal side effects (heartburn, reflux). Naproxen may offer fewer cardiovascular side effects (high blood pressure, for example), but can lead to gastrointestinal side effects. Another NSAID, called meloxicam (Mobic), is long-acting and has less of an adverse effect on platelets. All NSAIDs can cause gastrointestinal-, cardiovascular-, renal- (kidney-), and bleeding-associated side effects. Talk to your doctor or healthcare provider about

customizing an NSAID for your specific situation.

An often-overlooked recommendation relates to the timing of NSAIDs and aspirin for patients who take aspirin daily to protect against myocardial infarction (MI), stroke, and death from cardiovascular disease. These patients should take their aspirin two or more hours before taking most NSAIDs. This prevents the NSAID from interfering with the protective effects of aspirin. (According to research findings, celecoxib does not interfere with aspirin's effectiveness so timing is not a concern.)

Topical NSAIDs don't reach the bloodstream to the same extent as the oral ones; therefore, the exposure to the kidneys, heart, stomach, and platelets (the component of the blood that helps it clot) is much less. If you want to avoid taking oral NSAIDs, a topical prescription NSAID called diclofenac is available in gel form (Voltaren), for osteoarthritis of the joints in the arms and legs, and in solution form (Pennsaid), for osteoarthritis of the knee. You may think that applying medicine topically won't take away as much pain, but a large scientific review of many studies found that oral and topical NSAIDs provide equal relief. Topicals are applied directly over the painful site and absorbed directly into the tissue. Sometimes, a rash, burning, or itching develops, but in my experience, this has not proven enough of a problem for any of my patients to stop applying the medicine.

There are a number of over-the-counter topical pain relievers marketed for OA and pain that contain substances such as methyl salicylates (Salonpas), menthol (Bengay), camphor (Vicks VapoRub), salicylic acid, and trolamine salicylates. Some patients of mine have experienced a decrease in pain after using these. Menthol is found in the peppermint plant and in eucalyptus oil. It produces a coolness by stimulating cold receptors in nerve membranes. Camphor desensitizes nerves so they can't transmit pain signals as effectively.

If topical analgesics or oral NSAIDs don't help, duloxetine (Cymbalta) is usually the next medicine to try. Studies of duloxetine have shown both good pain relief and improvement in physical function. Duloxetine is FDA-approved for musculoskeletal pain. If you prefer herbals, you may want to think about boswellia. It improved pain and function in patients with knee OA according to a few recent studies. We discuss herbal remedies in depth in Chapter 20, Alternative Medicine and Pain Relief.

Afflicted joints can also be injected with steroids to reduce inflammation and pain. As we noted in Chapter 2, Joint and Soft Tissue Pain, steroids are beneficial when injected in the knee and shoulder, and patients report improvement for the hip too, even though the evidence is less strong for this joint. Less often, the hand joints are injected with steroid when patients don't respond well enough to other therapies.

When osteoarthritis occurs in the knee, doctors can inject hyaluronic acid (HA) to ease the pain and stiffness. As we discussed in Chapter 2, Joint and Soft Tissue Pain, hyaluronate is a thick liquid that occurs naturally in the synovial fluid that surrounds the knee; it becomes thinner in patients with osteoarthritis. Hyaluronic acid injections in the knee and shoulder can help augment the supply of fluid, better lubricating the joints. It looks like this also may be an option for OA hip pain based on studies showing reductions in pain, walking, and NSAID consumption. I've personally administered a series of three to five HA injections into the knee to patients who don't get relief from oral or topical NSAIDs or intra-articular steroid injections. The procedure is usually quick and relatively painless;

speak to your doctor if you think you may benefit from it.

Prolotherapy (the injection of high concentration dextrose, a sugar) is one of the cutting-edge therapies examined in Chapter 16, Regenerative Biomedicine. Physicians have used prolotherapy injections for the treatment of osteoarthritic joints of the hands or knee with positive results.

If osteoarthritis pain leads to major life changes and limitations and other therapies do not provide relief, a trial of opioids may be worthwhile. Opioids may also be an option for patients who are not surgical candidates. Opioid medications are discussed in more detail in Chapter 14, Pharmacological Therapies. The Centers for Disease Control recommends initiating opioid therapy for chronic non-cancer pain by starting short-acting opioids at the lowest dose and for the shortest period of time. As a result of this recommendation, you will likely see more healthcare providers using immediate release opioids (oxycodone (Percocet), hydrocodone (Vicodin), codeine) instead of extended-release opioids (OxyContin, MS Contin, Duragesic). Tramadol (Ultram), a weaker opioid used alone or in combination with acetaminophen or an NSAID is a good initial step. Other opioids (including extended-release opioids in certain circumstances) can be prescribed as well.

It's important to individualize the approach. A large scientific review studying opioid treatment for OA found that opioids provided some benefit on pain and function coupled with an increased risk of side effects. Ultimately, the benefits of opioid therapy need to outweigh the potential harms to a patient to warrant their use.

Although the American College of Rheumatology does not favor them, many patients have turned to nutritional supplements such as glucosamine and chondroitin. Some practice guidelines in Europe recommend these supplements. In fact, some European studies have shown that prescription doses of 800 mg of chondroitin and 1500 mg of glucosamine daily (available in Europe) can reduce osteoarthritis symptoms. In the United States, glucosamine and chondroitin are considered nutritional supplements and are sold over-the-counter, and most studies have not shown much benefit. This may be because the doses tested have been too low. A recent investigation of chondroitin (400 mg) together with glucosamine (500 mg) given three times daily compared to celecoxib (200 mg) given daily showed that both groups of patients benefited when surveyed. That is, the two supplements were as effective as celecoxib in significantly reducing pain, improving stiffness, and facilitating function in patients with moderate to severe knee pain after six months of treatment. I encourage my patients to try these supplements because they may help and side effects are minimal, if any. Some of my patients have waited a month or more before noticing an effect. Both clinical experience and research findings tell us that glucosamine and chondroitin are slow in their onset, but can provide extended pain relief and functional improvement.

Many of my patients get some pain relief when they apply heat (heating pad, heat packs, hot water bottles) to their back, neck, or joints. Indeed, heating and cooling techniques have been used to treat OA for many years. Heat decreases muscle spasm, raises the pain threshold, and acts directly on the nerves to produce relief. Just make sure the temperature isn't too hot; burns can definitely occur. Not as many of my patients use cooling therapy, but ice packs can also increase pain threshold and inhibit muscle spasm.

Other non-traditional therapies that benefit many patients with osteoarthritis are discussed in Chapter 19, Mind-Body Techniques for Pain Relief, including biofeedback, cognitive behavioral therapy (CBT), and hypnosis. Acupuncture, tai chi, meditation and massage, yoga, and Pilates can also be extremely helpful to increase blood flow to the joints, increase range of motion, and calm the mind. Tai chi, the practice of combining slow, graceful movements and meditative techniques has been shown to lower pain and facilitate function in several studies. Tai chi is inexpensive and patients of mine have enjoyed the social benefits of this mind-body practice as well as the physical benefits.

If you like spa therapy as much as I do, you'll be happy to know that mud-pack therapy in concert with mineral baths, knee massage, and exercises outperformed exercise alone in a study examining almost 400 patients with knee OA. Also, topical essential oils can soothe arthritic pain. We discuss these therapies in more detail in Part 3, Integrative Therapies for Pain, and specifically in Chapter 20, Alternative Medicine and Pain Relief, and Chapter 21, Aromas, Music, and Pain Relief.

### Osteoarthritis Pain and Surgery

When a patient's quality of life is significantly diminished by osteoarthritis that cannot be effectively controlled, it may be time to consider joint replacement. Patients considering this procedure should find a surgeon who is well trained in joint replacement; the surgeon should perform several such replacements each month.

## Innovative Treatments for Osteoarthritis Pain

Cutting-edge treatments utilizing stem cell paste grafts allow patients to regrow articular cartilage in the knee. Coupled with meniscus transplants, this option is allowing people to delay knee replacement surgery or forgo it altogether. Best of all, these biologic techniques allow patients to remain much more active than they could with an artificial knee. Scientists are working to make these procedures available for other joints as well.

Clinical trials are currently under way for a class of drugs that prevent the structural progression of osteoarthritis once it has been diagnosed; this will have a disease-modifying effect. Drugs of this type are referred to as biologic therapies. The type that are being developed for arthritis are monoclonal antibodies. Monoclonal antibodies are laboratory-made cells that attach to substances in the body and aid in treating diseases. Monoclonal antibodies are also discussed in Chapter 12, Cancer Pain and Caregiving, and Chapter 14, Pharmacological Therapies.

Another exciting therapy on the horizon targets the biological pain pathways that lead to osteoarthritis. Specifically, this treatment involves an antibody that binds to a molecule called nerve growth factor (NGF). NGF is released from cells in inflamed joints and causes nerves to sprout. As people age, NGF sensitizes sensory nerve fibers and causes normal activity such as hiking or jogging to hurt when they shouldn't. Clinical studies are currently underway for use of these anti-NGF drugs in patients with osteoarthritis, low back pain, and bone cancer pain. You can read more about NGF in Chapter 8, Skeletal Pain, and Chapter 12, Cancer Pain and Caregiving, as well as Chapter 16, Regenerative Biomedicine.

Regenerative biomedical therapies, such as prolotherapy and stem cell therapy, which are covered in Chapter 16, may also offer exciting potential for altering the disease process in OA.

## Understanding Rheumatoid Arthritis Pain

Kiki, the teenager confined to wheelchair, was diagnosed with rheumatoid arthritis. Rheumatoid arthritis (RA) afflicts about two million Americans, and its symptoms are similar to those of osteoarthritis (OA). Rheumatoid arthritis, however, is not caused by wear and tear; it is an autoimmune disease that can strike at any time of life, even in childhood. In healthy people, our body's immune system protects us from disease and infection. But for people who have an autoimmune disease, the immune system attacks healthy cells in the body by mistake. Rheumatoid arthritis is considered an inflammatory polyarthritis (an arthritis that occurs in multiple joints). Like Kiki, RA patients are more likely to experience swelling in the joints, and RA progresses much more rapidly than osteoarthritis. Unfortunately, RA often becomes quite severe within weeks or months of the onset of symptoms.

The medical community still has a lot to learn about rheumatoid arthritis. We know that the immune system of the patient causes the synovial fluid of the joint to be infiltrated by inflammatory cells, which negatively affects the lubricating properties of the cartilage. This process causes a synovitis—an inflammation of a synovial membrane—to develop inside the joint. The synovitis acts like a tumor that erodes the cartilage, bone, and even the muscles. Researchers are not sure why this condition persists after its initial onset, nor why the medications used to treat it can only put it into

remission rather than cure it. Unlike OA patients, patients diagnosed with RA routinely get initial and periodic x-rays or MRIs of the hands, wrists, and feet. This allows their healthcare providers to follow the disease's progression and remission during treatment.

Most of the time, rheumatoid arthritis begins in the small joints of the feet and hands: the wrists, knuckles, and first joints of the fingers. Within weeks, it progresses to other parts of the body, almost always in a symmetrical fashion. RA typically travels from the large joints of the upper extremities such as the neck and shoulders and moves into the elbows, hips, and knees. Mercifully, it leaves the spine untouched. If inflammatory cells inside the joints destroy the bones in the wrist, nerve compression can occur, causing carpal tunnel syndrome. For this reason, symptoms of carpal tunnel syndrome can lead to a diagnosis of rheumatoid arthritis.

Rheumatoid arthritis can appear at any age, but we see it most frequently in adults in their thirties, forties, and fifties. Although RA is three times more common in women than men, sufferers who become pregnant frequently experience a remission of symptoms. It is not clear why this is the case, but the hypothesis is that the same immunological protection that prevents the mother's immune system from attacking the fetus also protects her joints from rheumatoid arthritis attack.

There is some evidence that smoking, gum infections, and poor oral hygiene may predispose people to develop rheumatoid arthritis, and there probably is an ill-defined genetic component. Some relatives of those with rheumatoid arthritis go on to develop it, but others do not. A blood test called the cyclic citrullinated protein antibody test (CCP test) is available to detect early rheumatoid arthritis. This test provides a more clear and specific biologic marker for the disease than the traditional marker in the blood (which is called rheumatoid factor). Unfortunately, the CCP test can be a false negative in up to 50% of patients when symptoms initially strike, so a complete history and examination is important.

In some cases, joint pain can occur from viruses (rubella, parvovirus B19, and hepatitis B virus, for example) and be mistaken for RA. Tests help differentiate these sources of multiple joint inflammatory pain symptoms, though

and most viral syndromes only last up to several weeks, whereas RA persists. Fibromyalgia, covered in Chapter 4, Neuropathic Pain, and Lyme disease, discussed in Chapter 11, Disease-Related Pain, can both resemble RA. Distinguishing features of fibromyalgia include reports of tender areas at non-joint locations (the trapezius muscle and down the spine, for example). Also with fibromyalgia, there are no signs of synovitis—warmth, swelling, or decreased range of joint motion. Lyme arthritis usually occurs in a few large joints, especially the knee and then the shoulder, ankle, elbow, or wrist. It's not commonly experienced in the small joints of the hands and feet either as RA is.

Rheumatoid arthritis is extremely painful, and although it can come and go, it leaves sufferers feeling fatigued and sickly, as if they were fighting a severe cold or the flu. The good news is that there are treatments that can bring it under control and even send it into remission.

## Treating Rheumatoid Arthritis

Diagnosed in the 1980s, Kiki was put on a therapeutic dosage of aspirin: 26 pills a day. She was also given steroids

and opioids to try to control the inflammation and pain. All these drugs caused very unpleasant side effects. Today, the most important class of drugs in the battle against rheumatoid arthritis (RA) is known as disease-modifying anti-rheumatic drugs, or DMARDs. DMARDs work by halting the progression of the disease and hopefully protecting joints from further damage. The oldest DMARD is Methotrexate, which has been used successfully for 30 years. Other important and conventional DMARDs include leflunomide (Arava) and sulfasalazine (Azulfidine). Hydroxychloroquine (Plaquenil) has also been shown to be mildly to moderately effective in treating rheumatoid arthritis, but it is not disease modifying. All of these are oral medications.

Biologic DMARDs are relatively new; they've been used since 1998. These drugs work by targeting the effects of inflammatory substances that our bodies produce naturally. Tumor necrosis factor (TNF) is an inflammatory molecule called a cytokine. TNF plays a key role in the inflammation associated with rheumatoid arthritis. Biologic agents—so called because they are proteins rather than chemical compounds—that are used for treating rheumatoid arthritis include TNF inhibitors such as etanercept (Enbrel), infliximab (Remicade), adalimumab (Humira), certolizumab pegol (Cimzia), and golimumab (Simponi).

There are other biologic DMARDs that block the receptor (docking station) for other cytokines such as Interleukin-1, and Interleukin-6. Because they have not produced equal benefit compared to other biologic drugs, these biologic DMARDs aren't prescribed very often. However, the FDA recently approved sarilumab (Kevzara) which blocks the Interleukin-6 receptor for patients not benefitting from other DMARDs.

Patient response to biologics is highly individual. One person may tolerate a particular drug well, while another experiences unpleasant or even unbearable side effects. This is why, if you have RA, it is important to work with your rheumatologist to find the right treatment for you. In general, for the most part, biologic DMARDs offer more effective relief from symptoms than conventional DMARDs. Patients can feel better in several days to weeks after starting biologic DMARDs. Although these drugs have revolutionized rheumatoid arthritis treatment (because they halt bone destruction so quickly) most of them must be injected by your doctor, making them less convenient. Whichever DMARD is chosen, realize that starting therapy as soon as possible after diagnosis leads to better outcomes. DMARDs can cause serious side effects too, such as liver abnormalities or infections (herpes zoster, known as shingles, for example).

Often, nonsteroidal anti-inflammatory drugs (NSAIDs), oral steroids (prednisone), or even joint injections with steroid are used to control pain for patients until DMARDs become effective or prescribed for patients experiencing flare-ups. Although long-term steroid use must be avoided, short-to medium-term use (for up to two years) does show slowing of RA progression. Opioids may be needed for disease flare-ups or for end-stage RA. There have been reports of infections requiring hospitalization in RA patients on opioids, perhaps due to the immunosuppressive effect of the opioids (that has been found in animal and laboratory experiments). RA patients are already vulnerable to serious infections because of the autoimmune disease itself as well as medications such as steroids and DMARDs that suppress the immune system. Since there is a *potential* association between opioid use and infection risk, it's prudent to use opioids only for short periods and at the lowest effective dose.

Thanks to the DMARDs, RA patients can look forward to a much greater chance of remission, less disability with more function, and less pain. There are also a variety of non-drug therapies that bring day-to-day relief to RA patients. It is important to keep in mind that these therapies will not stop bone damage, so they must be incorporated in addition to, not instead of, the disease-modifying anti-rheumatic drug treatments. Some patients have found dietary adjustments that include the addition of omega-3 fatty acids to the diet make a positive difference in symptoms. Ayurvedic medicine (a type of complementary or alternative medicine), yoga, and naturopathic medicine have all helped some patients find relief. You can learn more about these therapies in Part 3, Integrative Therapies for Pain. Integrative therapies along with NSAIDs can help to reduce the day-to-day flare ups of rheumatoid arthritis.

### Rheumatoid Arthritis Pain and Activity

Sedentary behavior makes rheumatoid arthritis worse, just as it does with osteoarthritis and many other conditions. Thus, physical activity is absolutely essential to managing RA effectively. Physical therapists and occupational therapists should be enlisted to help ensure that patients learn to use their affected joints correctly, keeping blood flowing to the area without damaging the joints further. Finding someone to help you exercise safely and often is an important step for anyone with RA.

## New and Innovative Treatments for Rheumatoid Arthritis Pain

Cutting-edge treatments for rheumatoid arthritis that we can look forward to seeing in the future include janus kinase (JAK) inhibitors. These are oral medications that behave like biologics which block inflammatory cytokines, but JAK inhibitors are chemical compounds and provide their benefits much more conveniently. They are also metabolized by the body very quickly, so any potential side effects are very short lived. These drugs block signals inside of cells that lead to the production of cytokines and other inflammatory molecules. In November 2012, tofacitinib (Xeljanz) became the first JAK inhibitor approved for RA use in the United States.

# Understanding Gout

Gout is often referred to as the King of Diseases and the Disease of Kings. It earned the name King of Diseases because of the crushing pain that patients experience during attacks, considered worse than any other form of arthritis. It is known as the Disease of Kings because attacks are often associated with the consumption of alcohol and rich foods such as lobster or foie gras. There are historical records that describe gout symptoms in people as long ago as 2600 BCE in ancient Egypt. King Henry VIII of England, Sir Isaac Newton, and Benjamin Franklin all suffered from gout.

## Causes of Gout

Gout affects between five and eight million people in the United States alone. The disease is becoming more prevalent in America and across the world perhaps from our increased longevity, particular medications used to treat chronic disorders, and increased consumption of food and food additives that lead to diabetes and obesity. Gout is the sudden acute inflammatory response to the accumulation of monosodium urate crystals in the joints. Humans and other primates do not produce uricase (also called urate oxidase), the enzyme that enables other mammals to metabolize uric acid. Uric acid is a byproduct of the breakdown of purines. Purines occur naturally in the body and are involved in DNA synthesis, but they are also found in many foods including lobster and other seafood, dairy products, anchovies, herring, organ meats, alcohol, asparagus, and mushrooms. Large meals rich in such foods are known to trigger gouty attacks.

Men between the ages of 40 and 50 are 20 times more likely than women to have gout, although post-menopausal women have been known to be afflicted. The risk of gout increases with the factors associated with metabolic syndrome, which include a large waistline, high blood pressure, high LDL ("bad") cholesterol, high blood sugar/pre-diabetes, and high triglyceride levels in the blood. A family history of gout or metabolic syndrome also increases risk. Trauma, surgery, fatty foods, and dehydration can all provoke an attack. Consuming alcohol raises the risk of attacks in men.

Patients experience gout attacks when their immune systems attack the crystals in their joints. An acute gout attack begins with a feeling of tightness and burning in a single joint, usually the base of the big toe or the knee. Within hours, the joint becomes swollen and red, and the pain level becomes unbearable. Many patients can't walk during the attack or even tolerate bed sheets touching the area around the joint. An attack can last for days or even weeks, but peak pain severity is reached within 12 to 24 hours. In addition to a meal rich in purines or alcohol, weather and temperature changes and trauma have all been known to

trigger attacks. The attacks usually occur at night and in the early morning. Less commonly, the attacks can manifest in multiple joints, but this typically happens later in the disease among patients who remain untreated.

As excruciating as the pain of gout may be, individual attacks are not actually that dangerous. Single attacks do not damage the joints, tissues, or bones. However, recurrent attacks can. If gout is not effectively managed, the number of joints involved can increase. Those who are not diagnosed or treated will likely have another episode within two years. Unlike other forms of arthritis, which tend to spare particular areas of the body, no joint is safe from gout. About 10 years or so after the initial onset of gout, some patients may develop tophi—lumps in the skin formed by collections of crystalized uric acid—if the disease is not controlled. Surgery may be necessary to remove tophi in order to improve joint mobility.

### *Diagnosing Gout*

A doctor can make a preliminary diagnosis of gout based on the nature of the attack. Gout is diagnosed definitively when a rheumatologist performs an arthrocentesis by inserting a needle into the affected joint and extracting synovial fluid. If the rheumatologist identifies uric acid crystals in the fluid (by looking under a microscope), the patient is confirmed to have gout. Ideally, the arthrocentesis should be performed during an acute attack, but even a "dry tap" (on a joint that is not swollen with fluid) that yields uric acid crystals is sufficient for a positive diagnosis.

Other tests associated with gout include measuring the uric acid levels in the blood. Although higher uric acid levels in the blood are associated with an increased risk of gout, most people with high levels will not necessarily develop the disease. In addition, the presence of uric acid levels in the blood during an acute attack may be normal or low. Thus, a blood test alone cannot serve as a diagnosis. The best time to examine uric acid blood levels is two weeks or so after an acute attack is over. Gout attacks occur when the immune system attacks the uric acid crystals causing pain from inflammation and tissue damage. A fracture or traumatic event to the bone or joint can mimic an acute attack as can a disorder called pseudogout. Most of the time, analysis of the synovial joint fluid distinguishes these and other conditions from gout.

## Treating Gout Pain

Dietary changes, such as reducing alcohol intake, avoiding shellfish, organ meats, and dairy products, can lower the risk of gouty episodes by limiting uric acid levels. Realistically, most patients with gout find it hard to modify their diet, so knowing about effective medical treatments is important.

As with many other pain conditions, the first treatment to try is over-the-counter nonsteroidal anti-inflammatory drugs (NSAIDs), such as ibuprofen (Motrin), naproxen (Naprosyn, Aleve; 500 mg twice per day), or indomethacin (Indocin) (50 mg three times per day). Aspirin is not used to treat gout pain because it increases levels of uric acid. You can take NSAIDs for several days until the pain and inflammation are gone.

If NSAIDs do not bring sufficient relief or they can't be used for medical reasons, your doctor may try injecting steroids into the joint to bring down the swelling. While the injection of local anesthetic into the joint provides immediate pain relief, the steroid effect is not immediate. Removing fluid from an affected joint with a needle also reduces pain. For patients with symptoms in the big toe joint, a nerve block around the posterior tibial nerve located in the ankle along with a steroid injection around the joint itself (periarticular injection) can provide relief. Occasionally, oral steroids (prednisone) may be provided for acute, painful gout attacks. Rarely, intravenous or intramuscular steroids are injected.

For some people who cannot tolerate NSAIDs or for whom NSAIDs are ineffective, oral colchicine (Colcrys) can be a good option if taken within 12 to 24 hours of the outset of an attack. Colchicine blocks the cells causing inflammation from uric acid build up and works fast to reduce inflammation and pain. Some patients experience unpleasant gastrointestinal side effects (diarrhea, cramping), but others tolerate colchicine well. Patients continue to take colchicine for the duration of the attack. This drug can even stop acute attacks if taken early enough.

If patients start having more frequent attacks or there is evidence of joint injury, then doctors may consider preventive medications that lower uric acid levels such as probenecid. Probenecid (Probalan) increases uric acid excretion through the kidneys to reduce the number of gout attacks. It's not commonly used but can be helpful in patients with normal kidney function. Lesinurad (Zurampic), which just entered the market, promotes the excretion of uric acid too. Lesinurad is taken with allopurinol (Aloprim) or febuxostat (Uloric). At this point, many doctors will also reach for allopurinol, a drug that reduces the amount of uric acid our bodies produce. A new drug, febuxostat, works in a similar fashion and can be used for those intolerant to allopurinol or who have chronic kidney disease. Both allopurinol and febuxostat are oral medications.

It's important to control uric acid formation in the body because kidney stones composed of uric acid can develop and sometimes impair kidney function. In general, the goal with preventive therapy is to lower the blood uric acid level to less than 6 mg/dL. Bear in mind that acute gouty flare ups can still occur when a patient is taking any of the medications that lower uric acid levels.

For gout sufferers who cannot tolerate oral medications or who have advanced gout, pegloticase (Krystexxa), a type of uricase enzyme, can be injected intravenously every two weeks to reduce uric acid levels and prevent gout attacks. It is remarkably helpful for dissolving tophi, which may otherwise need to be removed surgically.

Three other injectable, biologic medications in development for acute gout (anakinra (Kineret), canakinumab (Ilaris), and rilonacept (Arcalyst)) have also been shown to bring about pain control for those unresponsive to typical medications. These three medications block a cytokine called Interleuken-1 or its receptor and at least one may be available soon.

Canakinumab is approved for use in Europe and patients have responded well to anakinra in clinical trials.

Although gout can be an unbelievably painful disease, it is manageable, and new therapies are offering increasing hope as well as a dramatic reduction in chronic gouty arthritis.

## Hope for Arthritis Pain Relief

After years of being confined to a wheelchair, Kiki now not only walks on her own, but she also travels over 200,000 miles a year to speak all over the world. Although she once found it very difficult to discuss her pain, she is now an internationally recognized patient advocate, author, speaker, and educator. She has had 16 surgeries and 12 joint replacements, but she has been able to stop taking many of the medications that were causing unpleasant side effects. Rheumatoid Arthritis no longer dictates every aspect of her life.

Kiki works daily to balance getting enough rest with enough of the physical activity that she knows is essential to protecting her joints. She has learned to ask for help from those around her. Most of all, Kiki has overcome arthritis and has taken control of her life.

To learn more about various self-care and pain treatment options and therapies, read the chapters in Part 1, Understanding and Treating Your Pain, and Part 2, Medical Therapies for Pain: Traditional and Innovative. There you will find more information and ideas for working with your physician and other healthcare providers to find ways to prevent, manage, and address your pain.

You can learn more about arthritis pain by listening to the arthritis pain episodes of my weekly radio program, *Aches and Gains*. You can find the broadcasts on arthritis pain at the following URLs.

**Osteoarthritis**
http://paulchristomd.com/osteoarthritis

**Rheumatoid Arthritis**
http://paulchristomd.com/rheumatoid-arthritis

**Gout**
http://paulchristomd.com/gout

## Suggested Further Reading

Arden, Nigel, Hunter, David, Prieto-Alhambra, Daniel. *Osteoarthritis: The Facts.* (n.p.): Oxford University Press, 2014. The book helps patients and their carers better understand the condition, empowering patients with the knowledge and skills to actively take charge of their own health. http://tinyurl.com/ycpbgvxw

Arthritis Foundation. *Good Living with Osteoarthritis.* (n.p.): Arthritis Foundation, 2006. The Arthritis Foundation presents tools for living with osteoarthritis, from relieving pain to popular supplements, alternative therapies and simple exercises. https://tinyurl.com/yafnba8z

Bales, Peter. *Osteoarthritis: Preventing and Healing Without Drugs.* (n.p.): Prometheus Books: 2008. Orthopedic surgeon Peter Bales highlights the nutritional connection to osteoarthritis with a focus on new genetic research. https://tinyurl.com/y9ya74yv

Blum, Susan. *Healing Arthritis: Your 3-Step Guide to Conquering Arthritis Naturally.* (n.p.): Scribner, 2017. Dr. Blum offers a science-based, drug-free treatment plan for arthritis patients. https://tinyurl.com/ycl5fgec

Cooper, Grant. *The Arthritis Handbook: Improve Your Health and Manage the Pain of Osteoarthritis.* (n.p.): DiaMedica, 2008. This book offers a blend of advice, dietary info, targeted exercise, and tips to avoid the use of medication, injection therapy, and surgery. https://tinyurl.com/yb2j6799

Konshin, Victor. *Beating Gout: A Sufferer's Guide To Living Pain Free*. (n.p.): Ayerware Publishing, 2015. This book covers all aspects of gout from its progression, diagnosis, and treatment to research on diet and lifestyle choices. https://tinyurl.com/y7vqeooy

Schoffro Cook, Michelle. *Arthritis-Proof Your Life: Secrets to Pain-Free Living Without Drugs*. (n.p.): Humanix Books, 2016. A study of natural sources for helping arthritis sufferers including diet, herbs and vitamins, exercise and other natural pain relieving methods. https://tinyurl.com/y8px6x2m

Shiotzhauer, Tammi L. *Living with Rheumatoid Arthritis*. (n.p.): Johns Hopkins University Press, 2014. This book explains the causes, symptoms, and treatment options for people with rheumatoid arthritis while offering practical strategies for coping with the pain, fatigue, and emotional toll of a chronic illness. https://tinyurl.com/y7wqjunm

Wiley, Mark V. *Arthritis Reversed: 30 Days to Lasting Relief from Joint Pain and Arthritis*. (n.p.): Tambuli Media, 2014. Dr. Wiley presents a powerful, integrated mind/body approach to arthritis relief and prevention by identifying underlying sometimes hidden-causes. https://tinyurl.com/ybzxy8z7

---

# Other Resources to Explore

Arthritis.org is the official website of The Arthritis Foundation. The foundation has a Helpline to answer questions over the phone: 1-844-571-4357. https://tinyurl.com/ybdky2mq

ArthritisResearchUK.org is similar to The Arthritis Foundation, publishing up-to-date research in their news section.

Creakyjoints is an Online Patient Community for those suffering from arthritis. It is part of the nonprofit Global Health Living Foundation.

RheumatoidArthritis.net provides patients with tools and resources to help manage their disease, including articles contributed by physicians and a community forum.

# 4

# Neuropathic Pain

## Understanding Neuropathic Pain

Perhaps nothing is more frustrating for pain sufferers than to have friends, family members or even doctors fail to take their pain seriously. Patients not only struggle to get effective treatment, but are also accused of exaggerating or imagining their pain. Unfortunately, many people suffering from neuropathic pain find themselves in exactly that position—misunderstood, misdiagnosed, or even disbelieved. Neuropathic pain affects as much as 8% of the general population, impairing daily function, sleep, and mood.

The word "neuropathic" in the term neuropathic pain implies that nerves are injured or dysfunctional, sending the wrong signals to the spinal cord or brain. In contrast, nociceptive pain (such as the pain caused by arthritis) comes from the activation of normally functioning nerves by certain molecules such as cytokines or other inflammatory or pain-producing substances.

Neuropathic pain can manifest as discrete or widespread areas of pain; sensory deficits (decreased sensation or numbness); burning, tingling, electric-like pain provoked by light touch; and/or pain attacks without a known trigger. Neuropathic pain is a disease or injury of the nerves themselves. We classify neuropathic pain according to its location. For example, we say it is peripheral—in the nerves of the arms, legs, or chest. Or we say it is central—in the spinal cord or brain. It can also be classified based on the cause of pain: infectious (HIV or shingles), traumatic (nerve injury), metabolic (painful diabetic neuropathy), or toxic (chemotherapy neuropathy). (Recall that, as we explained in Chapter 1, Headache Pain, peripheral nerves are part of the peripheral nervous system. They make up the large network of nerves that connect the brain and spinal cord—central nervous system—to the body.) Another term we use when we are talking about this kind of pain is "neuralgia," which refers to intermittent bursts of pain rather than the more typical continuous type of neuropathic pain.

Many of my patients want to know why they feel this type of pain. Any number of the following mechanisms may cause neuropathic pain in a given patient:

* When nerves are injured, they become overexcited and fire when they shouldn't. Physicians refer to this as ectopic nerve activity.

* Peripheral nerves can become sensitized after injury, leading to more overexcitability and the ability to fire much more easily. This is called peripheral sensitization.

* Peripheral pain signals from impaired nerves can trigger reversible changes in the spinal cord and brain of the central nervous system. This leads to the magnified pain response called central sensitization.

* Nerve injury can weaken the body's natural ability to inhibit pain (also known as impaired inhibitory modulation).

* Microglia are cells that play a role in the immune defense of the brain and spinal cord. It's thought that mistakenly activated microglia may contribute to pain hypersensitivity or chronic pain conditions by releasing cytokines and other pain-inducing substances.

Nerves are always involved in pain, but with neuropathic pain, the nerve cells themselves are damaged or not functioning properly. While neuropathic pain can be a signal of a serious underlying illness, people can also experience neuropathic pain in a part of the body where there is no obvious damage to the muscles, bones, or connective tissues. This can make correct diagnosis much more challenging, since a problem may not show up on a scan or in a blood test.

The symptoms of neuropathic pain can be relatively mild: an ache, an itch or a tingle that just doesn't seem to go away. Or symptoms can be severe: a stabbing, burning, or searing sensation that makes life unbearable without being obviously connected to an illness or injury. Many sufferers experience allodynia—the reaction of extreme pain from a stimulus, such as the pressure of a bed sheet or clothing on the skin—that shouldn't cause pain at all. Other people with neuropathic pain may experience hyperalgesia—disproportionate intense pain from something, such as a pinprick, that ordinarily causes pain.

Patients can find themselves frustrated or even enraged, as healthcare providers suggest the pain is all in their head, and friends and family grow weary of their complaints. But there is hope. With the correct diagnosis and treatment, for a limited number of people neuropathic pain goes away completely, while other patients are able to manage the pain effectively and regain control of their lives. Bear in mind that the diagnosis of neuropathic pain is mostly based on history and physical examination rather than special tests.

In this chapter, we'll discuss seven major types of neuropathic pain: painful diabetic neuropathy, complex regional pain syndrome, trigeminal neuralgia, fibromyalgia, persistent shingles pain, multiple sclerosis, and neurogenic thoracic outlet syndrome. As well as being considered a neuropathic pain syndrome, fibromyalgia is also categorized as a central sensitivity syndrome (CSS). Central sensitivity syndromes are a group of conditions in which patients experience a magnified pain response in the central nervous system. They include migraines, chronic Lyme disease (post-treatment Lyme disease syndrome), and irritable bowel syndrome.

## Treating Neuropathic Pain

Several classes of medications have proven helpful in the treatment of neuropathic pain. It is important to keep in mind that response to pain medications is highly individual, so what works for one person may not work for another, even when both people suffer from the same condition. It is therefore always important to work closely with your doctor and keep a journal of your symptoms when trying any course of treatment. If you don't find relief after a month or two of any treatment, it's probably time to try something else. Along with medications, patients with neuropathic pain may need combined therapies incorporating nerve blocks, rehabilitation, psychological support, integrative approaches, or neurostimulation.

Anticonvulsant medications such as gabapentin (Neurontin) and pregabalin (Lyrica) and tricyclic antidepressants (TCAs), such as nortriptyline (Pamelor), amitriptyline (Elavil), and desipramine (Norpramin), often provide good, but not necessarily complete, relief for neuropathic pain. It's particularly important to try these medicines for two to three weeks or more at the proper dose before concluding that they are not effective. If they don't work, serotonin–norepinephrine reuptake inhibitors (SNRIs) such as duloxetine (Cymbalta) and venlafaxine (Effexor) are typically the next drugs to try. The antidepressants can reduce chronic pain; don't discount them because of the mistaken impression they are only used for depression. Antidepressants such as TCAs and SNRIs are prescribed for many forms of pain and can secondarily improve depression and sleep disturbances, which I feel make them an additional asset.

In my practice, I have found greater success with the anticonvulsants and the TCAs rather than SNRIs. As a matter of fact, the TCAs have proven effective in many published trials for neuropathic pain conditions such as painful diabetic neuropathy, postherpetic neuralgia (chronic shingles pain), and post-stroke pain. This is also true for gabapentin (Neurontin) and pregabalin (Lyrica).

Topical anesthetics, such as lidocaine (patch or gel), EMLA cream (combination of lidocaine and prilocaine), ketamine, or capsaicin creams/patch, can also provide relief when applied directly to the affected areas. There is less evidence for the effectiveness of these treatments, though. Lidocaine blocks sodium channels in nerves causing them to spontaneously discharge less often.

Capsaicin, the active ingredient in hot chili peppers, depletes a pain-producing neurotransmitter, called substance P, from pain-sensing nerve endings. Unfortunately, capsaicin also causes a burning sensation during the initial weeks of application, which prevents some patients from using it.

If all the mediations previously mentioned in this section fail to bring sufficient relief, doctors may prescribe opioids such as morphine, oxycodone, or hydrocodone. Tramadol (Ultram), a medication that shares some properties with opioids, is often used before the stronger opioids just listed. Morphine, oxycodone or hydrocodone have a higher risk of misuse, abuse, and overdose, and there is also a lack of long-term evidence of effectiveness. That being said, there is evidence for short-term benefit in neuropathic pain and certain patients may be candidates for these drugs if their pain is severe enough to affect their function and quality of life.

## Interventional Procedures for Neuropathic Pain

A fair number of patients don't experience enough relief from the medications just described or the integrative therapies discussed in the following material.

For this reason, it's important to be aware that interventional procedures are available for neuropathic pain or neuralgias. For instance, targeted nerve blocks using local anesthetic and/or steroid can help with head pain and headaches from occipital neuralgia, groin pain from ilioinguinal neuralgia (pain experienced post-hernia repair surgery), chest wall pain from intercostal neuralgia (pain experienced after thoracic surgery or mastectomy), facial pain from trigeminal neuralgia, leg or arm pain from complex regional pain syndrome, and radicular pain in the arm or leg from disc herniation or stenosis. Recall that when nerve blocks are used for pain treatment and management, a local anesthetic medication is injected around a specific nerve in the body.

Pulsed radiofrequency (PRF) treatment is beneficial for reducing pain for several months in patients with occipital head pain from occipital neuralgia or groin/genital pain from ilioinguinal neuralgia, for instance. In PRF, doctors place a needle near the nerve. The needle transmits a low intensity electrical field around the nerve to reduce the firing of pain signals in that nerve. Similarly, alcohol or other chemicals can be injected around specific nerve bundles (in the sympathetic nervous system) for therapeutic benefit in patients with severe cancer pain, substantially improving their quality of life. Spinal cord stimulation (see Chapter 15, Pain-Relieving Devices) or peripheral nerve stimulation can improve neuropathic pain in the back or down the legs in patients whose pain persists or changes following spine surgery (failed back surgery syndrome), in patients with arm or leg pain from complex regional pain syndrome, and in those with other painful neuropathic conditions.

Another therapy provided by pain pumps (intrathecal drug delivery systems), which involves placing small doses of medicine into the spinal fluid, can ease disabling neuropathic pain from cancer. Spinal cord stimulation and pain pumps are covered more extensively in Chapter 15, Pain-Relieving Devices.

## New and Innovative Treatments for Neuropathic Pain

An interesting and fairly new neurostimulation treatment called Scrambler Therapy has been FDA-cleared since 2014 for treating chronic neuropathic and cancer pain. Scrambler Therapy had been used in Europe for about 20 years to treat a condition known as chemotherapy-induced peripheral neuropathy (CIPN). This condition causes burning, stabbing, and tingling sensations in the hands and feet in up to 40% of patients undergoing cancer chemotherapy using classes of drugs called antineoplastic agents.

The Scrambler Therapy device, which is discussed in more detail in Chapter 15, Pain-Relieving Devices, uses nerve stimulation to relieve pain by transmitting low frequency electrical stimulation. It is believed that this process targets pain receptors in the periphery, spinal cord, and brain to inhibit pain impulse transmission, thereby reducing the intensity of the pain. Skin surface electrodes are placed above and below the area of pain for ten 30–45-minute sessions, during which some patients report a tingling or stinging sensation.

Research studies of Scrambler Therapy show benefit in patients with visceral pain (pancreatic cancer, colon cancer, gastric cancer) as well as conditions such as failed back surgery syndrome and brachial plexus neuropathy. Many patients in these studies had dramatic relief without side effects.

About 8%–10% of neuropathic pain originates form the peripheral nerves. A minimally invasive stimulation device called StimRouter, designed to treat peripheral nerve pain, is available for patients with certain kinds of neuropathic pain in the arms, legs, pelvis, and trunk. The technology delivers small pulses of energy to specific nerves believed to be causing pain such as the axillary nerve in the shoulder or the ilioinguinal nerve in the groin. The StimRouter uses a very thin and short lead (wire) that is positioned next to a pain-generating nerve, which is connected to a power source (receiver) on top of the skin. Patients use a wireless programmer to control the settings. A couple of clinical studies have shown good pain relief and safety. So far, I've seen pain relief and functional improvement in patients of mine with post-stroke shoulder symptoms. A more extensive discussion of these types of treatments is found in Chapter 15, Pain-Relieving Devices.

Botulinum toxin (Botox) is also showing promising results in patients with peripheral neuropathic pain disorders. For example, patients have experienced relief with trigeminal neuralgia, postherpetic neuralgia, complex regional pain syndrome, and diabetic peripheral neuropathy.

Smoked or oral cannabis (marijuana) is growing in popularity for treating chronic pain. Specifically, the literature is demonstrating the value of this therapy for neuropathic pain from multiple sclerosis and HIV neuropathy. Almost half the states have legalized the use of cannabis for chronic pain and cancer patients. Many questions linger concerning the best method of cannabis delivery (oral, smoked, vaporized), dose, frequency, and long-term safety, not to mention legality at the federal level. Nevertheless, medical marijuana may soon become a more common treatment option given that a variety of cannabinoids, the term for all compounds structurally related to the active compound in cannabis, tetrahydrocannabinol (THC), are in development for ultimate approval by the FDA. Medical marijuana is covered in Chapter 14, Pharmacological Therapies.

Medications aimed at stimulating nerve re-growth also offer promising therapies for patients with neuropathic pain. These treatments are reviewed in Chapter 16, Regenerative Biomedicine. Another exciting therapy has been seen in animal research on transplanting stem cells to the site of spinal cord injury. These sorts of transplants may help to repair damaged nerve cells in humans in the future.

## Integrative Treatments for Neuropathic Pain

In addition to conventional medications, many people suffering from neuropathic pain may find relief from integrative treatments such as cognitive behavioral therapy (CBT), hypnosis, acupuncture or even topical essential oils, such as peppermint, clove, lemongrass, eucalyptus, and German chamomile.

CBT makes patients aware that changing how they think and feel about pain can make a meaningful difference in their lives. It's provided benefit in HIV neuropathy and spinal cord injury pain among several other pain conditions. Hypnosis has been found helpful for people with phantom limb pain—a type of neuropathic pain that sometimes occurs in amputees. Acupuncture can reduce pain in diabetic peripheral neuropathy and a combination of cupping (an alternative medicine practice using suction on the skin), Chinese herbs, acupuncture, and nerve blocks were shown to reduce pain among those with postherpetic neuralgia.

Similarly, the validation and encouragement of support groups have allowed patients of mine to feel better about themselves and their condition; the positive reinforcement of others with similar struggles has fostered hope and the belief that they can get better. All these kinds of therapies are discussed in much more detail in Part 3, Integrative Therapies for Pain.

# Understanding Painful Diabetic Neuropathy

Anyone who watched television during the '50s and '60s will remember actor Jerry Mathers as the inquisitive and loveable titular character on *Leave It to Beaver*. It's hard to believe that iconic little boy is now in his sixties and, like many older Americans, is facing some health challenges. After decades of successful acting, Mathers acquired a catering company in the 1990s and in his new food-oriented environment began overeating. Within a couple of years, the five foot eight inch actor had ballooned to 250 pounds. He also began experiencing a pins and needles sensation and sharp pain in his feet, along with shoulder pain that became so severe he was unable to lift his arm.

Like too many others, Mathers ignored these symptoms for a very long time. Finally, at the urging of a family friend who was also a physician, he agreed to a get a physical. At his doctor's office, he was shocked to learn he had developed diabetes and that the pain he was feeling in his shoulder and feet was painful diabetic neuropathy (also called diabetic peripheral neuropathy or DPN). His doctor informed him that if he didn't make some lifestyle changes, he would be dead in three to five years.

## Causes of Painful Diabetic Neuropathy

Diabetes is a metabolic disease in which the body loses its ability to regulate blood sugar levels. When a person has diabetes, the body's ability to produce or respond to the hormone insulin is impaired, resulting in high levels of glucose in the blood and urine. Diabetes affects hundreds of millions of people worldwide, and about half of them experience neuropathic symtoms. For up to 20% of diabetics, the pain is severe. There are two type of diabetes—type 1 and type 2—and different mechanisms are responsible for the two types. Type 2 diabetes accounts for up to 95% of diabetes. This makes type 2, or adult onset, diabetes the most common cause of painful diabetic neuropathy, which is also referred to as diabetic peripheral neuropathy (DPN).

In the early stages of diabetes, patients may not exhibit symptoms of DPN. Over time, however, diabetes damages the peripheral nerves (the nerves outside the brain and spinal cord) causing numbness, tingling, burning, stabbing, and cramping pains. How does diabetes damage peripheral nerves? The prevailing theory suggests that high glucose levels that result from diabetes produce stress on nerves. When blood sugars are high, they diminish blood flow to the nerves, which sensitizes the nerves to pain and can lead to numbness, weakness, and falls (due to loss of sensation in the feet). Among its many functions, insulin acts as a growth factor and actually has receptors on nerve cells. So insulin deficiency together with glucose toxicity leads to insulin resistance and degeneration in the nerve cells themselves.

A neurologic exam, quantitative sensory testing (which identifies injury to small nerves), skin biopsy (examining the small nerves under a microscope of a tiny piece of skin), and electromyogram/nerve conduction testing (EMG/NCT) can all be used to diagnose DPN. However, a new, noninvasive five-minute test called confocal microscopy, which involves looking at nerve supply to the cornea, may soon serve as a sufficient indicator of the condition. Although currently just in the research trial phase, it looks promising.

## Symptoms of Painful Diabetic Neuropathy

Most patients experience pain first in the feet. Pain will often spread symmetrically up the legs and to other parts of the body. This is why doctors refer to the distribution of pain as a "stocking-glove": the abnormal sensations appear in an area of the body that could be covered by a stocking or glove. The pain is worse at rest and improves with walking.

Other common symptoms of DPN include weakness, difficulty balancing, and even difficulty with the autonomic nervous system, which controls bowel and bladder function, sweating, blood pressure, and other involuntary processes. Patients may also experience restless leg syndrome and carpel tunnel syndrome.

## Treating Painful Diabetic Neuropathy

The first priority for anyone with painful diabetic neuropathy, or diabetic peripheral neuropathy (DPN), is to get the diabetes under control by controlling blood sugar and body weight.

Controlling triglyceride levels and hypertension is also vital to prevent DPN from progressing. Once patients begin exhibiting symptoms of diabetic neuropathy, it's extremely difficult to reverse the process. This highlights the importance of prevention.

To address the pain of DPN, doctors turn to the classes of medications described at the beginning of the chapter such as the anticonvulsants, antidepressants, topicals, and sometimes opioids. Pregabalin (Lyrica), gabapentin (Horizant), duloxetine (Cymbalta), tapentadol (Nucynta), and the lidocaine patch are FDA-approved treatments for DPN. The scientific literature points to pain relief from the tricyclic antidepressants (TCAs) (amitriptyline (Elavil), desipramine (Norpramin)), duloxetine, pregabalin, and maybe gabapentin. Some doctors use topical capsaicin in different formulations (cream, lotion, gel, patch) with varying degrees of success, and lidocaine patches can reduce pain as well. Combining drugs from different medication classes can be more effective than prescribing one drug alone; this is one strategy used to better control pain.

Antioxidants are another option. For instance, alpha-lipoic acid has shown the ability to reduce pain, numbness, and pins and needles sensations in DPN at doses of 600 mg by mouth daily.

For those who don't respond to conventional strategies and continue to suffer, some studies have demonstrated 50% relief of pain for prolonged periods of time with spinal cord stimulation (SCS). SCS is also discussed in more detail in Chapter 15, Pain-Relieving Devices. SCS is probably an underutilized technique in DPN patients who do not have good results with other therapies. Published studies do report favorable results with SCS in treating neuropathic pain from diabetes. But because DPN often progresses to other parts of the body, patients may find their pain moving to areas outside the coverage provided by SCS, rendering the treatment less effective over time. SCS can provide a valuable option for managing pain alone or in addition to conventional therapies. Pain pumps delivering medications directly to the spine can also be helpful, though they are rarely used for DPN patients.

There is also promising research being conducted on actually regrowing peripheral nerves after injury. For instance, researchers are targeting certain genes that will give even small nerves in the body the capacity to sprout and reconnect if they are damaged. When nerve cells are injured, the nerve activates certain genes called regeneration-associated genes (RAGs) to support re-growth. Groundbreaking research using electrical stimulation at the site of nerve damage in animals and humans has shown the ability to accelerate nerve regeneration by "activating" RAGs. Further, studies have found that nerves treated this way recover better than they would without treatment or even if the nerve were reattached surgically.

Studies in animals have revealed that transcutaneous electrical nerve stimulation (TENS) also stimulates nerve regeneration following nerve injury. Electrical nerve stimulation in the form of a TENS transmits electrical current to the skin using skin surface electrodes. You can learn more about TENS in Chapter 15, Pain-Relieving Devices, and more about nerve regeneration in Chapter 16, Regenerative Biomedicine. These developments in nerve regrowth are particularly exciting because nerves injured from diabetes are less likely to cause neuropathic pain if they can re-grow.

Infrared light therapy (monochromatic infrared energy) may or may not alleviate pain due to DPN according to clinical studies. It reportedly releases nitric oxide, dilates blood vessels, and then reduces pain by increasing oxygen delivery to nerves. It has few side effects, though, so even if it is less likely to be effective, it may be worth it to try it.

Other new therapies on the horizon for DPN include methods of altering metabolic pathways for sugars, strategies to increase blood flow directly to nerves, and drugs that manipulate or block sodium and calcium channels (ion channels) in nerves to reduce neuropathic pain.

Jerry Mathers went to Jenny Craig for help with weight loss; he was determined not to starve himself but to try instead to live a healthier lifestyle. By modifying his portions and walking an hour a day five days a week, he dropped nearly 90 pounds over the course of about a year. In addition to bringing his diabetes under control, Mathers found that the more weight he lost, the further apart his episodes of neuropathic pain were. Today, the pain is gone and hasn't come back.

Mathers now spends much of his time raising awareness of diabetes by telling his story and sharing about the risks of letting the disease go uncontrolled. In both public appearances and educational videos, Mathers urges people to get regular physicals and not to ignore any pain they may be feeling. He encourages those trying to lose weight to learn more about healthy food preparation and portion control, and to take it one day at a time. "It won't happen overnight," he said on my radio program, "but your life will be so much better in the long run."

## Understanding Complex Regional Pain Syndrome

Almost everyone deals with a minor fracture or sprain at some point. A slip on icy pavement, a fall that results in a twisted ankle, or any other trivial accident is a normal part of life. Most of us experience some moderate pain, ice the injury, take some ibuprofen, and expect a full recovery within a couple of days. But for the small group of people who have complex regional pain syndrome (CRPS), a minor injury like this can becomes a life-altering experience that plunges them into the depths of pain and despair.

CRPS remains poorly understood. It generally follows musculoskeletal trauma but also can be triggered by surgery, inflammation, stroke, crush injury, myocardial infarction, neoplasms (tumors), and sprains. Immobilization or disuse of a limb may also lead to the onset of CRPS.

There are two major forms of CRPS. A person with CRPS Type I (also known as reflex sympathetic dystrophy syndrome, or RSD) has experienced an acute injury and the injury has caused them spontaneous pain far out of proportion to the original trauma. For instance, a CRPS Type I scenario might involve having surgery on your big toe, which was painful to the touch, red, swollen, and hard to move, and four months after the surgery, instead of resolving, the symptoms have expanded to involve your entire foot. In an instance like this, we can't pinpoint an exact nerve that was injured.

In CRPS Type II (also known as causalgia), patients show evidence of a specific nerve injury (revealed by nerve conduction testing) such as the ulnar nerve (funny bone), but they report pain that extends beyond the territory of the injured nerve.

The clinical features are the same for both subtypes of CRPS; we see the symptoms expand beyond the confines of the injury in both situations. Studies indicate that CRPS is three to four times more common in women than in men, and there are at least 50,000 new cases of CRPS-I occurring annually in the United States.

A frequent question that arises is when does CRPS develop? Based on the mechanisms involved and a study of many patients following fractures, it seems that CRPS typically develops during a three to four month period after the initial injury. It's not likely that CRPS can be diagnosed earlier because injuries (from sprains, surgery, or trauma along with tissue infections, for example) can all present with the same features of CRPS, and yet they are clearly part of the normal healing process.

Patients of mine also want to know whether CRPS will spread to other limbs. While spread is not universal, 48% of patients in one study described spreading of symptoms to another limb. This occurred 19 or more months after the onset of symptoms, and more than a third of these instances of spread were related to another trauma.

Spreading symptoms of CRPS can be contiguous, expanding beyond the injured area to nearby areas (for example, it starts in the big toe and travels up to the thigh); mirror image, manifesting in the opposite extremity (it starts in the right arm and then presents in the left arm); or independent, moving diagonally across the body (it starts in the right arm and then presents in the left leg). In my experience, I see more contiguous spread, but other experts report mirror image spread more often.

CRPS is typically associated with two presentations—warm and cold. That is, patients may present with one or the other, although both can be seen in any patient. Warm CRPS patients exhibit a warm, red, swollen limb, while cold CRPS patients display a cool, dusky, sweaty limb. There is a suggestion that if a patient is diagnosed with warm

CRPS initially, it is more likely to resolve within a year. Patients with an initial diagnosis of cold CRPS typically do not see resolution this quickly. Furthermore, studies suggest that there may be a transition point from warm CRPS to cold CRPS beginning during the first year of injury, establishing a possible transition marker from acute to chronic CRPS.

CRPS has profound effects on patients. CRPS is thought to be a disease of the central nervous system, peripheral nervous system, and the sympathetic nervous system. It appears that multiple mechanisms are involved: nerve injury, central and peripheral sensitization, altered sympathetic nervous system function, inflammation and immune dysfunction, brain changes, and psychological distress.

It's estimated that about one third of patients with CRPS may suffer from sympathetically mediated pain, which is pain that is worsened by the release of catecholamine neurotransmitters such as norepinephrine and epinephrine from the sympathetic nervous system. Catecholamines produce pain when they are released into the bloodstream from emotional or physical stress in these patients because these neurotransmitters attach to pain-sensing nerves.

Functional MRI studies show a reorganization of the parts of the cerebral cortex that process pain in CRPS patients. There is a loss of gray matter in areas of the brain involved with emotion. Recall that gray matter loss has also been detected in patients with chronic low back pain too (see Chapter 2, Joint and Soft Tissue Pain). Fortunately, studies have shown a reversal of these cortical changes with therapies that reduce pain. There may also be an autoimmune component to CRPS based on preliminary studies.

## Symptoms of Complex Regional Pain Syndrome

CRPS is characterized by intense, excruciating (aching, burning, shooting, stabbing) pain usually in one extremity or part of an extremity. Other common CRPS symptoms include excessive sweating and changes in the color, temperature, dryness, swelling or shininess of the skin in the affected region. Patients may also experience spasm, tremor, twitching, weakness, or atrophy in the affected extremity. As with to other chronic pain conditions, patients with CRPS often experience depression, anxiety, fear, disuse of the painful body part, and social withdrawal. The emotional toll cannot be overemphasized. I've heard patients say, "life as I know it is over," because

the pain, immobility, and isolation of the syndrome changes their life so drastically.

One CRPS patient of mine had to wear an oven mitt over her hand to protect it from coming into contact with anything, even the wind. It is not uncommon for a person with CRPS to present with an arm curled up like a claw, because the pain of movement is so great. I've also seen patients with an affected leg or arm that is half the size of the normal limb because of atrophy. Other patients describe a bed sheet touching their painful limb being akin to 50 sharp knives stabbing them.

Unfortunately, if CRPS is not recognized early enough, the body may lose the ability to "turn off" the pain. Patients delaying treatment for longer than six months may have a poorer long-term outcome. There is some indication, however, that early stage CRPS may be reversible, and identifying the syndrome and then starting treatment as early as possible are key to recovery.

## Diagnosing Complex Regional Pain Syndrome

Because no definitive test exists for CRPS, doctors must rule out other diseases that share similar symptoms, including thoracic outlet syndrome (covered later in this chapter), discogenic disease, deep vein thrombosis, cellulitis (skin infection), and various disorders of the circulatory and lymphatic systems. There are a number of tests that can help exclude these and other sources of pain, but none of these tests make the diagnosis of CRPS. Therefore, doctors need to make sure that no other disease better explains the signs and symptoms.

Most importantly, the diagnosis is made by a thorough clinical evaluation of symptoms and signs. The "Budapest Criteria" are considered the standard means of diagnosing the condition and were adopted as such by the International Association for the Study of Pain (IASP) in 2012. For example, pain specialists look for patients to report at least one symptom* in three of the four categories listed below and to display one sign in two or more categories:

1. *Sensory:* Increased sensitivity to a sensory stimulation (hyperesthesia); evidence of hyperalgesia (exaggerated response to something painful like a needle) or allodynia (pain from something that shouldn't cause discomfort such as clothing)

2. *Vasomotor:* Temperature asymmetry or skin color changes

3. *Sudomotor/edema:* Edema (swelling) or sweating changes

4. *Motor/trophic:* Decreased range of motion or weakness, tremor, dystonia (continual muscle contraction) or trophic changes (hair, nail, skin changes)

## Treating Complex Regional Pain Syndrome

Treatment for complex regional pain syndrome (CRPS) should take into account not just the physical symptoms but also the emotional distress most patients experience. This means that an effective approach should include cognitive behavioral therapy (CBT) to improve coping and minimize the impact of the condition. (Cognitive behavioral therapy is covered in Chapter 19, Mind-Body Techniques for Pain Relief.) Better coping skills can lead to better function with a renewed ability to self-manage pain. Psychological support also targets learned disuse of affected limbs, life stress, and emotional distress that can worsen the disorder.

Because CRPS lacks precise diagnostic criteria, it has been omitted from many

---

* "Symptoms" are experienced and reported by patients, while "signs" are discovered by doctors through medical exams or tests.

medication studies on neuropathic pain. Consequently, multiple medications are currently used to ease the pain of CRPS with incomplete results. These include corticosteroids, nonsteroidal anti-inflammatory drugs, calcitonin, dimethyl sulfoxide (DMSO), N-acetylcysteine, antidepressants, antiepileptics, and opioids. Topical medications such as 5% lidocaine patch, EMLA cream (local anesthetic mixture), and DMSO have demonstrated relief, especially for skin sensitivity. Topical ketamine also shows promise in limiting allodynia and hyperalgesia.

Oral steroids can be effective for acute CRPS with significant inflammation (probably during the first 13 weeks of symptoms), and a drug called calcitonin given intra-nasally, or the bisphosphonates (alendronate and clodronate, for example) have been found to reduce pain and inflammation and improve range of motion. These drugs are probably most helpful when bone scans shows active breakdown of bone, although they may have a role in prevention of bone breakdown and treatment of the disease. For example, we are awaiting the results of a large clinical trial using a bisphosphonate called neridronate (given intravenously) specifically studied in patients with CRPS Type I over a one-year period.

Injection therapies, such as sympathetic nerve blocks, can relieve pain and restore motor function through physical therapy. They also help patients tolerate de-sensitization procedures to the skin while undergoing physical therapy. These blocks are performed if the clinical evaluation demonstrates that the sympathetic nervous system is contributing to the patient's painful symptoms. Epidural and brachial plexus blocks (blocking the nerves in the neck or armpit that provide sensation to the arm) that interrupt the sympathetic nerves can also help facilitate physical therapy, though these are performed less often.

Several studies indicate that spinal cord stimulation (SCS) helps reduce pain in patients with CRPS-I, especially when combined with physical therapy. (SCS is discussed in more detail in Chapter 15, Pain-Relieving Devices.) SCS devices also appear to improve daily function and are associated with improvements in mood and anxiety. Some experts are now advocating that clinicians consider SCS much earlier (for example, at three months) as a treatment for CRPS. The National Institute of Clinical Excellence and British Pain Society support the use of SCS for both CRPS and other neuropathic pain conditions. In my clinical experience, SCS can make a meaningful difference in the lives of those using this therapy.

For patients with severe muscle spasms leading to dystonia (continual muscle contraction), a muscle relaxant called baclofen (Gablofen, Lioresal) placed into the spinal fluid using an implanted pump has shown good pain relief with functional restoration.

The fascinating use of mirror therapy (mirror visual feedback) has shown some benefit in those with early to intermediate CRPS. This technique was initially applied to patients with phantom limb pain and requires patients to move their healthy limb in front of a mirror while hiding the painful limb. The theory is that moving the healthy limb in front of the mirror tricks the brain into seeing the diseased limb move normally. In turn, the sensory part of the brain corrects the abnormalities in pain processing induced by a chronically painful arm or leg.

Many specialists treating CRPS have seen the benefits of functional restoration. This incorporates getting patients to move the painful arm or leg, desensitize the painful area, and normalize movement. The approach ideally requires an interdisciplinary team consisting of physical therapists, occupational therapists, recreational therapists, and vocational therapists. Specifically, physical therapy is critical to enhancing range of motion, flexibility, and then strength. Most patients tolerate restoration much better when they get relief from the pain therapies previously mentioned. I have found that a multifaceted approach that includes medications, psychological support, functional restoration, and sometimes spinal cord stimulation offers the best benefit.

Alternative therapies can also be useful for patients battling CRPS. Some of my patients have benefited from auricular (ear) acupuncture, discussed in Chapter 20, Alternative Medicine and Pain Relief. You can read more about CRPS and cognitive behavioral therapy in Chapter 19, Mind-Body Techniques for Pain Relief. Physical therapy and forms of alternative medicine discussed in Parts 2 and 3, have also given patients the tools they need to get their lives back and conquer this debilitating disease.

## Emerging Treatments for Complex Regional Pain Syndrome

When all the measures outlined in the previous sections have failed, some physicians have had success with a less conventional method involving ketamine, a drug most often used for the purposes of general anesthesia. Ketamine blocks a key pain receptor, reduces cytokine levels, and can alter symptoms of central sensitization (such as magnified pain responses like allodynia and hyperalgesia). When this treatment is chosen, a pain specialist administers a sub-anesthetic intravenous dose of ketamine typically for four hours a day for several days in an outpatient facility. Sometimes this is enough to reduce the severity of pain and symptoms of CRPS. Although ketamine is a promising treatment for this severe syndrome, repeated use can cause liver problems and side effects include hallucinations, nausea, headaches, and elevated blood pressure. Ketamine is also a drug with a potential for abuse. This treatment is not usually covered by insurance and can cost approximately $2000 per session.

If a patient still doesn't find lasting relief and all other therapies have failed, a highly controversial approach is to allow the patient to go into a ketamine coma. In this case, the patient is intubated (with a breathing tube inserted into the trachea) and rendered unconscious for five days in the intensive care unit. This treatment is risky, but some patients have reportedly gone into remission, going off all their pain medications and leading completely normal lives afterwards. Unfortunately, many of these patients also had infections from their stay in the ICU, while others experienced a relapse in pain within a few months.

Naltrexone (Vivitrol, Revia) is a medication typically prescribed to help patients with opioid addiction or alcohol dependence. It blocks opioid receptors. Interestingly, it may help ease pain in CRPS in oral, low-dose form by blocking the activity of immune cells in the brain and spinal cord known as microglia. A study in CRPS patients is currently ongoing. I've had one patient with severe CRPS tell me that this drug helps with symptoms.

Botulinum toxin (Botox) administered subcutaneously or intramuscularly along the area of pain has shown to improve allodynia, pain, and dystonia in preliminary studies.

### Preventing Complex Regional Pain Syndrome and Relapse

How about preventing CRPS from ever happening? This is certainly an area of ongoing interest. Research suggests that taking vitamin C (500 mg per day for at least 45 days following wrist fracture) can reduce the risk of CRPS-I from developing. On the other hand, another study demonstrated that vitamin C was associated with an increase of CRPS development at six weeks after fracture. It's therefore unclear until further studies clarify these contradictory findings. I do recommend to anesthesiologists and surgeons that minimizing tourniquet time on limbs may aid in prevention since ischemic reperfusion injury represents another possible mechanism of CRPS.

And how about preventing relapse? If a patient with CRPS needs surgery and can't postpone it until signs and symptoms are minimal, it may make sense to consider regional anesthetic techniques (epidural, or brachial plexus block for the arm), sympathetic blocks (stellate ganglion block for the arm, or lumbar sympathetic block for the leg), or even daily subcutaneous injections of salmon calcitonin (100 units daily from the time of surgery until four weeks after). Studies point to the beneficial effects of these strategies in offering some protection against relapse.

Overall, acute CRPS usually resolves with limited treatment, but a subset of patients progress to chronic CRPS and need more aggressive management. It's encouraging to see more effective therapies beginning to emerge.

## Understanding Trigeminal Neuralgia

Trigeminal neuralgia (TN)—intermittent bursts of pain—is so excruciating that some have called it the suicide disease; I have actually had patients express the desire to end their lives if they couldn't find a way to control the pain from this condition. Typical symptoms include sudden, brief, stabbing electrical shock sensations radiating from the ear down one side of the face. Attacks can be triggered by something as simple as washing the face, brushing the teeth, applying makeup, receiving a kiss on the cheek, or even feeling a gentle breeze. Victims are often left unable to eat or talk without pain. It is a rare condition, affecting women more than men and lasting weeks or months at a time.

### *Causes of Trigeminal Neuralgia*

The trigeminal nerve is the largest cranial nerve and transmits feeling from the face to the brain. This nerve also controls the chewing muscles. It begins just in front of the ear and then splits into three branches: the first (the ophthalmic) continues along the forehead to about an inch below the hairline; the second (the maxillary) extends from just below the inner part of the eye to the back of the temple region; and the third (the mandibular) encompasses the remainder of the face and the jaw. Most of the time, the pain occurs in the maxillary or mandibular branches. It's thought that trigeminal neuralgia is generated by demyelination, damage to the protective covering around the nerve. As a matter of fact, multiple sclerosis—a demyelinating disease—can cause TN.

In patients with TN, the trigeminal nerve sends waves of pain signals to the brain in the absence of painful stimuli. In other words, areas of the face supplied by healthy branches of the nerve can trigger the symptoms. The condition is attributed to three causes: tumors can irritate the trigeminal nerve; a pathogen, such as HIV, can infect the nerve itself; or a blood vessel can touch and irritate the nerve. The last—vascular compression of the trigeminal nerve root—is by far the most common cause of the condition.

### Diagnosing Trigeminal Neuralgia

A growing number of patients in recent years have been preliminarily diagnosed with trigeminal neuralgia by dentists. Dentists see patients for dental pain who recognize the symptoms as neurological in nature and refer them to a pain specialist or surgeon. The specialist will often order an MRI to rule out other causes and to get a closer look at the blood vessels near the trigeminal nerve.

## Treating Trigeminal Neuralgia

About 70% of trigeminal neuralgia patients respond to the anticonvulsant carbamazepine (Tegretol). Carbamazepine is considered the drug to try first given its long history of effectiveness; carbamazepine is approved by the FDA for TN treatment. If carbamazepine doesn't work, doctors typically try oxcarbazepine (Trileptal). There is strong evidence that both of these medications are effective.

Baclofen, an antispasmodic medication, and lamotrigine (Lamictal), another anticonvulsant, have both shown benefit in research trials and are implemented when patients are not responding to carbamazepine and oxcarbazepine. The topical medications such as lidocaine can also be very helpful, and even the over-the-counter medication Anbesol, applied to the gums has helped patients desensitize that area of the mouth so that they can brush their teeth or talk for longer periods of time.

When medications fail to bring TN pain under control, more invasive interventions may be indicated. Microvascular decompression, in which a thumbnail incision is made on the side of the head, moves blood vessels away from the nerve. Many surgeons believe this procedure is the best for healthy trigeminal neuralgia patients. It's the most frequent choice for treating this condition due to its safety, efficacy, and longer duration of pain relief. The risk of facial numbness, leakage of cerebrospinal fluid, or hearing problems is low, and there is little risk of developing a side effect called anesthesia dolorosa (constant burning and itching from injury to the trigeminal nerve).

Minimally invasive procedures that can bring relief for trigeminal neuralgia include glycerol injections or radiofrequency ablation, both of which work by damaging the trigeminal nerve to prevent it from transmitting unwanted pain signals. The success rate for glycerol is good—about 80%—but about half of the patients who undergo this treatment find that pain returns within 18 months. Radiofrequency ablation heats the nerve to the point of facial numbness. Pain relief from ablation typically lasts about 10 years, but some new studies show that, for some patients, pain may return in as little as five to seven years.

Another treatment, called balloon compression, works by squeezing the nerve to reduce sensation; about 80% of patients find near complete relief from this procedure, although a little less than a third will find pain returning in about six years.

As noted earlier, many surgeons believe microvascular decompression is the best for healthy trigeminal neuralgia patients. In contrast, glycerol rhizolysis, balloon compression, and radiofrequency ablation carry a 2%–3% risk of the side effect known as anesthesia dolorosa. These last three interventions often cause facial numbness along with pain relief while microvascular decompression has a very low risk of numbness. The incidence of facial numbness after balloon compression can reach 20% because this procedure damages the nerve more than the glycerol injection, which has a relatively low risk of permanent numbness.

Radiation surgery (gamma knife) uses a cobalt beam to damage the trigeminal nerve. Pain relief is slower with this treatment than with the glycerol injection, radiofrequency ablation, or balloon compression, requiring four to 12 weeks before onset. Fortunately, with the other interventional treatments, patients often feel better the day of the procedure. Similar to microvascular decompression, the risk of anesthesia dolorosa from radiation surgery is very low.

Some integrative therapies have shown success in treating trigeminal neuralgia as well. Acupuncture seems to provide sustained relief to about 65% of patients, although consistent sessions may be needed to keep the pain at bay. Chiropractic treatments have been shown to provide relief for up to seven to 10 days. Some researchers are also exploring the efficacy of administering B complex vitamins in large doses (50–100 mg per day). Botulinum toxin (Botox) injected into the skin along areas where pain is experienced has shown substantial reductions in pain for patients not responding to conventional therapies. The doses are small and side effects are minimal.

Repetitive Transcranial Magnetic Stimulation (rTMS), an exciting therapy which uses magnetic energy, holds great promise for treating trigeminal neuralgia based on three separate scientific studies. This noninvasive treatment uses pulses of magnetic energy to activate particular areas of the brain. A motor cortex stimulator—a surgical device that emits tiny pulses of electricity—can also be implanted for controlling unyielding facial pain. A small electrode (paddle) is placed on the brain and delivers small "doses" of energy that interrupt pain sensing nerves. Although not approved by the FDA for pain, motor cortex stimulation (MCS), which is discussed more in Chapter 15, Pain-Relieving Devices, is particularly promising for trigeminal neuropathic pain as well as pain following a stroke.

Finally, gene therapies may eventually allow us to change the way nerves respond to painful stimuli. Researchers are doing just that in animal studies today. Furthermore, early research into injecting stem cells around the trigeminal nerve in patients with trigeminal neuropathic pain is showing encouraging evidence of effectiveness. We cover regenerative therapies more broadly in Chapter 16, Regenerative Biomedicine.

In short, patients with trigeminal neuralgia have several paths to pain relief and many reasons to be hopeful. They should also be sure to access the TN national support group for treatments and specialists (www.tna-support.org).

## Understanding Fibromyalgia

Fibromyalgia (FM) is not universally recognized as neuropathic in nature, but it shares enough characteristics with other such diseases to be discussed in this chapter. Fibromyalgia affects about 4%–8% of the population, and leads to widespread body pain, fatigue, sleep disturbance, sexual dysfunction, and even memory problems. Women are six times more frequently affected than men, and onset can occur at any time in life, including childhood or adolescence. However, it more commonly strikes middle-aged women.

Because patients present with no obvious physical illness, they are often accused of faking or exaggerating their pain. Yet, it's estimated that 10% of the general population suffers from chronic widespread body pain, much of which is compatible with FM. Even more astounding is that greater than 40% of patients referred to a pain clinic meet the diagnosis for FM. The rare spreading of complex regional pain syndrome (CRPS) symptoms to the entire body may instead represent a diagnosis of FM.

We used to believe the FM was a discrete disease entity. On the contrary, it exists on a continuum with multiple types of symptoms. The condition can be disabling and involves both sides of the body above and below the waist. I've had patients say, "I hurt all over," or "it feels like I have a never-ending flu." The pain is mainly in the muscles, but many experience it in the joints and some report joint swelling. There is an increased sensitivity to pressure and light touch with some patients displaying allodynia (experiencing pain from something that shouldn't cause discomfort such as clothing touching the skin) and hyperalgesia (experiencing 10 times the typical amount of pain from sensations such as an ordinary pinprick). These are clinical features of neuropathic pain and that's why FM reflects the process of central sensitization (magnified pain response).

FM patients commonly suffer from depression and sleep disturbances as well. They wake up unrefreshed even after sleeping for eight to 10 hours, or alternatively may experience insomnia. As one of my patients said, "I have unending fatigue." A lot of FM patients talk about how they struggle to pay attention and think quickly on their feet. "Fibro fog" is the term I've heard them use. Migraine and tension type headaches occur in more than 50% of FM patients, and it's not surprising for them to suffer from other associated conditions such as abdominal pain, pelvic pain, and bladder problems.

## Diagnosing Fibromyalgia

Though previously diagnosed with a tender point exam, new diagnostic criteria for fibromyalgia have made that exam unnecessary. Patients are now diagnosed either by physician assessment or by a self-report questionnaire. Part of the reason for the change is our growing understanding of the relationship between FM and clinical symptoms such as fatigue and cognitive changes.

A scoring system has replaced the tender point exam. The scoring system combines a widespread pain index (WPI) and a symptom severity (SS) scale for making the diagnosis. The WPI measures the number of painful body regions, such as the shoulder girdle, hip, jaw, arms, legs, and back. There's a list of 19 defined areas. The SS score includes an estimate of the degree of fatigue, waking up tired, trouble thinking, and abdominal pain, for example. The symptoms need to be present for at least three months for a positive diagnosis. A physician makes a diagnosis of FM if the WPI and the SS scores add up to specific numbers. However, other conditions should be ruled out before patients are diagnosed with fibromyalgia, because there are many disorders that can mimic its symptoms (lupus, hypothyroidism, headache disorders, or rheumatoid arthritis, for example).

## Causes of Fibromyalgia

Unlike some of the other disorders discussed in this chapter, the pain of fibromyalgia originates predominantly in the central nervous system (brain and spinal cord) but the peripheral nervous system and autonomic nervous system seem to be involved too. Although the causes of fibromyalgia are uncertain, we know that the blood levels of pain-inducing neurotransmitters, such as substance P, glutamate, and nerve growth factor, are higher in people with fibromyalgia, while other neurotransmitters that dampen pain, such as serotonin and norepinephrine, are lower. The net result of this imbalance is that the "volume control" of the central nervous systems is set far too high. Just like turning a hearing aid up would make a whisper sound unbearably loud, a fibromyalgia patient feels the softest touch like a painful slap. There's additional evidence that the release of inflammatory molecules (cytokines and interleukens, for example) produce peripheral nerve inflammation that results in swelling, skin discoloration, and unpleasant sensations to the touch in particular parts of the body.

Brain imaging also supports the "volume control" explanation. For instance, functional magnetic resonance imaging (fMRI) studies have shown that certain regions of the brain are more active in patients with fibromyalgia undergoing painful stimuli. It seems that patients with fibromyalgia sense more pain than those without fibromyalgia when given the same type of unpleasant stimulus.

A number of genes have been identified over the past few years that appear to be linked to this increased pain sensitivity. There is also a growing body of evidence that a significant percentage of people suffering from other conditions such as rheumatoid arthritis and osteoarthritis may also suffer from this "volume control" problem in their central nervous systems. Stress, traumatic events, repetitive injuries, Lyme disease, lupus, ankylosing spondylitis (a type of arthritis affecting the low back), HIV infection, and Hepatitis B and C have all been linked to the development of fibromyalgia.

## Treating Fibromyalgia Pain

The FDA has approved pregabalin (Lyrica), duloxetine (Cymbalta), and milnacipran (Savella) for use in treating fibromyalgia (FM) symptoms. Some of my patients report improvement in their pain and function with these medicines, but others have been disappointed. The other class of medications that should be considered is the tricyclic antidepressants and specifically, amitriptyline (Elavil). This drug has been thoroughly studied and found to reduce pain and sleep disturbance in FM patients. A recent analysis found that it outperformed duloxetine and milnacipran in pain relief, fatigue, and quality of life. Anti-inflammatories and opioids are rarely helpful for FM pain. Both tizanidine (Zanaflex), which is considered a muscle relaxant, and tramadol (Ultram) can be beneficial in managing aspects of fibromyalgia. Cyclobenzaprine (Flexeril) another muscle relaxant taken in low dose can also help.

### New and Innovative Treatments for Fibromyalgia Pain

A new drug, mirogabalin, that works like pregabalin (Lyrica) is showing promise. Researchers are studying mirogabalin in patients with FM and neuropathic pain with the expectation that it will offer pain relief with fewer side effects compared to similar medications currently on the market. Low-dose naltrexone, mentioned as an emerging treatment for complex regional pain syndrome (CRPS) earlier in this chapter, may also help patients manage FM symptoms. This drug may work by blunting inflammation and blocking immune receptors in the central nervous system. When the immune defense cells in the brain and spinal cord (called the microglia) are activated, they produce cytokines. These cytokine molecules along with activated microglia may be responsible for the symptoms we see in FM. It's thought that naltrexone may block the functioning of migroglia and thereby help to control the syndrome.

Oral cannabis-based medicine may also help this type of pain, but we don't have enough evidence yet. Some people with FM pain have found relief from Scrambler Therapy and Repetitive Transcranial Magnetic Stimulation (rTMS), mentioned previously in this chapter; rTMS has shown positive effects on quality of life about a month after initiation.

## Integrative Treatments for Fibromyalgia Pain

When managing fibromyalgia, don't forget the importance of sleep. Sleep disturbances in fibromyalgia patients can worsen symptoms and the syndrome itself leads to disrupted sleep. It seems like an impossible situation, but help exists. We cover some helpful strategies for restoring sleep in this book in Part 2, Medical Therapies for Pain: Traditional and Innovative, and Part 3, Integrative Therapies for Pain.

Maintaining a healthy weight and diet is also very important in overcoming fibromyalgia. Excess body weight leads to the production of the inflammatory molecules referenced earlier called cytokines. Cytokine production leads to inflammation and then pain. Shifting your diet from inflammatory-producing foods, such as fried foods, fast foods, and high-fat animal proteins, to healthier, pain-fighting foods, such as plant based proteins, fish, and dark berries, can make a difference in your pain.

Aerobic exercise, as well as resistance training and flexibility training have brought benefits to FM patients in clinical trials. In larger scale analyses, aerobic exercise alone has been proven to boost global well-being, pain, and physical function. Aquatic exercise offers similar benefits. For these reasons, it's important for patients to incorporate exercise into their FM care plan. You can read more about the importance of eating well and exercising regularly in Chapter 17, Weight Control, Exercise, and Diet.

Many fibromyalgia patients obtain surprising relief from cognitive behavioral therapy (CBT). CBT is a proven therapy for insomnia and demonstrates positive effects on long-term pain reduction in FM. You can learn more about CBT in Chapter 19, Mind-Body Techniques for Pain Relief. Biofeedback is another strategy that has proven successful with fibromyalgia pain that is discussed in Chapter 19.

Acupuncture and, in particular, electroacupuncture has the ability to manage pain and improve stiffness for people suffering from FM. Electroacupuncture is a form of acupuncture where a small electric current is incorporated. It does, however, often require eight to 10 sessions before achieving results. This topic is discussed more extensively in Chapter 20, Alternative Medicine and Pain Relief.

Jin Shin Jyutsu, a Japanese form of acupressure, which is discussed in more detail in Chapter 22, Harnessing the Human Biofield, has helped fibromyalgia patients where traditional therapies have failed. Practitioners of chakra healing note that clients with fibromyalgia feel better after these energy-healing sessions.

Music therapy, and movement-based therapies such as Revolution In Motion, Qigong, tai chi and yoga, which are discussed in more detail in Chapter 21, Aromas, Music, and Pain Relief, and Chapter 23, Pain Relief through Movement, have made notable differences in some patients'

symptoms. For example, Qigong and tai chi seem to show benefits in pain and sleep quality while yoga offers improvement in many symptoms such as pain, fatigue, mood, and acceptance, according to the literature. These are inexpensive, quite safe, and I recommend them. The Feldenkrais Method focuses on correcting unhealthy posture, and although the scientific literature is still developing in this area, studies show pain relief, better sleep, and less fatigue in fibromyalgia patients. Practitioners notice an improvement in quality of life as well.

Patients feel reassured to hear that FM is not life threatening. Managing stress, sleep hygiene, and exercise all come together to lessen the impact of the syndrome. Most importantly, the majority of patients live normal and active lives despite the waxing and waning symptoms.

## Understanding Postherpetic Neuralgia (Persistent Shingles Pain)

When Donald, a successful attorney, starting visiting doctors in 2008, he looked like a photograph from a medical school textbook. At age 56, he had developed lesions on the right half of his forehead, eyebrow, and eye that began oozing a substance that looked like melted butterscotch. At the same time, swelling engulfed his right eye until he was unable to see out of it. The oozing lesions on his forehead turned into scabs while massive swelling also engulfed his left eye, leaving him blind for nearly a week.

"You won't believe this," Donald said on my radio program, "but at one point, my right eyebrow just fell off into my hand." He was not only afraid for his health, but feared that his work as an attorney would suffer if his appearance didn't improve. After some misdiagnoses from well-meaning doctors, Donald's condition was finally correctly identified as shingles. He received treatment, and, in time, the rash cleared up. (His eyebrow also grew back!) But unfortunately, Donald's suffering was far from over.

Postherpetic neuralgia (PHN) affects patients who have previously had shingles, which is caused by the same virus responsible for chicken pox (varicella zoster virus). This neuropathic pain syndrome is the most debilitating complication of the viral infection. The pain can diminish a patient's quality of life and ability to function as much as major diseases such as myocardial infarction, heart failure, type 2 diabetes, and depression. There are roughly over 1 million people in the United States with PHN.

## *Causes of Postherpetic Neuralgia*

Most of us had chicken pox as children. When people recover from chicken pox, the virus, unlike other viruses, travels up sensory nerves into the nerve cell bodies, which are clustered in little knots on either side of the spinal cord. These knots of nerve cell bodies are called ganglia

(more specifically, dorsal root ganglia), and the chicken pox virus lies dormant in them for years. For some of us, the virus wakes up at some point and become shingles (herpes zoster). Although not considered life threatening, a study from Great Britain found that shingles increased the risk of heart attack by 10% and mini-strokes (transient ischemic attacks) by 15%. This may result from the virus spreading from the nerves to the blood vessels and triggering an inflammatory response.

The older we get, the greater our risk for developing shingles becomes. For instance, shingles occurs in more than half of all people older than 60 years, and there is an overall 32% lifetime risk of developing shingles. Most of the time, a shingles outbreak goes away within four weeks, but about 10% of patients develop postherpetic neuralgia, which is defined as pain lasting more than three months after the onset of the rash. PHN leads to considerable suffering, impairing the ability to function on a daily basis, negatively impacting quality of life, and eroding psychological health. The severity and frequency of PHN increases with age, which means we will see more of it in the future as the worldwide population is aging at an unprecedented rate. Among the developed nations, people 65 years and older are projected to reach 30% of the total population by 2050. Therefore, the individual and public health costs related to PHN will likely grow. And despite the significant burden of PHN, it's often underdiagnosed and poorly managed.

## Symptoms of Postherpetic Neuralgia

Once the chicken pox virus "awakens" in the sensory ganglia, shingles patients experience a painful skin rash that appears as vesicles (fluid-filled blisters) on one side of the body. The blisters turn into scabs, and then clear up. For most people, the pain fades as they recover from shingles, but some patients find their nerves unable to recover from the damage, leading to PHN. PHN pain can range from mild to very severe and can last for months, years, or even for the rest of the patient's life. Patients describe the pain in

different ways—constant aching or burning, episodic and shooting, or allodynic like Donald's.

Donald's dull, achy, itchy sensations continued for months after his shingles had successfully resolved. And unfortunately the pain got worse: aches became lightning bolts and itches grew fiery hot. PHN suffering is individual: Some patients find the water pelting their skin from the shower unbearable, but Donald actually found cold water soothing. He couldn't feel a light touch on the right side of his forehead, but the slightest amount of pressure caused an explosion of pain.

While other patients may not have pain on their foreheads like Donald did, they may experience allodynia. Allodynia involves hypersensitivity, experiencing pain from something that shouldn't cause discomfort. For example, a patient with allodynia may find the sensation of fabric touching one side of the chest or abdomen to be unbearable. For others, the breeze of cool air on the forehead when playing tennis causes a burning sensation that forces them to give the sport up. It's like having a bad sunburn that never goes away. Allodynia can be so intense that patients may have to stay home without clothes on with the heat cranked up to make it through the day.

Some may even have to stop driving because they can't bear the pressure of car upholstery fabric or a seatbelt against their chest or abdomen. They soon become isolated and often depressed.

## Preventing Postherpetic Neuralgia

While there is no sure way to prevent PHN, there are important steps you can take to lessen your risk. When we are healthy, the shingles virus remains dormant because our immune system prevents the virus from multiplying. Anything that suppresses the immune system (HIV infection, or steroids used to prevent rejection of transplanted organs, for example) also increases the risk of a shingles outbreak.

For the same reason, age increases our risk and the severity of the symptoms we are likely to experience. In people who are over 60 years of age, the ability to suppress the virus weakens. By age 85, there is a 50% chance of developing shingles, and there is a 20% chance of developing PHN for people who live to 80 or longer. Older adults should ask their doctors about getting vaccinated against shingles. Zostavax has been shown to reduce the risk of shingles by 51% and PHN by 66%. Those are impressive numbers, and the study involved more than 38,000 patients who were 60 years old and over. Importantly, the Shingles

Prevention Study (SPS) showed that the vaccine neither caused nor induced the development of shingles.

The vaccine is FDA-approved for adults age 50 and over and should be considered at that age, even though the risks of getting shingles and PHN are significant lower in healthy people at age 50. Unfortunately, the vaccine is not covered by insurance until age 60 and the cost ranges from $160 to $200.

Patients often ask if they should bother to get vaccinated. PHN causes unyielding and often debilitating pain that disrupts sleep, alters daily activities, and restricts social life, so prevention is key.

It is important to note that shingles can occur even once you have been vaccinated, and it can occur more than once. Even though PHN can also occur after vaccination, one study found that vaccination is associated with a lower risk of PHN in women but not men. More studies are needed because it is not clear when patients should get re-vaccinated or how long they should wait to get vaccinated after a bout of shingles. It is also not known if people should bother to get vaccinated once they have received a diagnosis of PHN.

A novel and more powerful shingles vaccine (Shingrix) targeting immune-compromised patients and those over 50 has shown impressive results in preventing shingles and significantly reducing the risk of PHN. It's currently awaiting approval by the FDA. Patients will need two injections of the new vaccine, administered six months apart.

## Treating Postherpetic Neuralgia (Persistent Shingles Pain)

When the shingles virus wakes up, it does tremendous nerve damage, killing many nerve cells and causing hemorrhaging. This is why it is very important to get shingles diagnosed and properly treated quickly. The virus replicates and injures various parts of the nerve, leading to pain and skin changes seen on one side of the body, usually on the chest or the forehead and eye. Due to the constant transmission of impulses from the damaged nerve to the spinal cord along with direct injury of the cord, pain pathways become disorganized and create the symptoms of PHN. These disturbances of the peripheral and central nervous systems (called peripheral and central sensitization) amplify pain responses and create discomfort and pain.

Beginning a course of antivirals such as acyclovir (Zovirax), valacyclovir (Valtrex), or famciclovir (Famvir) within 72 hours of the appearance of the rash can help resolve shingles and may lessen the risk of PHN. Antivirals prevent the virus from multiplying and further damaging nerves, which can reduce the chances of developing PHN. The shingles virus is more sensitive to valacyclovir and famciclovir, which are better absorbed, reach higher blood levels, and therefore achieve greater antiviral activity. Even if treatment is delayed beyond three days, the evidence suggests that patients still benefit from antiviral therapy.

Most studies indicate that patients who experience prodromal pain (pain before the shingles rash appears) may also be at greater risk of PHN. Controlling the pain as early as possible is therefore critical. Interestingly, a misdiagnosis of myocardial infarction (heart attack) or disc herniation can occur during this prodromal period because the pain is sharp, stabbing, and can shoot across the chest.

There are several FDA-approved medications for PHN including gabapentin, pregabalin, topical capsaicin, and topical lidocaine patch. The FDA has also approved two extended-release forms of gabapentin called Gralise and Horizant for patients to take just once a day. I usually recommend gabapentin or pregabalin (Lyrica) to start because they don't interact unfavorably with other medicines that patients may be using to control other medical conditions. Pregabalin generally has a quicker onset than gabapentin, which patients appreciate. I've had some patients tolerate the extended-release gabapentin drugs better than the immediate release formulation and pregabalin.

The tricyclic antidepressants (TCAs) are also helpful for pain, sleep, and mood, but they can lead to more side effects, especially in older adults. But there is ample evidence from the literature that TCAs can effectively reduce the pain of PHN. Because of this, if pregabalin and gabapentin don't provide sufficient relief, I urge patients to consider the TCAs.

Opioids should be reserved for pain that is unresponsive to other treatments given their general risks and specific risks of falls and hip fracture in older adults. Tramadol (Ultram), a weak opioid, can be used initially and then stronger opioids (oxycodone, morphine) if needed. A weaker opioid in patch form, buprenorphine (Butrans), is a consideration for around the clock dosing in patients who may benefit from longer duration therapy.

Topical lidocaine patches help patients with sensitized skin due to allodynia.

There is no associated skin numbness either. Capsaicin applied to the skin as a liquid or a patch (below the jaw) is effective too. The FDA has approved a high dose capsaicin patch called Qutenza. Despite the positive outcomes from the clinical studies on the capsaicin patch, I have not seen comparable improvement in patients I've treated.

Some patients with unrelenting pain have found relief from spinal cord stimulation (SCS), and botulinum toxin (Botox) injected over the painful area is a promising therapy for limiting pain intensity and improving sleep quality. There are limited but encouraging results from clinical trials on SCS and botulinum toxin for PHN. In my experience, I've seen mixed results from SCS, but this therapy is an option when more conventional therapies fail. Botox is discussed in Chapter 1, Headache Pain, and SCS is discussed in more detail in Chapter 15, Pain-Relieving Devices.

Patients have more trouble with PHN when they're not busy, so distraction acts as a key alleviator of pain. Activities such as walking, golf, playing card games, listening to music, reading, or socializing can all help.

For Donald, Botox has lessened both the frequency of shooting pain episodes as well as his constant pain. It's made a noticeable difference in his life. Some of the anticonvulsants mentioned earlier in the chapter have also helped Donald keep the pain under control, but he still suffers daily. He has tried alternative therapies such as acupuncture and vitamins but hasn't had much success with them. What Donald has found extremely helpful is staying busy at work, having a full social life, and keeping a sense of humor. Like many other PHN sufferers, he has found that staying as active as possible and focusing on life rather than the condition is very good therapy.

## Understanding Multiple Sclerosis

Multiple sclerosis (MS) is an autoimmune disease that attacks the central nervous system. It's an inflammatory and degenerative chronic disease. There are at least 350,000 people with MS in the United States alone. Symptoms include pain, loss of muscle tone, spasms, loss of coordination, blurred vision, and depression. Depression, in fact, is three to 10 times greater among MS patients than in the general population. The National Multiple Sclerosis Society reports that 50% of all people with MS suffer from chronic pain; current estimates from the literature find that the figure is closer to 63%. MS patients list pain as one of their most concerning symptoms. The risk of developing pain seems to increase with age, longer duration of having MS, and more severe disability.

In 1996, country music superstar Clay Walker—then just in his twenties—began experiencing double vision, numbness, and a facial spasm that continued for eight weeks and left a blister on his eyeball. Walker was diagnosed with multiple sclerosis. Walker had seen his self-titled album go platinum, but his promising career, which demanded great physical exertion on stage, hung in the balance as he learned how to manage his disease.

### Causes of Multiple Sclerosis

Multiple sclerosis strips the myelin sheath, which surrounds nerve cells the way insulation surrounds wires, from the nerves around the brain and/or spinal cord. This leads to misfiring neurons, which causes spasticity (a condition in which certain muscles are continuously contracted), pins and needles sensations, and an inability to relax certain muscles, not unlike Charley horse–type cramps. The exact cause of MS is not clear, but the theory is that it begins as an inflammatory and immune-related disorder that later progresses to activation of migroglia (immune defense cells in the central nervous system) and chronic nerve degeneration. Environmental factors such as viral infections, sunlight exposure, and vitamin D levels appear to influence the risk of MS as well.

### Symptoms of Multiple Sclerosis

There is no set pattern in the way multiple sclerosis appears; the pain can come early or late in life, it can get continually worse, or it can appear to remit for a while. Pain is often widespread in the body and changes over time. Neuropathic pain in the limbs and headache are the most prevalent. Some patients report burning or aching pain around the body, and others suffer from spasms that lead to muscle cramps, tight and achy joints, and back pain. Musculoskeletal pain arises from immobility or paralysis as well.

Pain can appear acutely, causing intense but brief shock-like pain, similar to trigeminal neuralgia (covered earlier in this chapter). Trigeminal neuralgia (TN) can be a symptom of MS and sometimes leads to the diagnosis of multiple sclerosis. Less frequently, patients might experience a brief, electric shock sensation that runs down the spine into the limbs. The medical term for this is the Lhermitte's sign. Looking down usually provokes this pain. If it happens frequently and without any new spinal cord lesion, gabapentin (Neurontin) or pregabalin (Lyrica) can help.

---

## Treating Multiple Sclerosis Pain

Clay Walker experiences pain in his right hip and ankle as well as in the groin area, virtually every morning when he wakes up. Because of the spasticity that multiple sclerosis (MS) causes, stretching and exercise are an absolutely vital part of treatment. Walker credits daily stretching and biking with greatly reducing the pain he experiences with MS. Swimming and other forms of aquatic therapy get blood flowing to the affected areas, reducing pain and helping to build and maintain muscle mass.

In addition to exercise and stretching, MS can cause neuropathic pain that requires certain medications listed at the beginning of the chapter: anticonvulsants, antidepressants, and rarely the opioids.

Botulinum toxin (Botox) injections can be very helpful when the spasticity from MS is focused in a specific area. For example, MS patients struggling with incontinence may find relief with Botox injections into the bladder muscle. It can reduce muscle tone and facilitate passive movement in those with arm and leg spasticity too. When large tracks of muscle are in spasm, however, Botox is less useful. A muscle relaxant called baclofen can ease painful spams when given by mouth. Tizanidine (Zanaflex) is another first line, oral muscle relaxant for spasticity, although it can't be given into the spinal fluid.

In more severe cases where the disease has progressed significantly, causing spasticity or rigid muscles, baclofen can be administered directly into the spinal fluid through an implantable pump (intrathecal pump). This can ease the discomfort and exhaustion of muscles that are constantly tight, improve mobility, and enhance quality of life. Benefits of the pump therapy also include improvements in wheelchair seating, better sleep, and easier body positioning for care giving. These pumps are probably underutilized based on a survey study showing that only 1% of MS patients receiving spasticity treatment had an implanted pump compared to an estimated 13% of all MS patients who may be candidates. In my experience, pump therapy with baclofen offers very good improvement in selected patients with lasting effects. One study found very good control of spasticity and painful spasms five years into treatment. Drug side effects are minimal but patients can experience drowsiness or weakness. Pump-related side effects involve the catheter, and the pump does need replacement in four to seven years after activation. These pumps are covered in Chapter 15, Pain-Relieving Devices.

Medical marijuana is a politically and socially charged topic, but a growing body of research into the use of cannabinoids for neuropathic pain and muscle spasticity has shown benefits. For instance, the pill or oral spray forms can ease spasticity and pain in patients with MS. The oral spray is licensed in countries outside the United States for spasticity and neuropathic pain linked to multiple sclerosis as well as cancer pain. Some of the more frequent side effects of cannabinoids include dizziness, light-headedness, dry mouth, fatigue, and muscle weakness. Like certain other analgesics, medical marijuana can lead to dependence and withdrawal, but fatal overdose has not been reported. Medical marijuana is discussed in more detail in Chapter 14, Pharmacological Therapies. Research studies also suggest that aromatherapy massage over the painful area in MS patients may offer relief too. Aromatherapy is discussed in Chapter 21, Aromas, Music, and Pain Relief.

Immune system suppressants such as corticosteroids can help influence the symptoms and maybe progression of MS, but suppressing the immune system for a long time with steroids has negative side effects (osteoporosis, hypertension, mood changes, and stomach ulcers, for example). Walker receives a daily injection of copaxone (Glatiramer). It's thought that copaxone modifies abnormalities of the immune system that contribute to MS. There are other immune-modulating treatments for different forms of MS too.

Doctors who treat MS are very hopeful that the future will bring ways to reset the immune system—shutting down the inflammatory response—so it no longer attacks the central nervous system. There are even very early investigations into using stem cells to treat MS. Regenerative therapies such as stem cell therapy are covered in Chapter 16, Regenerative Biomedicine.

Fortunately for himself, his friends and family, and country music fans everywhere, Walker has maintained an incredibly positive attitude and kept his MS in remission for many years. He has received a humanitarian award for his charitable work related to the disease and his career has been virtually unaffected. He now has four platinum albums to his name and says that when he is on stage, he forgets that he has MS.

While on my radio program, Walker explained the essence of his hopeful outlook: "The disease is part of what you have to deal with, but it doesn't define who you are."

# Understanding Neurogenic Thoracic Outlet Syndrome

Neurogenic thoracic outlet syndrome (NTOS) is not a particularly well-known neuropathic disorder, but it may affect up to 8% of the population. Those at risk include data entry personnel, assembly line workers, athletes, professional musicians, and even office workers who hunch over their computers or use repetitive overhead arm motion.

The broad term, thoracic outlet syndrome, involves the compression of nerves and/or blood vessels that causes a narrowing between the base of the neck and the armpit—the area known as the thoracic outlet. This space is naturally smaller in women, who are three to four times as likely to be diagnosed with thoracic outlet syndrome than men. The neurogenic form of thoracic outlet syndrome does not impair the blood vessels, just the nerves. The narrowing causes pain in the neck, shoulders and arms, numbness or tingling in the fingers, arm weakness or swelling, headache, changes in the color of the skin, or muscle spasms in the upper back, particularly when the arm is lifted above the head.

If ignored, this syndrome can impair function of the arm as well as quality of life, not to mention lead to a great deal of emotional distress. Almost all patients are left feeling frustrated or even hopeless until they get a correct diagnosis and treatment. Studies have shown that NTOS sufferers whose pain is uncontrolled lead lives as severely limited as individuals with chronic heart failure. Since many people are diagnosed in their thirties or forties, these limitations can be devastating.

## Symptoms and Causes of Neurogenic Thoracic Outlet Syndrome

Like repetitive arm use or work related injuries, whiplash and neck injury can lead to this painful condition. Almost any injury that causes chronic neck muscle spasm can lead to NTOS. Many patients exhibit a history of trauma or repetitive stress to the scalene muscles (a group of muscles located on the side of the neck), and chronic stress of the anterior and middle scalene muscles is linked to the development of NTOS and chronic pain. (The anterior and middle scalene muscles elevate the first rib and laterally flex [bend] the neck to the same side; the action of the posterior scalene is to elevate the second rib and tilt the neck to the same side.) Extra ribs located in the neck can on rare occasions narrow the thoracic outlet and cause symptoms too.

A focal point of NTOS is the anterior scalene muscle, which is a posture muscle in the neck. It attaches to the first rib and primarily helps to bend and rotate the neck, although it also aids somewhat with respiration. When this muscle is tense for too long or becomes injured, scar tissue can compress the brachial plexus nerves beneath the muscle. Studies have shown that injury to the anterior or middle scalene muscles contributes to most of the pathology in NTOS. Muscle fibrosis (scar tissue) shows up three times more often than other changes in these muscles. When muscle spasm or scar tissue put traction on the brachial plexus, this leads to muscle and nerve swelling which limits the space within the outlet, causing symptoms.

Two relatively rare forms of NTOS involve the blood vessels. In venous thoracic outlet syndrome, the vein forms clots as the scalene muscle gets bigger, pressing against the nerves. Most people who suffer from arterial thoracic outlet syndrome have an extra rib that pushes against the artery, causing it to clot, which can be life-threatening. However, 95%–98% of thoracic outlet syndrome cases are neurogenic, although some neurogenic cases also involve arterial irritation.

## Diagnosing Neurogenic Thoracic Outlet Syndrome

Early diagnosis is very important for NTOS, because the longer the pain persists, the more the nerves become damaged. Unfortunately, many doctors may not consider thoracic outlet syndrome when evaluating a patient, because it is complex disorder without a definitive test to confirm its presence. X-rays, MRIs, CT scans, and electromyograms/nerve conduction tests (EMG/NCT) tend to be normal in a patient with NTOS. They are often performed to make sure that other medical conditions are not causing the same symptoms, though.

A special test called the medial antebrachial cutaneous (MAC) nerve conduction test can identify milder cases of NTOS and may help provide more objective evidence of the syndrome. However, more research is needed to validate the MAC before we can use it routinely.

In addition to listening carefully to a patient's history and performing an examination, I usually do an anterior scalene block with CT imaging to see if it reduces the pain. If it does, it appears to assist in confirming the diagnosis of NTOS. The theory is that the block temporarily paralyzes the muscle in spasm and allows the first rib to move down, which decompresses the thoracic outlet. A positive response to this intramuscular injection correlates with good surgical outcomes and may help predict whether patients will benefit from injecting botulinum toxin (Botox) into the muscle as a therapeutic tool.

## Treating Neurogenic Thoracic Outlet Syndrome

Physical therapy is recommended for patients initially diagnosed with neurogenic thoracic outlet syndrome. If caught early enough, some cases of NTOS can be resolved with physical therapy. Typically, postural correction, ergonomic changes (chair height, computer monitor position), and stretching exercises help restore muscle balance in the neck.

Short-term medicines such as muscle relaxants and nonsteroidal anti-inflammatory drugs (NSAIDs) are helpful for the musculoskeletal component of pain, and anticonvulsants or antidepressants ease the neuropathic aspect. Trigger point injections with local anesthetic into the trapezius muscle helps quite a bit for patients presenting with overuse or spasticity in this muscle.

### *Botox and Neurogenic Thoracic Outlet Syndrome Pain*

I have been using an innovative treatment for NTOS, performing a single injection of Botox into the anterior scalene muscle under CT scan guidance. This relaxes the muscle, reduces the spasms, and decreases nerve irritation. After studying different methods of imaging for injection, we have found that CT guidance minimizes side effects when compared to ultrasound or x-ray-guidance, for example.

Muscle tension and pain ease for approximately three to four months with Botox. Botox may also decrease pain and inflammation by inhibiting the release of substances involved with pain transmission and sensitization of the spinal cord and brain. Current evidence demonstrates that injecting Botox into the anterior scalene muscle alone, or in combination with other scalene muscles and even upper chest muscles, reduces symptoms of NTOS. An exciting possibility yet to be fully studied concerns the ability of Botox to actually improve wound healing and reduce scar tissue in injured muscles. This may be critical since scarring of the scalene muscles that are targeted for injection probably contributes to the development of the syndrome.

Published studies on Botox injections, including those I've authored, show good pain outcomes of greater than 50%, but there are mixed results related to the duration of relief. Many of my patients report good pain relief with improved function for several months. During this time, they are often able to return to a near-normal lifestyle and also do proactive physical therapy to help ensure that if the pain returns it will not be as severe. I find that repeating these injections every three months provides continued benefit for most patients, but there is variation to the frequency; some require slightly more frequent treatment and others spread the injections out across four to five months.

### Surgery and Neurogenic Thoracic Outlet Syndrome Pain

In the case of venous and arterial thoracic outlet syndrome, or cases in which the neurogenic form of the syndrome have progressed significantly, it may be necessary to surgically remove part of the anterior scalene muscle and/or the first rib. Success rates for surgical decompression can be as high as 90% with low complication rates, but other reports cite persistent disability in 60% of patients with more than 30% complication rates.

Many patients who have surgery and successfully complete their physical therapy afterwards find lasting relief, but having a minimally invasive approach to alleviating the burden of pain with Botox can be invaluable to those living with this condition. Furthermore, patients who are not surgical candidates, need to wait for surgery, or prefer to avoid surgery have a minimally invasive alternative in Botox.

---

## Hope for Neuropathic Pain Relief

Neuropathic pain can be as frustrating as it is excruciating, but patients should never give up. The medical understanding of the central and peripheral nervous systems is growing every day, and new treatments are on the horizon, which promise to bring relief to millions. If you are experiencing neuropathic pain, find a pain-literate doctor who will listen carefully to your symptoms and story and who will work with you to find the treatments that will help you the most.

To learn more about various self-care and pain treatment options and therapies, read the chapters in Part 1, Understanding and Treating Your Pain, and Part 2, Medical Therapies for Pain: Traditional and Innovative. There you will find more information and ideas for working with your physician and other healthcare providers to find ways to prevent, manage, and address your pain.

You can learn more about neuropathic pain by listening to the neuropathic pain episodes of my weekly radio program, *Aches and Gains*. You can find the broadcasts on neuropathic pain conditions at the following URLs.

**Painful Diabetic Neuropathy**

http://paulchristomd.com/painful-diabetic-neuropathy

**Complex Regional Pain Syndrome**

http://paulchristomd.com/complex-regional-pain-syndrome

http://paulchristomd.com/not-in-my-head

**Trigeminal Neuralgia**

http://paulchristomd.com/trigeminal-neuralgia

**Fibromyalgia**

http://paulchristomd.com/fibromyalgia

**Postherpetic Neuralgia**

http://paulchristomd.com/postherpetic-neuralgia

**Multiple Sclerosis**

http://paulchristomd.com/multiple-sclerosis

**Neurogenic Thoracic Outlet Syndrome**

http://paulchristomd.com/neurogenic-thoracic-outlet-syndrome

## Suggested Further Reading

Bested, Alison, and McCrindle, Louise. *The Complete Fibromyalgia Health, Diet Guide and Cookbook.* (n.p.): Robert Rose, 2013. This book offers tools that will help fibromyalgia patients help themselves. It uses The SEEDS of health approach: Support, Environment, Exercise/Pacing, Diet/Drugs, Sleep. https://tinyurl.com/y9wdho2u

Boroch, Ann. *Healing Multiple Sclerosis: Diet, Detox & Nutritional Makeover for Total Recovery.* (n.p.): Quintessential Healing, Inc., 2013. This book describes the author's journey with MS in addition to case histories, personal treatment programs, a nutritional makeover, a vitamin and supplement protocol, and tools to conquer stress. https://tinyurl.com/yamt2qnf

Brady, David M. *The Fibro Fix: Get To The Root Of Your Fibromyalgia And Start Reversing Your Chronic Pain and Fatigue in 21 Days.* (n.p.): Rodale Books, 2016. A 21-day detox, diet and movement program to relieve symptoms of fibromyalgia. https://tinyurl.com/yaj6vd6a

Jelinek, George. *Overcoming Multiple Sclerosis: The Evidence-Based 7 Step Recovery Program.* (n.p.): Allen & Unwin, 2016. This book explains the nature of MS and outlines an evidence-based 7 step program. https://tinyurl.com/ybgyut62

Juris, Elena. *Positive Options for Complex Regional Pain Syndrome (CRPS): Self-Help and Treatment.* (n.p.): Hunter House, 2014. This book explains CRPS in an accessible style providing medical treatments, complementary therapies, and holistic coping strategies. https://tinyurl.com/y825kv8l

Liptan, Ginevra. *The FibroManual: A Complete Fibromyalgia Treatment Guide for You and Your Doctor.* (n.p.): Ballantine, 2016. Dr. Liptan's program incorporates clinically proven therapies from both alternative and conventional medicine, along with the latest research on experimental options. https://tinyurl.com/ybt4l46k

Lyons, David, and Sloane, Jacob. *Everyday Health and Fitness with Multiple Sclerosis: Achieve Your Peak Physical Wellness While Working with Limited Mobility.* (n.p.) Fair Winds Press, 2017. This book is designed to help readers with MS maintain a healthy lifestyle and includes anecdotes from real people with MS. https://tinyurl.com/y9jcg6fz

Moulin, Dwight E, and Toth, Cory, eds. *Neuropathic Pain: Causes, Management and Understanding.* (n.p.): Cambridge University Press, 2014. Written by an international team of experts in the field, this book gives readers an in-depth understanding of the multitude of conditions causing neuropathic pain. https://tinyurl.com/y73p8ft8

Rymore, Robert. *Diabetic Neuropathy: Symptoms, Treatments, Diet, Management, Natural Remedies, Vitamins and Exercises.* (n.p.): IMB Publishing, 2014. A guide to Diabetic Neuropathy including symptoms, treatments, diet management, natural remedies, vitamins and exercises to relieve pain. https://tinyurl.com/y9tl4ed5

Teitelbaum, Jacob. *The Fatigue and Fibromyalgia Solution: The Essential Guide to Overcoming Chronic Fatigue and Fibromyalgia Made Easy.* (n.p.): Avery, 2013. A practical and concise guide to restoring health and energy. https://tinyurl.com/y729kmgj

## Other Resources to Explore

ActiveMSers.org was founded by Dave Bexfield to encourage those with MS to stay active. It features tips and tricks, exercises and a forum.

BartsMS Blog is for the Barts and The London Neuroimmunology Group to post their latest research in MS.

MSWorld is the official message board and chat center for the National Multiple Sclerosis Society.

MS Focus is the official website of the Multiple Sclerosis Foundation located in Florida. They also publish a magazine.

National Fibromyalgia & Chronic Pain Association's website provides support, education, research, and advocacy for fibromyalgia and chronic pain conditions.

The National Multiple Sclerosis Society's website offers information about symptoms and treatments as well as resources and the latest research.

# 5

# Pelvic and Sexual Pain

Ellen began to experience burning in her genital area at the age of 22. After testing negative for yeast and bacterial infections, as well as a host of STDs, Ellen had an ultrasound, which also failed to reveal any abnormalities. Her pain remained a mystery.

Without a diagnosis, Ellen's frustration grew as her pain worsened. Soon she was suffering not just during sexual intercourse, but during everyday activities, such as urination. Finally, an OB/GYN diagnosed her with vulvodynia (chronic pain in the vulva) but offered her no treatment plan. To add insult to injury, her primary care doctor told her that vulvodynia wasn't a real condition and that she should see a therapist for "psychological issues."

## Understanding Pelvic and Sexual Pain

Imagine working up the courage to seek treatment for a disease you found both terrifying and humiliating, only to be told it was all in your head. Unfortunately, that is the reality for far too many women who suffer from sexual pain that does not arise from cancer or a sexually transmitted disease (STD).

Slightly more than 20% of women have experienced sexual pain during their lives, a larger percentage than adults with asthma, cancer, or heart disease. Yet countless numbers have suffered in silence because of the fear and shame surrounding their symptoms. And when they have had the courage to seek treatment, far too many have been dismissed even by their own obstetrician-gynecologists.

Screening for sexual abuse in women with pelvic pain is important given that

30% of women worldwide have experienced sexual or physical violence by a partner. Equally alarming is the connection between sexual abuse and the onset of chronic pelvic pain and sexual pain disorders.

There's social stigma related to male sexual disorders as well, so underreporting is also common; however, a study examining over 4000 men found that 5% of men suffer from painful sex. In men, the causes range from painful ejaculation and chronic prostatitis to hernia repair, pudendal nerve compression (cyclists syndrome or pudendal neuralgia), and psychological trauma.

While temporarily painful intercourse isn't necessarily a cause for alarm, women who find sex painful or even significantly uncomfortable for an extended period of time should seek help from an obstetrician-gynecologist (OB/GYN) who understands sexual pain. Similarly, men experiencing painful sex should reach out to a knowledgeable urologist for guidance. Unfortunately, too many doctors are like Ellen's. They are only trained to recognize STDs, cancer, and other more common disorders. And like so many physicians, their patient load often makes it difficult for them to spend the needed time investigating pain that doesn't fit in the typical mold.

Sexual pain can be incredibly isolating. Ellen was fortunate to have close relationships with her mother and girlfriends and was able to share her suffering with them. Even so, she did not feel comfortable sharing her condition with the man she was dating. After her pain had persisted for months, the very thought of intercourse was painful. They broke up, and Ellen finally withdrew from the dating scene altogether.

To make matters worse, her doctor prescribed a pain medication that caused weight gain and made her lethargic, which made performing her job extremely challenging. Yet how could she explain her situation to her boss? While others suffering from cancer or even depression could be open about what they were dealing with, Ellen continued to suffer in silence.

For five years, Ellen, like many others in her situation, felt defined by her pain. Although she remained social and continued to go to work, she felt her life revolved around her medications: a pain pill that left her groggy and creams and suppositories that she applied to her genitals each night in order to be able to sleep. Ellen's pain was real. It had a specific cause and required a specific course of treatment. It simply took the right doctor with the right training to diagnose it.

Chronic sexual pain can take a tremendous emotional toll. Some doctors who do not understand sexual pain may assume the patient has a psychological aversion to sex. Sufferers often fear they have an STD, even if tests are negative. They may feel unattractive in a way that those with other kinds of chronic pain do not.

Some patients may withdraw from friends and family because of pain and embarrassment. Many may pull away from their husbands or partners, often feeling guilty because they are unable to be intimate. Patients even feel traumatized from having their sexual organs examined by so many doctors. Suicide fantasies are shockingly common. Ellen never told her boyfriend about her condition. Instead she gave no reason for her apparent discomfort with sexual intimacy, leaving him confused and distraught.

## Symptoms of Pelvic and Sexual Pain

Pelvic and sexual pain occurs in the pelvic region, which is between the navel in front and the lower spine in back and travels down to the upper thighs. It can involve the pelvic floor muscles, the ligaments, the nerves, and the organs such as the bladder, intestines, uterus, prostate (in men), and sexual organs.

Endometriosis, the presence of endometrial tissue outside the endometrial cavity and uterine muscle, causes distressing and sometimes debilitating pelvic pain, intensely painful periods, and painful intercourse. Hormone changes, nerve sensitization, and inflammation may all contribute to the symptoms.

The cultural taboos surrounding the discussion of sexual matters and the complex anatomical interconnections in the pelvis make sexual pain particularly difficult to diagnose. Beyond the typical problems doctors are trained to look for, there can be several causes of pelvic and sexual pain, which we discuss in the following sections of the chapter.

## Spasm in the Pelvic Floor Muscles

The muscles of the pelvic floor, as the name suggests, stretch across the bottom of the pelvic cavity. This is a bowl-like region between the public bone in front and the sacrum in back. There are muscles, tendons, and ligaments that hold the bones of the pelvis together. The pelvic floor provides vital support for the bladder, ovaries, fallopian tubes, and uterus and is often strained during pregnancy and childbirth. When the pelvic floor muscles spasm, they can cause unbearable pain in the genitals.

## Dermatologic Irritation and Inflammation

Sexual pain can be caused by damage to or inflammation of the skin of the vulva, labia, clitoris, or vagina. The skin of the genital area can break down causing burning and itching that make wearing underwear or even pants unbearable, not to mention intimate sexual contact. Diagnosis can be tricky, however, when the cause of the irritation isn't a common problem such as yeast, viruses, or bacteria. Causes may include the following:

- Hormonal changes, especially those that lower estrogen levels, can lead to vulvar (the external organs such as the labia and clitoris) or vaginal inflammation.

- Vulvar and anal cancer from human papillomavirus (HPV) can present as painful skin or skin that feels bumpy, rough, or bleeds.

- Less serious skin conditions such as eczema or psoriasis may appear in the vulvar region, making the area red, dry, and irritated.

- Chemicals in perfumes or those used in washing or drying clothes, bed linens, or sheets can lead to contact dermatitis and subsequent itchy, tender, skin.

- There are also specific conditions that can cause more chronic and inflammatory changes to the vulva and vagina that require the expertise of a gynecologist for proper diagnosis and treatment.

## Hormonal Imbalance

Our reproductive tracts are profoundly affected by the delicate balance of hormones in the bloodstream. Estrogen is central to the sexual well-being of women. When fluctuations occur, women can see drying, thinning, or shrinking of the vulva, sexual secretions, and pelvic floor muscles. Menopause can be a major factor in sexual pain. Surgically induced menopause due to a complete hysterectomy or the removal of both ovaries causes a drastic hormonal shift, which can have incredibly painful side effects from atrophy of the vulva or vagina. Other causes of hormonal imbalance include pregnancy and childbirth.

Even birth control pills can shift female hormone levels in a way that causes sexual or pelvic pain.

Women being treated for any kind of cancer may be surprised to experience pelvic or sexual pain as one of the side effects. Chemotherapy, radiation, and surgery can disrupt the hormonal balance and can bring about changes in the vulva. In particular, chemotherapeutic drugs for breast cancer often cause vaginal or vulvar pain by substantially reducing estrogen levels.

## Nerve Disorders

The sensory nerves in the pelvis are subject to damage and dysfunction just like any other nerves. Male and female patients often describe this sort of nerve pain as burning, shooting, stabbing pain, or pain that's caused by a light touch, such as clothing.

The pudendal nerve, the main nerve of the vulva, is often a culprit with vulvodynia, and the iliohypogastric and ilioinguinal nerves can cause clitorodynia (pain in the clitoris). Vulvodynia is persistent nerve-like pain along the parts of the vulva such as the mons pubis, labia, vaginal opening, and perineum. The branches of the pudendal nerve provide sensation to the rectal area, perineum (region between the anus and the vagina), labia, and clitoris.

Along with sensation to the rectal area and perineum, this nerve supplies the back of the scrotum and penis. Nerve pain can result in these areas of the body if the pudendal nerve or its branches become compressed, injured, entrapped, or inflamed, leading to an underestimated source of sexual pain. Both the iliohypogastric and ilioinguinal nerves travel along the groin and can cause pain in the frontal aspect of the vulva and pubis. Even the genitofemoral nerve that passes along the groin can induce pain in the labia or top of the vulva if it becomes damaged or irritated.

Sometimes a Cesarean section or other abdominal surgery accidentally damages these nerves. Other patients may have a neuropathic pain disorder (see Chapter 4, Neuropathic Pain) specifically in the pelvic area. Pudendal neuralgia, which we discussed earlier in the chapter, can be a source of pelvic pain in women and men. This condition results from injury to the nerve, usually causing intermittent stinging pain felt in the rectal, perineal, scrotal, labial, penile, or clitoral regions. Prolonged sitting, bike riding, or changes in the muscles of the pelvic floor can precipitate this nerve pain. One of the classic diagnostic features is that the pain is experienced when sitting and relieved by standing.

## Skeletal Abnormalities

Fractures, bone spurs, or bruises in the bones of the pelvis can also cause pelvic and sexual pain. For example, if the bones of the pelvis, such as the lumbar spine, sacrum, coccyx (tailbone), pubic bone, or hip bones, become misaligned or injured, pelvic pain can result. More specifically, women can feel vulvar or vaginal pain from pelvic joint abnormalities or muscular or tissue strain. Even low back pain can radiate to the vulva and rectum. When all other causes have been ruled out, doctors should consider an MRI of the pelvis to determine whether skeletal problems are at the root of the pain, especially if hip abnormalities are suspected. MRIs provide good visualization of musculoskeletal anatomy and help identify changes to the hip joint and surrounding soft tissues.

Ellen had actually experienced hip pain her senior year of college, but it wasn't until she visited Dr. Deborah Coady, an OB/GYN specializing in the treatment of sexual pain, that she even entertained the possibility that her hip pain could be connected to her vulvar pain. An MRI of her hipbone revealed bone spurs that were tearing into the cartilage of her hip joint. This, in turn, had activated trigger points in her pelvic floor muscles, causing them to tense and spasm and causing her unbearable genital pain. Muscles that are close to the hip and low back, such as the iliopsoas, piriformis, and gluteal muscles, can trigger radiating pain to the vulva or rectum.

After visiting Dr. Coady and getting a specific diagnosis, Ellen finally began to feel hopeful again. Although her road to recovery would prove a long one, she could finally begin treatment and take control of her life again. Fortunately, Ellen followed a course of treatment that allowed her to regain her sexual identity and heal her sexual pain.

## Treating Pelvic and Sexual Pain

Although chronic sexual pain can be incredibly distressing, the good news is that the overwhelming majority of women and men will get better with the right treatment. The proper treatment for sexual pain depends almost entirely on the cause. Infections can most often be cleared up with antibiotics, antivirals, or antifungals. Dermatologic problems are also highly treatable with the right medication, often including topical steroid ointments, anesthetic ointments, or hormone creams.

Hormonal problems can be more challenging to address: Creams or oils combining estrogen with testosterone applied topically or intra-vaginally have been successful in healing pain and discomfort due to hormonal imbalance, especially from estrogen deficiency. Natural oils, such as vitamin E or olive oil, applied to the skin of the vulva can assist in hydration as well as strengthen any weakened or dry tissue.

Several medicines used to treat neuropathic pain (see Chapter 4, Neuropathic Pain) such as the anticonvulsants and antidepressants should be considered for treating nerve pain of the genital area (pudendal neuralgia, for example).

Hypnosis, meditation, and relaxation exercises can also be very useful for patients in their recovery. Some patients also report that acupuncture has reduced their pelvic and sexual pain. Certain essential oils provided by medical aromatherapists either applied topically or taken orally have been an effective adjunct in soothing pelvic pain conditions in women like premenstrual syndrome and dysmenorrhea. Chaste tree berry taken orally can also be helpful to normalize hormone levels and is especially beneficial for women with premenstrual syndrome (PMS). Other oils include yarrow, sage, German chamomile, or Moroccan chamomile. For more immediate relief, these oils can be mixed with almond oil or olive oil as a carrier agent and then massaged into the skin for five minutes or so. Some oils can even be prepared as a vaginal suppository for chronic conditions. These oils may assist in balancing estrogen and progesterone levels, act as an anti-inflammatory and antihistamine, and ease overactive nerves. Aromatherapy is covered in Chapter 21, Aromas, Music, and Pain Relief.

Many doctors also recommend that patients with pelvic and sexual pain avoid propylene glycol and parabens (common additives in moisturizers, conditioners, and other cosmetics) because they are neurotoxins and can make the problem worse.

## Physical Therapy for Pelvic and Sexual Pain

Pelvic floor muscles in spasm can be treated with physical therapy, although it is quite invasive. The therapist must access trigger points through the vagina, and sessions can be painful. However, once the trigger points are deactivated, most patients find tremendous relief. Pelvic physical therapy can improve blood flow to muscles and connective tissue, remove accumulated chemicals such as lactic acid that trigger pain, stretch contracted muscles, and restore strength to the pelvic floor muscles. Intra-vaginal diazepam (Valium) can also be a good local muscle relaxant, and very little is actually absorbed into the bloodstream. If pelvic floor muscles do not respond to physical therapy, botulinum toxin (Botox) injections can help to relax tight muscular areas for three months or so.

## Integrative Treatments for Pelvic and Sexual Pain

Acupuncture, yoga, and Pilates have also been shown to help with muscular disorders in the pelvis. For those with endometriosis causing diffuse pelvic pain or referred pain to the back from this condition, an innovative method of reshaping posture to limit stress, strain, and pain may be useful. The Gokhale Method of posture realignment (discussed in more detail in Chapter 23, Pain Relief through Movement) uses a straightforward series of steps to optimize sitting, bending, walking, and standing. According to the Gokhale Method, the key is to reposition the bones and muscles of the spine in a way that resembles our "primal posture," the one we used as a child, which

was natural and correlates with a pain-free structure.

## Diagnostic and Therapeutic Blocks for Pelvic and Sexual Pain

Neuropathic pelvic and genital pain can take longer to heal than other kinds of sexual pain, but patients should not give up. Doctors can perform diagnostic and therapeutic blocks of the pundendal, iliohypogastric, ilioinguinal, and genitofemoral nerves to determine where the pain is coming from and to calm nerve irritation.

The autonomic nervous system (sympathetic and parasympathetic) controls the fight or flight response and regulates bodily systems such as digestion, respiration, and heartbeat. This part of the nervous system is often involved in visceral pain of the pelvic organs, because pain-sensing nerves travel along with the sympathetic and parasympathetic nerves. A superior hypogastric plexus block, for instance, can ease pain related to the bladder, uterus, prostate, ovaries, testicles, or vagina. For pain in the rectum, anus, perineum, coccyx (tailbone), vulva, and outer part of the vagina, a ganglion impar block can be effective.

A lesser known injection that targets the inferior hypogastric plexus located on the inner part of the sacrum may help to reduce pain in the clitoris, vagina, and urethra in women or the prostate, penis, and scrotal contents in men. In most cases, repeated nerve blocks offer the best course of therapy rather than a single injection. In patients with cancer pain (discussed in Chapter 12, Cancer Pain and the Caregiving), pain specialists can inject alcohol or other neurolytic medications around these nerves to produce more long-term relief.

## Neurostimulation for Pelvic and Sexual Pain

For patients with unrelenting pelvic pain, neurostimulation (discussed in more detail in Chapter 15, Pain-Relieving Devices) can offer needed relief. Typically, one or more small wires known as leads are either placed next to the lower thoracic spinal nerves in the epidural space for pelvic pain (nerve root stimulation) or placed much lower in the back along the sacral spinal nerves for those with bladder, vaginal, or perineal pain (sacral root stimulation). Sometimes, placing a lead in the epidural space at the bottom of the spinal cord can control pelvic pain or unrelenting pudendal neuralgia (conus medullaris stimulation). If a trial of stimulation is successful, then the wires and a battery are both implanted by the pain specialist or neurosurgeon in the operating room.

There is emerging interest and data on the application of spinal cord stimulation (SCS) for pelvic pain along with innovations in this technology. For example, a novel method of neurostimulation called dorsal root ganglion (DRG) stimulation targets specific nerves to control pain in regions difficult to reach with conventional spinal cord stimulation such as the groin, foot, and perhaps the pelvis. There have been some preliminary reports of treating pelvic pain with DRG stimulation in the literature.

## Stress Reduction for Pelvic and Sexual Pain

Stress activates our defense system. It "turns on" the nervous, endocrine, and immune systems. Continual sexual pain in the pelvic or genital area acts as a threat to the body like any other stressor and elicits the same physiological responses that manifest as more pain, depression, and physical ailments, such as digestive problems, headaches, or low back pain.

No matter what your diagnosis is, it makes sense to take steps to limit stressors in your life that may perpetuate your pain. For instance, you can exercise even moderately, or participate in any kind of movement-based activity like yoga. Remember to cultivate caring, supportive relationships, and choose healthy foods. Read more about strategies to help manage stress and live a healthy lifestyle in Chapter 17, Weight Control, Exercise, and Diet; Chapter 22, Harnessing the Human Biofield; and Chapter 23, Pain Relief through Movement.

Although studied primarily for migraine headaches, biofeedback (discussed in more detail in Chapter 19, Mind-Body Techniques for Pain Relief) can be successfully applied to those with pelvic pain. This technique helps patients recognize their body's response to stress, minimize it, and reduce tension and pain.

Because of the tremendous emotional toll of chronic pelvic and sexual pain, many patients also benefit from cognitive behavioral therapy (covered in Chapter 19, Mind-Body Techniques for Pain Relief) and even a serotonin–norepinephrine reuptake inhibitor (SNRI) like duloxetine (Cymbalta) to help them recover emotionally.

---

Ellen's journey to conquer her sexual pain began with orthopedic surgery to remove the bone spurs from her hip. After surgery, Dr. Coady helped her wean off the pain medication that had caused her weight gain and lethargy as well as her creams and suppositories. Ellen then began a year-long course of physical therapy on her pelvic floor muscles, which was painful at first but ultimately left her virtually pain free.

Ellen found hope and was healed of her sexual pain because she found an OB/GYN who understood sexual pain, listened to her symptoms, and investigated every possible cause of her pain until she found the answer. Although they had been apart for many years, Ellen did finally communicate with her old boyfriend to let him know why she had resisted being physically intimate with him. "I wish you would have told me," he responded.

---

## Hope for Sexual Pain Relief

The discussion of sexual pain is not as taboo as it once was, but there is still much work to do in our culture and in the medical community to make sure that doctors, especially OB/GYNs, understand this common condition. Although it can be a challenge, women suffering from sexual pain must continue to pursue an accurate diagnosis and workable treatment plan. It may take a long time, but the results will allow women to reclaim a very significant part of their lives.

To learn more about various self-care and pain treatment options and therapies, read the chapters in Part 1, Understanding and Treating Your Pain, and Part 2, Medical Therapies for Pain: Traditional and Innovative. There you will find more information and ideas for working with your physician and other healthcare providers to find ways to prevent, manage, and address your pain.

You can also learn more about sexual pain by listening to the pelvic and sexual pain episodes of my weekly radio program, *Aches and Gains*. You can find the broadcasts on sexual pain at the following URLs.

**Sexual Pain**

http://paulchristomd.com/sexual-pain

http://paulchristomd.com/sexual-pain-2

**Pudendal Neuralgia**

http://paulchristomd.com/cyclists-syndrome

http://paulchristomd.com/cyclists-syndrome-2

## Suggested Further Reading

Goldstein, Andrew, Goldstein, Irwin, and Pukall, Caroline. *When Sex Hurts: A Woman's Guide to Banishing Sexual Pain.* (n.p.): Da Capo Lifelong Books, 2011. This book tackles the stereotypes, myths, and realities of sexual pain. https://tinyurl.com/ycl5hcxs

Prendergast, Stephanie A., and Rummer, Elizabeth H. *Pelvic Pain Explained: What Everyone Needs to Know.* (n.p.): Rowman & Littlefield Publishers, 2016. This book offers readers guidance on navigating a pelvic pain diagnosis and treatment, helping them to better understand their pain from a physiological perspective as well as how to digest the current treatment options available. https://tinyurl.com/y8d4p7mg

Stein, Amy. *Heal Pelvic Pain: The Proven Stretching, Strengthening, and Nutrition Program for Relieving Pain, Incontinence & I.B.S. and Other Symptoms Without Surgery.* (n.p.): McGraw-Hill Education, 2008. Natural cures, in the form of exercise, nutrition, massage, and self-care therapy for those suffering from pelvic floor disorder, including pelvic pain, irritable bowel syndrome, endometriosis, prostatitis, incontinence, or discomfort during sex, urination, or bowel movements. https://tinyurl.com/yd9tykmy

---

## Other Resources to Explore

Pain "Down There" is a series of video guides for women experiencing genital and sexual pain lead by a team of professionals. http://www.paindownthere.com

PelvicPain.org is the official website for The International Pelvic Pain Society.

Pelvic Pain Rehab is the official website for the Pelvic Health and Rehabilitation Center in San Francisco. Includes various educational resources and a blog.

When Sex Hurts There is Hope is a personal blog about experiencing sexual pain, including interviews with professionals and product reviews.

# 6

# Infant Pain

A young mother holds back tears as the nurse takes her baby, who barely weighs three pounds. The ophthalmologist inserts a lid speculum into the baby's tiny little eye; he screeches and writhes in pain as the metal device forces his eyelids open, exposing the entirety of the eyeball. Working as quickly as possible, the doctor administers a series of drops while examining the blood vessels around the eyeball. But to mother and baby, those minutes feel like an eternity.

This kind of eye exam checks for retinopathy of prematurity (ROP), a condition that can cause severe vision loss, and, unfortunately, it is a necessary and common procedure for many preterm infants. Before the tremendous advancements in neonatal medicine of the last several decades, infants born prematurely or with other complicated illnesses often died at birth. But today there is great hope that most of these babies will not only survive their first year, but also live to become healthy adults. The road to health for these babies, however, is often paved with great suffering.

## Understanding Infant Pain

Normal, healthy infants typically receive a heel lance at birth to screen for genetic disorders and routine immunizations every few months. In contrast, almost all ill and preterm infants have to endure multiple painful procedures—from blood draws to complicated surgeries—in order to ensure that they have the best odds to survive and thrive. Unfortunately, progress in infant pain control has not quite kept pace with the rest of neonatal medicine.

It's difficult to imagine, but until the 1980s, most doctors did not believe the newborn nervous system was developed enough for infants to feel pain. Because of this misconception, even painful procedures including surgeries were performed without anesthesia. Doctors assumed that any pain behaviors the baby exhibited—such as screaming and wincing—were simply reflexive.

Now neuroscience has progressed to the point where we understand that babies do indeed feel pain, even in the womb. Because their pain inhibitory pathways are less developed than those in older humans, we now realize that infants may actually feel more pain than adults given the same stimuli. Although infants cannot communicate with us through language, pediatric specialists have developed metrics to evaluate the amount of pain they are experiencing.

Many people have seen the Wong-Baker FACES Pain Rating Scale, which is a chart of facial expressions that each correspond to a certain number on the pain scale. Children three years and older and even adults use the Wong-Baker Scale to rate the magnitude of their pain. Similarly, the Premature Infant Pain

Profile (PIPP) measures acute pain in infants using several indictors of behavior, such as eye opening, facial movements, eye squeeze, and heart rate. This tool has been rigorously tested, and medical experts believe it is valid and reliable. The Neonatal Facial Coding System (NFCS) is a similar tool that incorporates multi-dimensional behaviors in newborn and premature infants. Professionals can also monitor behaviors such as cry volume and duration.

These are steps forward, but the practice of preventing pain and offering pain relief for infants, especially the sick and premature, is still not progressing as fast as we would like. In the majority of hospitals, sick and premature babies are exposed to large numbers of painful procedures with little attempt to control the pain. And there is mounting evidence that uncontrolled pain in infancy has both short and long term effects on physical, behavioral, and neurological development. It could potentially even lead to a lifetime of pain in adulthood. In this chapter, we'll look at the reality of neonatal and infant pain, and the best ways to prevent and control it.

When Jan was diagnosed with placenta previa—a condition in pregnant women in which the placenta covers all or part of the cervical opening—she knew her twins would have to be delivered early by Cesarean section. But nothing could have prepared her for the suffering her tiny twins would endure before they came home from the hospital. Born at just 25 weeks, the twins spent nearly five months in the Neonatal Intensive Care Unit (NICU), fighting for their lives.

In addition to countless IV placements and blood draws, little Justin and Jacob had issues with their lungs and suffered from multiple infections. Jacob even became septic, developing an extremely painful blood infection that could easily have proven fatal. The babies had eye exams like the one described at the beginning of this chapter and constantly needed intravenous medications and fluids. But their little veins collapsed so often that nurses were forced to place the IV lines into the veins of their heads.

Like many preemies, Justin and Jacob also needed Pediatric Peripherally Inserted Central Catheters (PICC lines): long flexible IV tubes inserted into a vein in the arm and advanced until the tip is positioned near the heart. Tubes in their noses and throats prevented them from crying, but Jan had to watch them wince, furrow their eyebrows, and offer silent cries that were absolutely heartbreaking for the new mother.

The normal discomforts healthy newborns experience such as gas pain, the occasional blood draw, or routine immunizations are not cause for concern. Babies feel the pain for a few moments and then forget about it. But for the first several months of their lives, Jan's twins fought nearly constant discomfort and pain. This kind of situation requires a comprehensive pain reduction strategy, coordinated with all the healthcare providers responsible for the babies as well as with the parents.

## Preventing and Treating Infant Pain

Although sick and preemie newborns are too young for many methods of pain control, there are several steps parents and healthcare providers can take to mitigate the pain associated with tests and treatments these little ones must endure.

The most important step is coordination between various healthcare providers and specialists to ensure that babies are not exposed to unnecessary painful procedures. For example, if three doctors need blood samples from a baby for various tests, those samples can be drawn all at once instead of with three different heel lances. This might seem obvious, but too many hospitals do not take these simple precautions on a routine basis.

Just cuddling and rocking infants—particularly when it is the mother holding them—is tremendously comforting. When the mother cannot be present for a procedure, nurses can place a piece of fabric containing the mother's scent near the baby's face, which will also soothe and calm the infant. A so-called cozy cloth can promote well-being among infants too. It's a triangular piece of flannel that a mother puts inside her shirt to absorb her scent. The cloth is placed against or near the baby's face in moments of distress or pain.

Skin-to-skin contact—known popularly as "kangaroo care"—is an innovative technique that is also surprisingly effective. The mother removes her shirt and holds the baby—usually naked except for a diaper—against her bare skin under a hospital gown. When done for 20 to 30 minutes before a heel lance or intramuscular injection, for example, and continued during the painful procedure and sometimes afterward, this intimate contact has been shown to significantly reduce the baby's distress and discomfort. Jan noticed that her twins settled faster following a procedure and slept longer after kangaroo care sessions. Interestingly, singing, talking, or offering a finger for sucking don't add further pain-relieving benefits.

Breastfeeding before or during painful procedures such as immunizations, heel lances, or placing needles into veins, has proven to be highly effective in reducing infant distress. A combination of factors probably contributes to the analgesic effect—endorphins in the breast milk, the act of suckling, skin-to-skin contact, and the pleasant taste. Other comforting techniques include distracting the newborn with the mother's voice, music therapy, inhaled aromatherapy, or even visual stimuli such as colors and lights. The pain-relieving benefits of smells and sounds are covered in Chapter 21, Aromas, Music, and Pain Relief. Newborns can also find comfort in tight swaddling, or facilitated tucking, where the baby is swaddled into the fetal position.

Sugar water (24% sucrose or 25%–50% glucose if sucrose isn't available) administered with a cotton swab or a dropper is another simple method of infant pain control that is highly effective. There have been many published reports and reviews showing the effectiveness of oral sucrose during a painful procedure. Sucrose on the surface of the baby's tongue actually stimulates the baby's endogenous opioid response, essentially allowing the baby to produce natural painkillers made by the body. The sugar water technique has been shown to work very well during the first six months of life for up to about five minutes after a painful procedure. The sugar solution should be given about two minutes before the procedure. It is effective in older infancy as well but the effects do not last quite as long and the technique is no longer effective by 18 to 24 months.

Many infants also benefit from topical pain relievers such as a combination of lidocaine and prilocaine (EMLA cream or ointment) and even non-prescription strength topical lidocaine cream. Most procedures in preterm babies and infants produce mild to moderate pain, but surgery and other major procedures, such as placing breathing tubes and managing ventilators (respirators), induce discomfort and require opioids (morphine or fentanyl). There is evidence from scientific findings that opioid pain relievers given intravenously effectively reduce pain during surgery, and improve the stress response postoperatively in infants.

Acetaminophen (Tylenol) is often the pain reliever of choice for infants and children, and it's used for postsurgical pain and pain from minor procedures, not to mention cuts and scrapes. However, research findings typically show little analgesic benefit in neonates and infants who are given this drug orally or rectally. IV use may be more effective instead, and it does reduce opioid requirements postoperatively. Of note, it is recommended not to provide acetaminophen to infants in community settings prior to immunizations because it can reduce the immune (antibody) response to the vaccination.

Thanks to the hard work of many doctors and nurses, Jan's twins are now doing well. They have gained weight, progressed tremendously in their occupational and physical therapy work, and are well on their way to healthy, happy childhoods. Jan's advice to other parents with sick or premature infants is to be an advocate for their children. Parents should ask what they can do during painful procedures to comfort their babies. Push the doctors and nurses to use known methods of easing pain. There are international and national evidence-based guidelines on managing pain in infants. Most of the time, just asking should be enough to prompt healthcare professionals to implement measures that bring significant relief.

## Hope for Infant Pain Relief

The tremendous advancements in neuroscience over the last several years mean that growing numbers of doctors and nurses are becoming better educated in the area of neonatal and infant pain control. As noted earlier, untreated pain in infancy may lead to developmental, behavioral, and cognitive problems and a lifetime of pain as an adult. It is critical. then, to take measures that will ensure the comfort of newborns. We have every reason to believe that infant pain control will continue to advance as neonatal care continues to improve, and that our miracle babies will be given even better pain management options in the future.

To learn more about various self-care and pain treatment options and therapies, read the chapters in Part 1, Understanding and Treating Your Pain, and Part 2, Medical Therapies for Pain: Traditional and Innovative. There you will find more information and ideas for working with your physician and other healthcare providers to find ways to prevent, manage, and address your pain.

You can also learn more about neonates and babies in pain by listening to the related episode of my weekly radio program, *Aches and Gains* that is nationally syndicated on Sirius XM Radio. You can find the broadcast on neonates and babies in pain at the following URL.

**Infant Pain**
http://paulchristomd.com/babies-in-pain

## Suggested Further Reading

Anand, K.J.S., McGrath, Patrick J., Stevens, B.J. (eds). *Pain in Neonates and Infants: Pain Research and Clinical Management Series.* (n.p.): Elsevier, 2007. A comprehensive resource with the latest information in the field for use by researchers and clinicians. http://tinyurl.com/ya5g3ozj

Blackett Schlank, Christina, Zeltzer, Lonnie K. *Conquering Your Child's Chronic Pain: A Pediatrician's Guide for Reclaiming a Normal Childhood.* (n.p.): William Morrow,

2005. A guide for parents managing a child's chronic pain including lists of effective medication, breathing, muscle relaxation and visualization techniques. http://tinyurl.com/y83drjm3

Coakley, Rachael. *When Your Child Hurts: Effective Strategies to Increase Comfort, Reduce Stress, and Break the Cycle of Chronic Pain.* (n.p.): Yale University Press, 2016. A resource for parents and caregivers to help comfort children with chronic or recurring pain. http://tinyurl.com/yd87qs85

Dickerson, Michelle, and Marko, Tara. *Clinical Handbook of Neonatal Pain Management for Nurses.* (n.p.): Springer Publishing Co., 2016, A clinical handbook providing comprehensive information on pain management for the vulnerable neonatal population. http://tinyurl.com/yd2b9lng

Law, Emily F., Palermo, Tonya M. *Managing Your Child's Chronic Pain.* (n.p.): Oxford University Press, 2015. Easy-to-implement strategies and practical instructions for pain management in children, with guidance on how to prevent relapse and maintain improvements. http://tinyurl.com/yb68kre9

Oakes, Linda L. *Compact Clinical Guide to Infant and Child Pain Management: An Evidence-Based Approach for Nurses.* (n.p.): Springer Publishing Co., 2011. This go-to resource is for primary care providers who assess and treat infants, children, and adolescents experiencing pain. http://tinyurl.com/y8wszdfd

## Other Resources to Explore

Harvard Health is Harvard Medical School's blog, which includes articles about pain in newborns.

University of Michigan's medical school article on infant pain caused by medical procedures, circumcision and teething.

WebMD guide to over-the counter pain relief for treating children's fever and pain.

# 7

# Sports Injury and Pain

Imagine being in so much pain you couldn't walk 10 feet from your bed to your bathroom, but getting up the next day to play football against some of the most brutal competitors in the world. That was life for Michael McCrary, two-time Pro Bowl defensive end for the Seattle Seahawks and later the Baltimore Ravens.

Known for his speed and ability to take down much larger opponents, McCrary had everything an athlete could dream of: professional success, wealth, and fame. Yet his life was one of silent, nearly constant suffering. At the peak of his illustrious 10-year career, McCrary was diagnosed with depression, a side effect of the excruciating chronic pain in his knees.

Many athletes, like McCrary, may force themselves to play through the pain, often making the injury worse. Rare is the athlete like Olympic figure skater Peggy Fleming, who in addition to the 1968 Olympic gold medal, won five U.S. titles and three world championships. She credits her longevity in such an intense sport to listening to her pain and taking care of injuries when they were small. Although she did have cortisone injections to relieve knee pain when she was in her early teens, she typically opted to rest minor injuries and return to full training when the pain was gone.

Unfortunately, there can be financial incentives to compete through the pain. McCrary and other National Football League players earn a substantial salary, and McCrary says that he can sympathize with other athletes who mask pain when competing for similar paychecks. He also noted that the camaraderie teammates have with one another made him feel like he was letting them down if he didn't play.

During the last two years of his career, however, McCrary had so much pain in his knees that he was excused from practice—almost unheard of in the NFL—and only played football during Sunday games. I asked McCrary on my radio program if any of the team trainers who took care of him ever advised him to stop playing.

"It's really not their job to tell me or other players to stop playing, and I think if they had, they would not be trainers for long," he answered. Many healthcare professionals working for professional sports teams are often pulled in two directions—the health of their players and the profits of the team. Unfortunately, these competing interests often result in the players' health and pain losing to the broader financial interests of the team. "I iced my knees before practice and after practice to dull the pain and keep the swelling down. I might have just as well lived in the freezer," he said. When McCrary was ultimately assessed by a couple of orthopedic surgeons, they said he needed two total knee replacements, which wasn't particularly shocking for him to hear.

## Understanding Sports Injury and Pain

Exercise is essential to good health and some pain (a certain degree of soreness after a workout, for example) is normal. There are many health benefits of physical activity; among them are improved aerobic fitness, muscular strength, bone health, and cognitive performance. The Centers for Disease Control and Prevention (CDC) recommend that school-age children participate in at least 60 minutes of physical activity per day, which can include games, sports, work, or recreation. For adults, they advise two hours and 30 minutes each week of moderate intensity aerobic physical activity (tennis or brisk walking), or one hour and 15 minutes each week of vigorous intensity aerobic physical activity (jogging or swimming), or a combination of these two.

Many of us fall short of these recommendations, but others overtrain and risk injury to achieve an advantage over competitors. Pushing the body too hard can result in both traumatic and overuse injuries. Traumatic injuries occur as a result of a single incident—a broken bone from a fall, a sprained ankle from twisting too quickly, or incorrectly planting a foot. These may be mild and heal quickly or be so severe that they require surgery. Overuse injuries, on the other hand, occur from repetitive motions—throwing thousands of pitches, shooting thousands of jump shots, or swimming thousands of laps. These kinds of actions can cause repeated microtrauma anywhere in the body. For instance, they can damage muscles, tendons, bone, nerves, and blood vessels.

Sometimes injuries are also due to poor mechanics. A pitcher who pitches incorrectly is at greater risk of throwing out his elbow, just as a long jumper or weightlifter with poor form is more likely to suffer an injury. In professional and higher level college sports, these issues are often addressed by coaches. But younger or recreational athletes may not have the benefit of this kind of expertise.

Chronic muscle-overuse injuries are common, occurring in about 30%–50% of all sports. In fact, 80% of all sports injuries are musculoskeletal. Professional and even many collegiate athletes train hundreds of hours a year to prepare for competition. The volume and intensity of the training alone leaves athletes vulnerable to overuse injuries. The nature of a particular sport can put athletes at risk for traumatic injuries. Contact sports such as football and rugby are obviously notorious for concussions, impact fractures, joint dislocations, and tendon and ligament tears. But sports with high risks of falling, such as gymnastics, figure skating, and "extreme" sports, can also pose similar risks.

While professional and college athletes are at greater risk of injury than recreational athletes, they usually have the advantage of state-of-the-art diagnostic equipment and world class medical care. Michael McCrary underwent four knee surgeries during his time with the Ravens to enable him to keep playing. Recreational athletes can easily push themselves too far as well, but they will typically have to rely on more conservative methods to ensure they can remain active and pain free.

### Child Athletes at Risk

One of the most disturbing trends in sports-related pain is the increasing number of young athletes experiencing traumatic or overuse injuries. A few decades ago, the only injuries orthopedists would expect to see in young children were the occasional broken bones from falls on the playground. Now sports medicine doctors are seeing young athletes with torn tendons and ligaments, bone fractures, and overuse injuries such as tendonitis, stress fractures as well as degradation of cartilage and other joint problems usually associated with much older individuals.

About half of all sports injuries in adolescents are due to overuse.

Why the recent increase in injured child athletes? Sports medicine doctors point to two trends. First, children are playing organized, competitive sports much earlier than ever before, some beginning as young as age three. Second, instead of playing a variety of sports throughout the year, children are specializing in one particular sport very early on, and they are practicing intensively for many hours, particularly when they show potential. This sport specialization means that for elite-level gymnasts, figure skaters, and even some dancers, spending 30 to 40 hours training in a single week. These intense training regimens, which are often extended throughout the year, don't provide sufficient time for microtrauma to repair itself. The volume of training in young athletes is directly correlated to their risk of overuse injury just as it is in adults.

However, there are several factors that make sports pain in children different from that in adults. From a physical standpoint, children often heal much more quickly than adults, but they are also vulnerable to injuries that adults are protected from. The growth plates—areas of growing tissue at each end of the long bones—are particularly weak and prone to injury in young athletes. A traumatic incident that might only cause a minor sprain in an adult will frequently cause a growth plate fracture in a child. Furthermore, evidence is mounting that some sports injuries can cause arthritic changes in the skeleton, leading to chronic pain in adulthood.

From a psychological standpoint, children are often able to describe pain to their doctors in a more straightforward manner than adults, because they are less prone to try to interpret what the pain means. However, depending on their relationships with the adults in their lives, children may hide pain from their parents and coaches for fear of disappointing the adults. Child athletes who are particularly driven may conceal their pain in order to avoid missing out on competitive opportunities. Some child athletes engage in sports to meet the expectations of their parents and are under extreme pressure to perform. By the time young athletes reach high school, they may see their sport as a central part of their identity, feeling devastated if they have to cut back their training for hours or even quit.

Parents understandably become very invested in their children's athletic activities. After all, they are the ones who pay the bills, drive to practices, and attend the competitions. Many parents, intentionally or unintentionally, encourage children to push through pain instead of resting for a full recovery. Some parents may simply be competitive, while others are entertaining the possibility of college scholarships or even professional careers. Parents who express too much disappointment at a loss, or even too much excitement at a win, may unintentionally make their children believe that their performance dictates their parents' happiness—a burden too great for any child to bear.

Pediatric orthopedists note that, unlike at the collegiate and professional levels, many youth sport coaches may have little to no training in injury prevention. This means that they may push children too far in an effort to improve performance as well as fail to recognize warning signs of overuse injuries. Some sports have no credentialing requirements at the recreational level, so parents need to be on guard.

Osgood-Schlatter disease is a painful condition that affects children—boys more than girls—by causing inflammation in the region a couple of inches below the knee cap where the patellar tendon attaches to the tibia bone. It causes knee pain and occurs more frequently in children participating in sports that require jumping and running. Sports that require frequent contraction of the quadriceps muscle lead to the problem. These sports include ballet, gymnastics, figure skating, and soccer. Osgood-Schlatter symptoms resolve when the growth plate fuses during skeletal maturity.

Other common overuse injuries from youth sports include stress fractures of the lamina (part of the spine), femur (thigh bone), patella (knee cap), tibia (shin bone), medial malleolus (inside of the ankle), and foot.

It is easy to forget that for every young Olympian or successful professional athlete we see on television, there are likely hundreds of others who were on the brink of such success but had to quit because of injury. Whitney Phelps, older sister of swimming legend Michael Phelps, was well on her way to similar Olympic achievements, and ranked number one in the nation in butterfly by the age of 10. Unfortunately, as she recounted to sports journalist and author Mark Hyman in his book *Until It Hurts: America's Obsession with Youth Sports and How It Harms Our Kids*, she was so plagued by overuse injuries that she shocked the swimming world by failing to qualify for the 1996 Olympics. And while she does not suffer from chronic pain today, she rarely swims, even recreationally.

## Preventing Sports Injury and Pain

Recreational athletes should focus on building a good foundation of cardiovascular fitness, strength, and flexibility, as well as remembering not to rush into any new activity. If you've never run a race before, train for a 5K or a 10K before signing up for marathon. Scheduling rest is also very important; muscles need time to recover, and no one should work out seven days a week.

Parents of child athletes, in addition to maintaining open communication about how the child's sport is going, need to keep an eye out for overtraining and other harmful coaching practices. They should watch their children for pain behaviors such as limping, muscle imbalance, disruptions in sleep, or problems with school performance. Children should be encouraged not to be afraid to tell their parents or coaches that they hurt. They should not be persuaded to continue to practice or play through the pain. Sports for children should be kept playful and fun for as long as possible, and parents should pay attention to coaches' credentials, track records, and styles. In addition, sport diversification should be promoted at younger ages. It may even be a better strategy for developing elite-level athleticism in a single sport from the transfer of skills of several sports.

## Treating Sports Injury and Pain

Sports injuries and the pain they cause can be treated in a variety of ways, depending on their nature and severity. The most conservative treatments involve rest, icing, and sometimes wrapping or taping. Broken bones (covered extensively in Chapter 8, Skeletal Pain) or even strained tendons and ligaments may require casting to allow for complete healing. Most stress fractures heal if the athlete rests, does rehabilitation, and gradually returns to the sport. Some breaks are high risk, though, and need to be followed by a specialist; otherwise, the bone may not heal properly, resulting in chronic joint pain.

The nonsteroidal anti-inflammatory drugs (NSAIDs) are the most frequently used analgesics worldwide. They are also the most often used to treat acute and chronic musculoskeletal disorders. Over-the-counter NSAIDs are a common method for treating minor sports pain. Over-the-counter acetaminophen (Tylenol) is a frequent first-line choice for acute pain. Adults should remember to stay below the maximum adult dose of 3000–4000 mg per day, while dosing for children is based on their weight or age. The rule of thumb is to use the lowest dose for the shortest period of time, but extended use for chronic therapy may be needed and should be monitored by your healthcare provider.

Topical medicines for treating pain are becoming more popular. For instance, the diclofenac patch (Flector 1.3%) can be used for acute sprains and strains, and evidence supports its pain-relieving and anti-inflammatory effects. Five percent ibuprofen gel or cream (not available in the United States) has also been found to reduce pain in soft tissue injuries like sprains.

Professional athletes who compete injured will often receive various kinds of injections, usually corticosteroids in sites where they are experiencing pain to both control the discomfort and decrease inflammation.

While in the NFL, Michael McCrary would use therapeutic ultrasound massage with the transcutaneous electrical nerve stimulation (TENS) device to warm up his leg muscles before a game, and would immediately ice his knees afterwards. He also used prednisone as needed to control inflammation and decrease pain along with other pain medicines. Many times, these were needed just to get through the day.

Both traumatic injuries and overuse injuries can lead to the need for surgery. Sometimes surgery is required to repair bones or reattach ligaments or tendons. For instance, anterior cruciate ligament (ACL) injuries (in the knee) are becoming particularly common in younger athletes. Similarly, overuse injuries of the elbow may require reconstructive surgery. As an example, ulnar collateral ligament reconstruction—more popularly known as "Tommy John" surgery after the Major League Baseball pitcher on whom the procedure was first performed in 1974—may be needed. In this procedure, a tendon usually from the wrist is transferred to the elbow to replace the damaged ulnar collateral ligament and reconstruct the joint. Unfortunately, some parents have started to view this surgery as a way to give their children a competitive advantage in pitching, a sign of how unhealthy attitudes toward youth sports can become.

## Integrative Therapies for Sports Injury and Pain

Practitioners of Jin Shin Jyutsu and the other healing techniques discussed in this section, which are covered in more detail in Chapter 22, Harnessing the Human Biofield, report that this form of energy healing can be quite effective for sports injuries and, specifically, overuse injuries. Esther Gokhale, founder of the Gokhale Method of posture realignment, believes that her strategy for restoring healthy posture can be effective for musculoskeletal problems. Dr. Edythe Heus has developed a unique system of conditioning and reorganizing muscles and nerves called Revolution In Motion. It's an exercise program that she asserts fine-tunes proprioception, a part of the sensory nervous system that gives us an awareness of our body parts in space. Dr. Heus has seen her program help to free clients from pain related to overuse injuries, and she's worked with world class athletes to optimize their performance.

## Stress Reduction for Sports Injury and Pain

Various stress-reduction techniques can improve persistent muscular pain. Biofeedback, discussed in Chapter 19, Mind-Body Techniques for Pain Relief, can be a useful strategy for reducing muscle pain, Similarly, patients using hypnosis can respond well to suggestions focusing on activities that can modify chronic musculoskeletal pain. Engaging in cognitive behavioral therapy (CBT) to positively change your thoughts, feelings, and behaviors can reduce the perception of pain. Mindfulness-based stress reduction

can dampen sympathetic nervous system arousal and pain. Additional useful techniques are discussed in Chapter 19, Mind-Body Techniques for Pain Relief.

Improving sleep hygiene by getting seven hours or so of sleep at night is discussed in Chapter 18, Sleep, Stress, and Emotional Health. Sleep is more important than you might imagine for improving pain, because sleep facilitates the production of protective antioxidants, conserves energy, and supports immune function. Sleep deprivation can lead to muscle aches or can worsen muscle pain and other conditions that already exist. Studies on slow wave sleep deprivation (lack of the deepest level of sleep) demonstrate that sleep-deprived patients not only develop muscle aches but have a lowered pain threshold. When injured, try to maintain good sleeping habits or even elevate your level of sleep. Animal studies validate that more sleep can speed recuperation.

There is also evidence that interactions with therapy dogs for just five to 15 minutes enhances healing environments by lowering stress hormones such as cortisol, increasing endorphins, and providing a distraction. In one study, patients with pain experienced relief and an improvement in mood after their encounter with a dog. Animal therapy is discussed further in Chapter 22, Harnessing the Human Biofield.

## Regenerative Therapies and Sports Injuries

If injured ligaments or tendons produce chronic musculoskeletal pain and instability, prolotherapy can offer a safe and simple means of repairing these tissues. Prolotherapy involves the injection of dextrose (sugar) and sometimes other chemicals into these ligaments or tendons for overuse injuries such as elbow epicondylitis (aka tennis or golf elbow; pain in the inner or outer part of the elbow from repetitive gripping or from wrist movements performed in sports like tennis or golf), sprained ankles, and whiplash injuries. Research on conditions such as tennis elbow and knee osteoarthritis as well as Osgood-Schlatter disease, indicate that prolotherapy shows benefit if pain persists and doesn't improve with nonsteroidal anti-inflammatory drugs (NSAIDs), ice, use of protective gear, and physical therapy.

A related regenerative therapy called platelet rich plasma (PRP) therapy is thought to enhance the ability of certain cells to regenerate tissue and promote healing. It's an emerging treatment for painful conditions such as plantar fasciitis (pain and tenderness located on the inner portion of heel), elbow epicondylitis (tennis or golf elbow) and Achilles tendinopathy (problems related to the Achilles tendon, such as swelling, inflammation, or tears). Specialists also inject PRP for acute muscle injury due to trauma in athletes. PRP promotes faster recovery as well as muscle healing. You can read more about regenerative treatment options in Chapter 16, Regenerative Biomedicine.

Today, Michael McCrary has successfully moved on from professional football. He still has discomfort while standing, but he has incorporated pain-relieving therapies to assist his mobility and enhance his quality of life. He says if he had it all to do over again, he would have retired sooner, but he still finds comfort in the support of his family and friends. "It's not only the individual who has to learn how to overcome the pain, it's the family around that individual. It's another team sport with the objective of getting through the pain every day," he said. McCrary takes his pain one day at a time and reminds himself that others have suffered worse than he has.

## Hope for Sports Injury and Pain Relief

Sports-related pain is a message from the body that should be heeded not ignored. Professional and college athletes should make sure they are being cared for by doctors who are not just concerned with their performance, but with their long-term health and well-being too. Recreational athletes should set realistic goals, pace themselves sensibly, and seek appropriate medical care when warranted. And parents of young athletes should ensure that their children's bodies are being preserved for a healthy and pain-free adulthood.

To learn more about various self-care and pain treatment options and therapies, read the chapters in Part 1, Understanding and Treating Your Pain, and Part 2, Medical Therapies for Pain: Traditional and Innovative. There you will find more information and ideas for working with your physician and other healthcare providers to find ways to prevent, manage, and address your pain.

You can learn more about sports pain by listening to my weekly radio program, *Aches and Gains*. You can find the broadcast on sports pain at the following URL.

**Sports Pain**
http://paulchristomd.com/sports-pain

## Suggested Further Reading

Albrecht, Jack. *Tennis and Golfer Elbow Relief in Only Days: Everything You Need to Successfully Treat Your Symptoms and Speed your Recovery.* (n.p.): Spectrum Ebooks, 2015. A guide to Tennis or Golfer elbow relief with fast and easy daily routines. http://tinyurl.com/y74cxzf7

Demirakos, George. *Fix My Shoulder: A Guide to Preventing and Healing from Injury and Strain.* (n.p.): Rowman & Littlefield Publishers, 2014. This book explores the anatomy and function of the shoulder, methods of preventing pain and injury, and treatments for healing. http://tinyurl.com/ya4z954d

Joyce, David, Lewindon, Daniel. (eds). *Sports Injury Prevention and Rehabilitation: Integrating Medicine and Science for Performance Solutions.* (n.p.): Taylor and Francis, 2015. Evidence-based best practices in all the core areas of sports injury risk management and rehabilitation. http://tinyurl.com/y8xps6cg

Langendoes, John, and Sertel, Karin. *Kinesiology Taping The Essential Step-By-Step Guide.* (n.p.): Robert Rose, 2014. Taping for Sports, Fitness, and Daily Life. A guide to taping for effective treatment of conditions like muscle pain, bruising, sore muscles, bad posture, swelling, strains, sprains, arthritic conditions and more. http://tinyurl.com/yaw9dzkp

## Other Resources to Explore

Spineandsports.com is the New York Spine and Sports Medicine's website including blog addressing pain treatment.

Sportsinjuryclinic.com includes a list of sports injuries, symptom checker, rehabilitating exercises, treatment therapies and a blog.

Spine-health.com has articles about sports injuries, back injuries and back pain.

Sports-health.com provides comprehensive, highly informative, and useful resources for understanding, preventing, and seeking appropriate treatment for sports injuries and related conditions.

# 8

# Skeletal Pain

Trevor's parents weren't too alarmed when he broke his leg at the age of six. He was an active little boy, and this seemed like a normal childhood mishap. But then he broke it the next year and then again the year after that. Trevor broke his leg 10 times between the ages of six and 16. His parents took him to specialist after specialist, no doubt fearing the worst.

Thankfully, Trevor didn't have cancer. He had fibrous dysplasia, a disease caused by a genetic defect that affects the body's ability to form new bone. It's like a fracture that never heals properly. Although this disease is rare, the pain experienced by patients with fibrous dysplasia has much in common with that felt by the millions of people who suffer from other kinds of skeletal pain every day.

## Understanding Skeletal Pain

We tend to think of our bones as hard and static, but bone is one of the most dynamic organs in the body. When our skeleton is functioning properly, it is very metabolically active and serves as a reservoir of minerals and growth factors that the body can draw upon in times of need including after injury, breaking a bone, after exercise, or during pregnancy.

Bone is made of three main layers. The periosteum is the outer membranous layer that provides blood flow to the bone. The cortical (calcified) bone is the hard part of the skeleton that supports the muscles and the rest of the body. Finally, the bone marrow is deep inside the bone; it produces all the red and white blood cells and platelets that circulate throughout the blood vessels.

## Aging and Bone Health

The stem cells inside bone marrow are constantly removing old bone and replacing it with new. This process is called remodeling. Healthy bone actually regenerates faster than cartilaginous structures such as joints, ligaments, and tendons. That is why a small bone fracture may heal faster than a severe sprain, especially in younger patients. As we age, this repair process slows down, leading to aches and pains. In fibrous dysplasia, Trevor's disease, the bone remodels itself incorrectly, producing a "woven" pattern, leaving the bone weak and vulnerable to fracture.

Before age 40, it takes our bodies about seven years to completely replace our entire skeleton. But as we age, our bodies take longer to break down old bone and replace it with new bone. We also experience an increase in our production of sclerostin, a protein that inhibits bone growth. Most of the skeletal pain associated with aging is likely due to wear and tear on the joints (osteoarthritis), microfractures which don't show up on x-rays, or just the pulling of tendons, ligaments, or muscles that attach to the periosteum.

## Causes of Skeletal Pain

Bone pain is felt more deeply in the body than almost any other pain, and it's often difficult for patients to pinpoint its location. Bone pain is also one of the most common reasons for doctor visits. Bone pain arises from common conditions such as osteoarthritis (see Chapter 3, Arthritis Pain), osteoporosis, and fractures. (Patients and doctors consider osteoarthritic pain to come from the joints, but we don't really know if the pain of osteoarthritis originates in the joint itself or in the underlying bone.) Bone pain can also be caused by some viral infections, diseases, such as sickle cell anemia, and more serious conditions, such as bone cancer.

For years, bone pain was not well understood on the cellular and molecular level, but that is changing. Fortunately, our growing understanding of the mechanism of skeletal pain is opening up many new possibilities for treatment. Today, we believe that improperly healed fractures and the degeneration of cartilage in the joints probably cause the sprouting of new nerve fibers into areas where nerve fibers should not be. This is referred to as "sprouting." (In fact, this same sprouting of nerve fibers into areas where they don't belong is associated with other painful disorders including cancer, irritable bowel syndrome, and endometriosis.)

Cartilage is found in joints, ligaments, and tendons. Healthy cartilage has no nerve endings or blood vessels and thus functions very effectively as a shock absorber for our joints. When sprouting nerves invade weakened or damaged cartilage, these nerves trigger pain signals during normal joint movement. This accounts, for example, for the pain felt in a knee or hip with arthritis.

As joints deteriorate and pain continues, a process called central sensitization can occur. This means that nerves in the spinal cord and brain become hypersensitive. The pain-sensing nerves in the joint become more active as well. When bone is injured, immune and inflammatory cells in the joint release chemicals, such as prostaglandins, that sensitize the nerves in the joint. When we walk normally and put pressure on the affected joint, these sensitized nerves are then activated and produce pain.

## Treating Skeletal Pain

Even very healthy individuals will almost certainly experience bone pain as they age. Perhaps the most important feature of healthy aging is maintaining the ability to move easily and stay active. Unfortunately, aging weakens the capacity of our skeletal system to remodel itself after wear and tear occurs, or after injury, often making exercise difficult or impossible. Researchers are striving to understand how our bones change with age, why we feel bone pain in the morning when we are 50 versus 25 years old, and how to develop therapies to help us remain active in life and age successfully.

### Neuropathic Bone Pain Treatments

The relatively new understanding of nerves growing where they don't belong (known as sprouting, which is discussed in the "Causes of Skeletal Pain" section in this chapter) in response to injury has opened up many therapeutic possibilities. This sprouting is triggered by nerve growth factor (NGF), a protein which—as the name indicates—stimulates nerve growth in bone and other tissues. Although NGF is critical to the survival of our nerves during our younger years (for children under five), as we age, NGF tends to sensitize our sensory nerves instead of protecting them. As a consequence, the normal motion of our bones or joints can be perceived by our bodies as painful. For example, as we age, we may experience hip pain following a gentle hike or short run due to the role of NGF. Scientists are working on medicines that can inhibit the production of NGF, which would prevent the painful sprouting of nerves into areas where they shouldn't be.

Skeletal sensation involves two major types of nerve fibers known as A-delta and C-fibers. They are distinguished mainly by the speed with which they conduct sensation: A-deltas conduct faster and C-fibers slower. Sharp, stabbing pain is believed to be associated with the A-delta nerve fibers and dull, aching pain with the C-fibers. These nerves exist in other parts of the body as well, but they lie along the periosteum, mineralized bone, and in the bone marrow of the skeleton. NGF binds to certain receptors located on these nerves, which then trigger pain in conditions like osteoarthritis (OA), fractures, and bone cancer. It turns out that 80% of the nerves that innervate (provide sensation to) the bone express NGF receptors, which is why researchers are investigating drugs like tanezumab, which block the NGF pain pathway.

As a matter of fact, tanezumab has shown great potential in clinical trials, which trials have indicated that it reduces OA pain and low back pain by 40%–50%. Some patients in these studies have needed to be told to slow down their activity level because they feel so much better. As of this writing, however, tanezumab is still in development for cancer pain and osteoarthritis.

Neuropathic pain results from nerve injury and nerve sprouting. Both injury and sprouting occur in bone pain, and this type of pain can respond to other medicines we use for neuropathic pain like the tricyclic antidepressants (TCAs), serotonin norepinephrine reuptake inhibitors (SNRIs), or the anticonvulsants such as gabapentin (Neurontin) and pregabalin (Lyrica).

## General Treatments for Skeletal Pain

Mild to moderate bone pain from arthritis, fractures, or cancer can be treated with nonsteroidal anti-inflammatory drugs (NSAIDs), such as ibuprofen (Motrin, Advil) or naproxen (Aleve). NSAIDs block the synthesis of prostaglandins so fewer of these molecules can sensitize nerves in the bone and joints. These medications are often very effective, but care should be taken with long-term use. Not only can NSAIDs cause problems for the stomach lining, blood pressure, and the kidneys, but they may also inhibit the remodeling of bone, which we need to heal properly. There are data from animal studies that demonstrate that NSAIDs slow the healing of fractures, but we aren't sure how much this occurs in humans yet.

Steroids can also be very effective against bone pain, especially when it is caused by cancer, but as with any medication that suppresses the immune system, doctors must help patients balance the risks and benefits of long-term use. Occasionally, opioids can also provide bone pain relief, though the NSAIDs often are more effective. With opioids, some patients find a decrease in mental sharpness over time as well as the usual concerns about tolerance, misuse, and abuse. Still, some patients with bone pain have found that opioids allow them to live their lives more fully, especially if cancer is the source of pain.

Bone pain sufferers can find relief with integrative therapies such as acupuncture, Pilates, and meditation, which are covered in some detail in Part 3, Integrative Therapies for Pain. Weight loss can be very helpful with bone pain, since it reduces the pressure on joints and bones. Chapter 17, Weight Control, Exercise, and Diet, discusses the advantages of being at a healthy weight when it comes to fighting pain. Take a look at your diet to ensure that you're consuming enough calcium for proper bone growth as well.

### Bisphosphonates and Skeletal Pain

For bone conditions such as osteoporosis, fibrous dysplasia, and metastatic bone cancer pain, a class of drugs called bisphosphonates (Boniva, Fosamax) can be very helpful. As we noted earlier in this chapter, in a process called remodeling, stem cells inside the bone marrow are constantly destroying old bone and replacing it with new. Bisphosphonates work by halting the body's process of remodeling bone. Although bisphosphonates are very good at halting the destruction of old bone, they also halt the growth of new bone, which can be a problem, especially in younger patients.

The bisphosphonate Pamidronate can offer relief, particularly when pain is felt in the long bones or the ribs. Denosumab (Xgeva, Prolia), a monoclonal antibody biologic therapy that acts like an extremely potent bisphosphonate virtually shuts down the cells that break down old bone. (Monoclonal antibodies are laboratory-made cells that attach to substances in the body and aid in treating diseases. Monoclonal antibodies are also discussed in Chapter 12, Cancer Pain and Caregiving, and Chapter 14, Pharmacological Therapies.) Denosumab is approved for the treatment of bone cancer, osteoporosis, and other disorders. Unfortunately, although it stops the destruction of old bone, denosumab is not able to promote the growth of new bone.

For patients with osteoporosis, bisphosphonates seem to be most effective when taken within the first two to three years of diagnosis. But, unfortunately, there are new concerns about their long-term use for any condition. This is because of rare but serious side effects that include osteonecrosis of the jaw, which is the painful and disfiguring death of bone cells in the jaw, due to lack of blood flow.

## Vertebroplasty, Kyphoplasty, and Skeletal Pain

For spinal bones that have collapsed due to cancer or osteoporosis, doctors can perform vertebroplasty or kyphoplasty, techniques that involve injecting bone cement into compressed bone. Both vertebroplasty and kyphoplasty help to stabilize bone and promote pain relief. Kyphoplasty uses an inflatable balloon that's placed inside the bone to help re-expand it before the cement is injected. These procedures are usually performed on an outpatient basis with light sedation. Bone cement is injected into the broken bone by the physician

under x-ray guidance to control pain and stabilize the spine. These minimally invasive procedures can be quite effective with a low risk of complications. A large scientific review examining many patients with cancer-related fractures of the spine found significant and rapid pain reduction with both of these techniques.

## New and Innovative Treatments for Skeletal Pain

There are several exciting treatments for bone pain on the horizon, including gene therapy. However, getting the gene to the correct target area on the bone in need of repair is tough to do. Gene therapies will most likely need to center on influencing sclerostin, which is only found in the bone and therefore can't be accessed by targeting other tissues. Sclerostin is a protein produced by osteocytes (bone cells) that blocks bone formation. Scientists are working on developing innovative biologic therapies that target inhibitors of bone formation, like sclerostin, in order to promote new bone growth even as we age. There is also mounting interest in the regenerative therapies, such as prolotherapy, for use in treating bone pain from chronic osteoarthritic conditions of the knee and finger, for example. You can read more about techniques like this one in Chapter 16, Regenerative Biomedicine.

Tissue regeneration looks promising and may play a role in healing torn tendons or ligaments and replacing cartilage. For example, the most common injury to the knee is a tear of the meniscus, the shock absorber of the knee. This often leads to arthritis and knee pain. Many orthopedists remove damaged tissue using arthroscopy, but a better option may be innovative methods of re-growing and then replacing the torn meniscus. Doctors believe it's more beneficial to save tissue rather than remove it, if possible, because the risk of arthritis may be reduced when there is more tissue present.

Many patients have received successful grafts of cartilage and tendon from other parts of the body to repair damaged joints, but this has the unfortunate consequence of weakening the part of the body from which the tissue was removed. Until recently, the only other option was to use human tissue from a tissue bank. Exciting new techniques include transplants from animal tissue—younger and stronger than human tissue—made possible by stripping away the carbohydrates that cause the human immune system to reject the tissue. Although animal tissue transplants are not routinely available in the United States, one recipient of an anterior cruciate ligament (ACL) transplant constructed from pig tissue won the Canadian Masters Downhill Ski Championship following this type of surgery.

Equally exciting is the potential of combining tenezamab to block pain with a drug to block sclerostin. In this case, we could reduce bone pain caused by NGF while building new bone by inhibiting sclerostin. This might allow us to limit the effects of joint and bone pain as we age.

Bones, joints, and muscles are often interconnected. A protein called myostatin inhibits muscle growth, and there are exciting clinical studies underway looking at drugs that will block myostatin and sclerostin in older adults with hip fractures and in those with multiple myeloma. This would open up the wonderful possibility of building muscle and bone in order to improve pain and function.

Despite all the progress that has been made in treating skeletal pain, we still have much to learn. Trevor's condition limited his life a great deal, causing him to spend much of his childhood in body casts and wheelchairs and on crutches.

As an adult, he had a major fracture at age 47, forcing him to have rods inserted into his femur.

To manage his daily pain, Trevor has used naproxen (Aleve) but found he needed too high a dosage to continue taking it. More recently, he has found relief with oxycodone, although he does find that it interferes with his concentration at times.

Yet Trevor has not allowed skeletal pain to control his life. As a sports lover, he served as the manager for the football and basketball teams in high school and college. He and his wife are very active in their church and find a great deal of support from their relationships. He's also an accomplished attorney. Trevor has found tremendous comfort in connecting with others who have the same condition. "Know that you're not alone," he says. That knowledge has the biggest impact on his life.

## Hope for Skeletal Pain Relief

To learn more about various self-care and pain treatment options and therapies, read the chapters in Part 1, Understanding and Treating Your Pain, and Part 2, Medical Therapies for Pain: Traditional and Innovative. There you will find more information and ideas for working with your physician and other healthcare providers to find ways to prevent, manage, and address your pain.

You can also learn more about skeletal pain by listening to my weekly radio program, *Aches and Gains*. You can find the broadcasts on skeletal pain at the following URLs.

**Skeletal Pain**
http://paulchristomd.com/skeletal-pain
http://paulchristomd.com/skeletal-pain-2

# Suggested Further Reading

Belkoff, Stephen M, Herve, Deramond, Mathis, John M. (eds). *Percutaneous Vertebroplasty and Kyphoplasty.* Springer, 2006. This book compares and contrasts data and claims that differentiate kyphoplasty from percutaneous vertebroplasty. http://tinyurl.com/yajy5vk9

Castleman, Michael. Lamou, Amy. *Building Bone Vitality: A Revolutionary Diet Plan to Prevent Bone Loss and Reverse Osteoporosis Without Dairy Foods, Calcium, Estrogen or Drugs.* (n.p.): McGraw-Hill Education, 2009. This book uses clinical studies to prove that a low-acid diet is the only effective way to prevent bone loss. http://tinyurl.com/y7wceb6d

Fraser, Ruthie. *Stack Your Bones: 100 Simple Lessons For Realigning Your Body and Moving with Ease.* (n.p.): The Experiment Publishing, 2017. Movement teacher Ruthie Fraser helps readers unwind and realign through 100 simple lessons in Structural Integration. http://tinyurl.com/ybfccytf

Isler, Jack. 21 Broken Bones: *A Guide to Understanding and Controlling Your Pain.* (n.p.): Green Ivy, 2016. This book describes the author's own journey against pain. http://tinyurl.com/y9u6zolj

Schneider, Diane L. *The Complete Book of Bone Health.* (n.p.): Prometheus Books, 2011. This book is a clear and accurate guide to improving bone health. http://tinyurl.com/yda2w5ej

# Other Resources to Explore

4BoneHealth offers evidence-based information about prevention and treatment of osteoporosis for all ages from experts in the bone health field.

The American Bone Health website offers practical and easy to follow advice for consumers through tools such as videos, downloadable materials, a fracture risk calculator and a hotline.

National Osteoporosis Foundation's official website with information on prevention, diagnosis and treatment of osteoporosis.

The New York Bone Blog by the NY Bone and Joint Specialists addresses shoulder, knee  back, neck, hip, ankle, foot and pelvic pain.

# 9

# Workplace Injury and Pain

Executive chef Mark Peel is an award-winning restaurant owner, author of several cookbooks, and a frequent judge on cooking competition shows like *Top Chef*. He joined me on my radio program to discuss the injuries—including sprains, strains and muscle tears—that constant standing, chopping, twisting, bending, and lifting cause in chefs. Peel himself was almost sidelined completely by carpal tunnel syndrome, neurogenic thoracic outlet syndrome (NTOS; covered extensively in Chapter 4, Neuropathic Pain), and low back pain (discussed in Chapter 2, Joint and Soft Tissue Pain).

During his first job as a dishwasher at the age of 17, Peel fell in love with the kitchen. The physical demands of cooking on the line, however, caused him to suffer from his first varicose vein at just 22 years old. Similar to stocking shelves, working in a factory, or on a construction site, cooking is physically demanding work but not particularly good exercise. Like many office workers, cooks may work at a table that is not quite the ideal height, leading to hours of hunching over and bad posture. Chefs often stand for 12 hours a day, six days a week, which can lead to chronic back and foot pain. The repetitive and rapid chopping that a skilled chef will engage in for hours can lead to overuse injuries in the wrists, hands, and fingers. All these factors led to the three separate pain problems Chef Peel experienced.

## Understanding Workplace Injury and Pain

Modern life, on the whole, is far more comfortable for human beings than at any other time in history. Most of us thankfully no longer have to endure hours of back-breaking physical work as many of our farming, hunting, and laboring ancestors once did. Even relatively dangerous jobs offer safety precautions to protect workers from catastrophic injury.

But, today, we face a new set of challenges that can lead to discomfort and pain. Medical and technological advancements help us live longer, but they can also have unintended consequences. Repetitive motions, the extended standing involved in manufacturing, food service, or retail jobs, and even the long periods of sitting that characterize many white-collar professions can all lead to chronic pain as well as overuse injuries. Fortunately, we are learning more about how to treat and prevent these problems.

## Treating Carpal Tunnel and Other Work-Related Injuries and Pain

Chef Mark Peel's neurogenic thoracic outlet syndrome (NTOS; discussed in Chapter 4, Neuropathic Pain) was most likely caused by frequently grabbing for cast iron skillets and pans stored on overhead racks. He often had to stretch his arm to hold a three-pound skillet over the stove while preparing food. When his symptoms first started, Peel thought he was having a heart attack because the pain was so intense. His work on the line was limited because the burning and numbness in his arm would return sporadically during the day. At home, he was afraid to bend down to lift his young children, thinking that he might drop them. Once diagnosed, Peel began arm stretches, ibuprofen (Motrin), and postural correction of his shoulders, all of which have made a big difference in managing his symptoms.

Peel's low back pain resulted from years of bending and twisting to pick up stock pots, which often weigh up to 60 pounds. Sadly, low back pain is likely quite prevalent in the food industry due to repetitive lifting, twisting, and bending with heavy pots and pans. Peel developed shooting numbness down his leg along with low back pain due to injury and age-related spinal stenosis, the narrowing around the spinal cord or spinal nerves. Similar to others with back and leg pain, Peel couldn't work, cook, or even drive for a while. Fortunately, better ergonomics, proper stretching, and occasional ibuprofen use have made the pain better, though Peel continues to have some numbness down his leg.

The years of chopping and slicing for hours a day almost certainly led to Peel's carpal tunnel syndrome. After six months of symptoms, which included numbness and burning in his hands and fingers, Peel's carpal tunnel was diagnosed by an EMG (electromyogram) and nerve conduction tests, tests that measure abnormalities in nerve function and muscle fibers. They are the gold standard for diagnosing median nerve entrapment at the wrist (carpal tunnel syndrome). The median nerve runs from the forearm into the palm of hand through the carpal tunnel, a passageway in the wrist. For people with carpal tunnel syndrome, this otherwise rigid space becomes compressed and inflamed by chronically sustained pressure, which can damage the nerve and cause abnormalities in the muscles supplied by that nerve.

Overall, there is about a 10% lifetime risk of developing carpal tunnel. Some occupations may put workers at more risk than others, especially those involving high repetition and hand force. In addition to workplace vulnerability, other risk factors for carpal tunnel include pregnancy, diabetes, hypothyroidism, and undergoing chemotherapy.

Fortunately, Peel was diagnosed early enough to avoid carpal tunnel surgery. He used ibuprofen and ice baths to soothe the inflammation and performed the regular stretches and exercises recommended by his physical therapist. He also wore a wrist splint—common in treating carpal tunnel—which prevented excessive flexion and allowed for the re-myelination of the injured median nerve. (Myelin is the insulation layer that surrounds the part of the nerve called the axon. The axon is a nerve fiber that conducts electrical impulses from the body to the spinal cord and brain. Think of the axon as a telephone wire and the myelin as the insulation surrounding the wire. Myelin allows impulses to travel across the nerve quickly.)

Other patients with carpal tunnel symptoms like Peel's can benefit from injections of a local anesthetic and steroid at the site of the pain as well as surgery when all else has failed. Some evidence suggests that surgery should be the first treatment offered because it is the most cost effective for resolving the condition compared to non-surgical treatments.

Alternative therapies, such as acupuncture, covered in Chapter 20, Alternative Medicine and Pain Relief, can also be quite helpful.

## Preventing Carpal Tunnel and Other Work-Related Injuries and Pain

Once he had recovered, Peel took several steps to keep his carpal tunnel as well as his low back pain and neurogenic thoracic outlet syndrome at bay. First, he cut back the number of hours he was working on the line. Second, he began taking breaks to stretch throughout the day. And third, he redesigned the kitchen in his new restaurant, Bombo, to prevent injury.

Bombo's new ergonomically correct design includes smaller pots and pans placed the correct distance from where line cooks work and protocols that include having two people carry larger pots. Peel doesn't store the heavy cast iron skillets above the workspace, greatly reducing the strain on those who must reach for them. Those heavy skillets are now placed closer to eye level or on the stove. Peel encourages the use of smaller containers for roasting and braising, and asks cooks to consider using two small pans in lieu of one large one.

Most of us spend 40 or more hours a week at work. Whether our work is physically demanding or sedentary, we need to pace ourselves. Taking time to stretch every hour or so can go a long way toward preventing pain down the road. If you are on your feet all day, consider wearing support stockings to promote blood flow, even if you don't have varicose veins. Make sure that desks or work tables are at the correct height to prevent hunching or straining the muscles of the shoulder and neck. Sit and stand with good posture, and avoid holding one position for too long. If your job involves standing, like those who cook professionally, try to work an hour or two less per day, stretch, and make of point of exercising several days a week.

As we age, it can be wise to cut back our hours if at all possible. Peel no longer works on the line, but enjoys teaching, tasting, and creating. He's found that the symptoms of his conditions, although still present, have receded into the background, and they certainly haven't prevented him from thriving in his career. Above all, all of us must deal with any workplace-related pain promptly instead of allowing it to drag on for too long. Seek medical attention and diligently follow any prescribed course of therapy to prevent the pain from returning or the injury from worsening.

## Hope for Workplace Injury and Pain Relief

To learn more about various self-care and pain treatment options and therapies, read the chapters in Part 1, Understanding and Treating Your Pain, and Part 2, Medical Therapies for Pain: Traditional and Innovative. There you will find more information and ideas for working with your physician and other healthcare providers to find ways to prevent, manage, and address your pain.

You can also learn more about work-related pain by listening to the work-related pain episodes of my weekly radio program, *Aches and Gains*. You can find the broadcasts on work-related pain at the following URL.

**Workplace Pain**

http://paulchristomd.com/kitchen-pain
http://paulchristomd.com/kitchen-pain-2

## Suggested Further Reading

Alstedter, Nikki, and Paviliack, Lora. *40 Dynamic Easy Exercises to Look and Feel Your Best.* (n.p.): Althea Press, 2016. This book shows readers active methods for improving alignment, reducing neck and back pain and techniques for practicing good posture at home and at work. http://tinyurl.com/yagwsabk

Bingham, Sandra. *Carpal Tunnel and Wrist Pain: Simple Relief Exercises.* (n.p.): Philip Gegan, 2013. Exercises to relieve wrist pain through Acupressure. http://tinyurl.com/yakk7c3n

Burden, Kent. *Workout at Work: 25 Exercises for Back Health to do at Your Desk.* (n.p.): MLF Press, 2013. This book helps improve your health and fitness through easy activities for the workplace. http://tinyurl.com/ybwtgfqu

Johnson, Jim. *Treat Your Own Carpal Tunnel Syndrome: Treatment and Prevention Strategies for Individuals, Therapists, and Employers.* (n.p.): Dog Ear Publishing, 2014. This book offers a complete, evidence-based, do-it-yourself program for people at risk or people already struggling with carpal tunnel. http://tinyurl.com/y72hlmsu

Pascarelli, Emil. *Dr. Parcarelli's Complete Guide to Repetitive Strain Injury: What You Need to Know About RSI and Carpal Tunnel Syndrome.* (n.p.): Wiley, 2004. How to prevent, treat, and recover from repetitive strain injury (RSI). http://tinyurl.com/y8lv46j6

Starett, Kelly. *Deskbound: Standing Up to a Sitting World.* (n.p.): Victory Belt Publishing, 2016. This book provides creative solutions for reducing the amount of time you spend sitting, as well as strategies for transforming your desk into a dynamic, active workstation. http://tinyurl.com/yb4wgp7w

## Other Resources to Explore

Carpel-tunnel.net is the project of Dr Jeremy D. P. Bland, consultant in clinical neurophysiology at the Kent and Canterbury Hospital and also at Kings College Hospital in London.

Orthoinfo is powered by the American Academy of Orthopoedic Surgeons, providing information about carpal tunnel syndrome. http://orthoinfo.aaos.org

# 10

# Postsurgical Pain

## Understanding Postsurgical Pain

Surgery has saved and improved the lives of countless millions. Ongoing improvements in diagnosing disorders and surgical techniques mean that more Americans are undergoing surgery than ever before. Worldwide, about 240 million surgeries are performed each year. This is great news; necessary procedures that were once risky and rare have become safe and commonplace.

But there is a risk with this increased number of procedures: Postoperative pain, left unchecked, can lead to persistent pain. The pain from the incisions made during surgery is supposed to go away as the incisions heal, and it often does. But more often than we'd like, such pain lingers past the time when the surgical wounds themselves are gone. The occurrence rate of chronic pain after surgery might be as high as 60%, depending on the type of surgery, and one of

many risk factors includes the intensity of immediate postoperative pain. The data tell us that many patients report severe pain not just after major surgical procedures, but after minor ones too.

Other reports suggest that as many as 10% of patients report severe, chronic pain a year after surgery. As one review states, "pain persists in every second patient months after thoracotomy (a type of chest wall surgery), amputation, or breast surgery. Although the risk of chronic pain after hernia repair hovers around 10%, long-term studies indicate that pain lasts up to six years in 8%–19% of patients." Given the volume of surgeries across the globe, these staggering numbers are the reason postoperative pain prevention has become a crucial concern.

Unfortunately, postoperative pain that lingers is often neglected. Studies demonstrate that problems managing the acute pain during and after surgery lead to a greater likelihood of lingering postoperative pain, which, in turn, often becomes chronic. And even mild chronic pain can have a substantial impact on our quality of life and how we function.

## Preventing a Lifetime of Pain after Surgery: Regional Anesthesia

Thankfully, an alternative approach to anesthesia during surgery has been shown to greatly reduce the number of patients with lingering postoperative pain. One study reports that regional anesthesia—epidurals and specific nerve-blocks—used during thoracotomy and breast cancer surgery may prevent chronic pain in up to 25% of patients. This is important since it is becoming apparent that one of the most important ways to prevent the transition from acute to chronic pain is to ensure postoperative pain control.

For decades, nearly all major surgeries were done using general anesthesia. For general anesthesia, patients inhale gases, such as isoflurane, sevoflurane, and desflurane that cause deep unconsciousness. Ether was one of the first anesthetic gases shown to be effective for surgery at the Massachusetts General Hospital back in 1846. Medications such as propofol (a sleep inducer) and fentanyl (an opioid pain reliever), given through an IV can also produce unconsciousness during surgery. General anesthesia provides pain relief by blocking pain receptors in the central nervous system. Regional anesthesia, in contrast, blocks pain transmission from the affected nerves themselves. It can be used during surgery and during the recovery period as well. When nerve blocks are used for pain treatment and management, a local anesthetic medication is injected around a specific nerve in the body.

### Regional Analgesia and Pain Control

Regional anesthesia is not appropriate for every surgery, but it can work for many common procedures, including joint replacements in the upper or lower body, arthroscopy, and rotator cuff surgery. Other procedures in which it can be successful include procedures that release compressed nerves, such as carpal tunnel surgery, hip surgery, amputations, hand or foot surgery, and open reduction and internal fixation procedures, which are used to treat compound fractures.

Most of us have heard of epidurals in the context of the pain relief offered to women during childbirth. The anesthesiologist or nurse anesthetist inserts numbing medication (local anesthetic) into the "epidural space" inside the spine, and just outside the sac of fluid surrounding the spinal cord. In a "spinal," the injection is made directly into the spinal fluid itself. For specific nerve blocks, the anesthesiologist injects the anesthetic around the nerve in question.

Regional anesthetic injections are often administered with ultrasound guidance, which helps the doctor avoid puncturing blood vessels, assists in visualizing the nerves, and reduces the risk of local anesthetic toxicity. Some anesthesiologists also use electric nerve stimulation to confirm correct needle placement instead of, or along with, ultrasound guidance. Some still use anatomic landmarks, but this is becoming less frequent.

A single injection of local anesthetic around the nerves may be used or in some cases, a catheter—a tiny tube that is about three inches long and about half the diameter of a toothpick—remains where the needle was inserted, delivering a continuous dose of local anesthetic pain medication during the surgery. Catheters are typically left in place for one to two days after surgery.

Anesthesiologists typically work to numb the patient one level above where the procedure will occur. For ankle surgery, they numb at the knee, and for knee surgery at the groin. Often this involves specific nerve blocks. For shoulder surgery such as rotator cuff repair, for example, doctors can numb the brachial plexus nerves in the lower part of the neck, and for knee surgery they numb the femoral nerve in the groin, or the lumbar plexus in the lower back.

Patients report feeling the affected areas of the body become warm and then heavy. Within 10 minutes, they are able to feel pressure but not pain. Maternity patients receiving epidurals for labor can typically move their legs, but patients getting specific nerve blocks for surgery feel that their affected body part is numb and very weak. This is normal. Sensation and strength return after the surgery is over and the body metabolizes the anesthetic (the block wears off).

There are many benefits of using regional instead of general anesthesia during surgery. First of all, patients do not need as much opioid medication for pain control, and some are able to avoid it altogether. This reduces opioid side effects such as grogginess, nausea, and constipation. Second, most patients report the pain control under regional anesthesia is far superior both during and after the procedure. Recovery is often much better with regional anesthesia as well. For instance, patients can perform more rehabilitation exercises in physical therapy because they aren't limited by pain, especially if a catheter remains in place after the surgery.

James—an army veteran—was in a serious car accident that shattered his left heel bone (calcaneus) and required two extensive surgeries to repair. He had general anesthesia for the first and was in horrendous pain for months afterwards. During his second surgery, his anesthesiologist opted for regional anesthesia instead of general and blocked his sciatic nerve, which supplies sensation to back of the thigh and the leg and foot below the knee.

After his second surgery, James felt an immediate difference between this procedure and his first surgery. Not only was he not experiencing any significant pain, he was able to sleep much better and go home much sooner with the catheter still in place. Instead of feeling sore and groggy, he was able to begin his physical therapy right away. After two days, he followed his doctor's instructions and removed the catheter himself instead of having to come back to the hospital. By his own account, the most painful part of James's postoperative experience was the medical tape pulling on his leg hair.

James's experience is quite typical for patients who have had regional anesthesia during surgery. Patients who have had similar procedures with both general and regional anesthesia very often prefer regional. In recovery, regional anesthesia patients report better pain relief, higher quality sleep, and greater range of motion of the area of the body affected by surgery, which allows them to do more physical therapy sooner.

For procedures compatible with regional anesthesia use, there are very few drawbacks to its use. Many patients may find the idea of needles scary and may fear that the procedure is too new and therefore risky. But regional anesthesia has been used for decades; its application is simply being expanded, made safer, and made more precise. There is a remote risk of nerve damage, between 1 in 1000 to 1 in 100,000, depending on the procedure. The risk of significant neurologic damage ranges from 1 in 50,000 to 1 in 150,000. Regional anesthesia is offering patients better satisfaction coupled with better outcomes from surgery. A growing number of studies are showing that blocking pain transmission before, during, and after surgery (the perioperative period) can protect against the development of chronic pain after surgery.

## Multimodal Analgesia and Pain Control

Regional anesthetic is a component of a larger effort to optimize pain control before, during, and after surgery. The name given to this strategy is Enhanced Recovery after Surgery (ERAS). Improving pain control and decreasing opioid-related side effects are central to most ERAS programs. The perioperative team aims to facilitate patient recovery by using multimodal analgesia—drugs such as acetaminophen (Tylenol), nonsteroidal anti-inflammatory drugs (NSAIDs), local anesthetics into the wound, gabapentin (Neurontin) or pregabalin (Lyrica), or ketamine. In addition to regional anesthesia, a patient may be given some of these medications to better control postoperative pain. There is good evidence that all of these therapies are effective for postoperative pain too.

## Hope for Postsurgical Pain Relief

There is a heightened interest in controlling pain after surgery. As a greater number of medical centers incorporate regional anesthesia and Enhanced Recovery after Surgery (ERAS) protocols, we hope to see fewer postoperative patients with chronic pain, better patient satisfaction with the surgical experience, and better resource utilization.

To learn more about various self-care and pain treatment options and therapies, read the chapters in Part 1, Understanding and Treating Your Pain, and Part 2, Medical Therapies for Pain: Traditional and Innovative. There you will find more information and ideas for working with your physician and other healthcare providers to find ways to prevent, manage, and address your pain.

You can also learn more about postsurgical pain by listening to my weekly radio program, *Aches and Gains*. You can find the broadcasts on postsurgical pain at the following URLs.

**Postsurgical Pain**
http://paulchristomd.com/postop-pain
http://paulchristomd.com/postop-pain-2

# Suggested Further Reading

Allport-Settle, Mindy J. *The Post-Surgical Pain Diary: Tracking Your Pain, Progress & Physical Therapy after Surgery.* (n.p.): PharmaLogika, 2011. This book is designed to collect comprehensive information tracking the process of healing after surgery with successful pain management. http://tinyurl.com/y8dzrxm7

Andrewes, Sue, William Casey, Michael Durkin, and Eltringham, Roger. *Post-anaesthetic Recovery: A Practical Approach.* (n.p.): Springer, 2013. This book describes the major complications liable to be encountered post-surgert and suggests how they may be avoided. http://tinyurl.com/yaux7vqn

Boachie-Adjei, Oheneba, Fischgrund Stanton, Andra, and Hiatt-Cobentz, Ruth. *Pilates for Fragile Backs: Recovering Strength and Flexibility After Surgery, Injury, or Other Back Problems.* (n.p.): New Harbinger, 2006. This book offers an effective program to help you manage pain and regain strength and mobility. http://tinyurl.com/y8pch9tr

# Other Resources to Explore

Cleveland Clinic is a nonprofit multispecialty academic medical center, article about pain control after surgery.

eMedicineHealth.com, a consumer health information site owned and operated by WebMD, including articles on pain after surgery.

WebMD article about dealing with post-surgery pain.

# 11

# Disease-Related Pain

Illness often causes pain and discomfort, but the pain and discomfort typically resolve when we recover from the original disease. Unfortunately, some infections cause pain that continues long past the time the illness resolves. We don't often think about infectious diseases leading to chronic pain conditions, but they can. HIV, for instance leads to chronic pain—expressed as "unbearable and intense"—in almost 80% of those with the diagnosis. Another example is transverse myelitis, inflammation of a portion of the spinal cord, which can occur after a lung or gastrointestinal infection, leading to some aspect of disability in 40% of patients. In addition, some inherited conditions can also cause debilitating chronic pain. There is no guaranteed way to prevent all disease-related pain, but there are important steps we can all take to lessen its impact and reduce risk.

## Immunizations and Pain Prevention

Whenever possible, it is best to prevent painful and potentially deadly diseases. Vaccines do this by introducing the body to a weakened form of the pathogen and allowing the body to build up its own natural immunity to the illness. After a vaccination, when the pathogen is encountered in the environment, the body is ready and able to eliminate it quickly. Besides maintaining good hygiene, nutrition, exercise and sleep habits, getting the standard courses of vaccinations recommended by your doctor is an important factor in preventing chronic pain from specific infectious borne illnesses.

The shingles vaccine (Zostavax), for example, substantially reduces the risk of developing shingles and the painful chronic neuropathic disorder postherpetic neuralgia (PHN). This condition is discussed at length in Chapter 4, Neuropathic Pain. Shingles is caused by the varicella zoster virus (VZV), which is the same virus that leads to chickenpox. PHN results from the reactivation of the VZV later in life and causes a great deal of physical and emotional distress. The shingles vaccine is FDA-approved for adults past age 50 and recommended for those 60 years of age and over. It can likely even help prevent recurrence in individuals who have already had shingles.

## Understanding Sickle Cell Disease

Imagine being 12 years old and in excruciating pain. Your mother takes you to the emergency room for treatment, but the doctors and nurses accuse you of being a drug addict and faking your symptoms, even though you have a documented genetic disorder that requires pain medication. That is exactly what happened to a well-known rapper who suffered from sickle cell disease and the agony that comes with it.

Albert Johnson, the American rapper better known by his stage name Prodigy, was diagnosed with sickle cell anemia—the most common form of sickle cell disease—before his first birthday. His mother brought him to the ER at the local hospital because he was screaming inconsolably. It turned out that Prodigy was suffering from a sickle cell crisis, a painful episode that can last for hours or even days. Children as young as six months can experience a painful crisis, which can manifest as irritability, poor feeding, and swelling of the hands or feet.

Our DNA is a biological databank containing millions of pieces of genetic information that dictate everything from our eye color to our shoe size. One tiny abnormality in our DNA can cause any number of rare but painful or even fatal disorders. Sickle cell disease is one such genetic disorder that affects millions worldwide and 1 in 365 African American children in the United States. It also occurs in ethnic groups from South and Central America, the Mediterranean, and India.

Normal red blood cells are soft and donut shaped, moving easily throughout the blood vessels, including tiny capillaries that are only about one cell thick. In the blood of people with sickle cell disease, an abnormality in the hemoglobin protein causes the red blood cells to become stiff, sticky, and crescent shaped.

This causes the cells to get stuck in the blood vessels and block blood flow. When there is less blood flow to tissues and organs in the body (ischemia), damage results from lack of oxygenation. This process initiates an inflammatory response and together with ischemic tissue damage, leads to extreme pain.

As recently as the 1970s, patients with sickle cell often died in childhood, but advancements in treatment now allow many to live well into adulthood. Sickling can still occur, though, causing painful throbbing and gnawing in the back, joints of the hands and feet, the long bones, and abdomen. Patients are also at risk for stroke and painful leg ulcers due to reductions in blood flow to those parts of the body.

## Treating the Pain of Sickle Cell Disease

There is currently no cure for sickle cell disease. (A procedure called hematopoietic cell transplantation offers the potential for cure, but experience is limited and there are several uncertainties about the risks and benefits.) However, there are a growing number of methods to prevent and manage the pain associated with it.

Prodigy remembered being in the hospital with painful crises many times throughout his childhood. Like many sickle cell patients, he exhibited a fever and unbearable pain in his legs, arms, stomach and back. Unfortunately, some of the ER doctors did not understand sickle cell disease well and did not take his pain seriously. Some accused him of being a drug addict who was faking his symptoms to obtain opioids. Other health care professionals forced him to wait for hours for medication, threatening to call the police if he didn't stop crying out from the pain.

Patients with sickle cell pain do not appear more likely to abuse opioid pain relievers, but many are undertreated because of an exaggerated fear of substance abuse. Studies show that the prevalence of addiction is lower for sickle cell patients than in other populations. As growing numbers of sickle cell patients reach adulthood, doctors are working to develop better life-long care strategies for them. Effective pain management is vital for sickle cell patients since more frequent crises are associated with worse health outcomes.

The pain from sickle cell can be debilitating and often becomes chronic, compromising quality of life. Therefore, treating acute sickle cell pain episodes early and aggressively may help control the development of chronic pain. Sickle cell disease presents as neuropathic pain in 20% of patients (discussed in Chapter 4), crushing headaches, and in males as priapism (an extremely painful prolonged erection). Many patients experience underlying pain all the time—particularly in the joints, bone, or from chronic ulcers—and then have episodes of severe acute pain that wax and wane. The disease can also affect the health of the kidneys, heart, and lungs. Fever in a sickle cell patient can be an indication of serious infection and must be evaluated promptly.

Doctors often use opioids to treat sickle cell pain, but some are now exploring the use of anticonvulsants as well. These drugs, such as gabapentin (Neurontin) and pregabalin (Lyrica), are used for neuropathic pain and are discussed in Chapter 4. A useful strategy for managing a crisis at home is to have a supply of short-acting analgesics on hand such as hydrocodone (Vicodin), and acetaminophen (Tylenol), as well as a nonsteroidal anti-inflammatory drug (NSAID) like ibuprofen (Motrin). By the time patients are admitted to the hospital, though, IV opioids are typically needed. Many patients believe that the IV PCA (patient controlled analgesia) device gives them better control over how much medication they receive and when they get it. When children are admitted to the hospital, parents should alert their pediatrician and make sure the treating doctors know which opioids or other pain medications have been the most helpful in the past.

Hydroxyurea—taken daily by mouth—can be an effective treatment for sickle cell pain. Babies are typically born with half fetal hemoglobin and half adult hemoglobin. As healthy babies grow, their fetal hemoglobin is gradually replaced by adult hemoglobin, but sickle cell patients continue to produce fetal hemoglobin into adulthood. Hydroxyurea increases the amount of fetal hemoglobin these patients produce, reducing the likelihood of their red blood cells sickling. Clinically, hydroxyurea can both reduce pain and limit the opioids patients often have to take to tolerate a sickle cell crisis.

Hydroxyurea has been well studied to benefit both adults and children. For example, adults have substantial decreases in the number of severe painful crises, the rate of vaso-occlusive events (blood flow obstruction), reductions in transfusion requirements, and hospital admissions. One study reported that adults taking this drug reduced their risk of dying from sickle cell disease by 40%.

Similar benefits have been seen in children as well. Side effects are possible but uncommon, even in the long term.

Staying well-hydrated is also extremely important to preventing sickle cell pain. Hydration helps to maintain the fluidity of the blood so that the red blood cells can travel throughout the body more easily.

Dehydration can also lead to a painful sickle cell crisis.

Alternative therapies such as biofeedback and hypnosis can also be very helpful for coping with the pain of the disease. These therapies are discussed in more detail in Chapter 19, Mind-Body Techniques for Pain Relief.

As an adult, Prodigy found a doctor who helped him manage the pain from his sickle cell anemia effectively. His strategy included drinking sufficient fluids and adhering to an anti-inflammatory diet. He also had opioid pain medications on hand so that he could treat a crisis immediately and prevent it from getting out of control.

Prodigy found that staying connected to supportive friends and family members as well as prioritizing his relationship with God were vital aspects of managing his sickle cell disease. He never hid his disease or the pain he experienced, writing about it in his music and talking publicly about it with his fans. His memoir, *My Infamous Life: The Autobiography of Mobb Deep's Prodigy*, has given hope to many suffering from sickle cell and other diseases felt to be out of their control.

## Understanding Lyme Disease

Lyme disease was first discovered in a group of children around Lyme, Connecticut, in the 1970s. The children came down with flu-like symptoms that just never seemed to go away. We now know that they were infected with the bacteria *Borrelia burgdorferi* transmitted from deer, mice, and other rodents to humans via the bite of a deer tick. Since then, Lyme disease has appeared across the country, although infections are concentrated in the northeastern and upper midwestern United States. Approximately 30,000 cases of Lyme disease are reported annually to the Centers for Disease Control and Prevention (CDC), but it is estimated that this number reflects just 10% of actual infections. The actual number may be more like 300,000 new cases per year. Although there is only about a 3.5% risk of infection with any given tick bite, people who spend a lot of time outdoors are at greater risk over their lifetimes because they can get repeated tick bites.

## Diagnosing Lyme Disease

Two aspects of Lyme disease make it easy to miss. First, its symptoms often mimic those of other disorders. Once the bacteria enter the central nervous system, symptoms can resemble those of multiple sclerosis, Alzheimer's disease, or Parkinson's disease. Lyme can also mimic fibromyalgia, chronic fatigue syndrome, Addison's disease, hypothyroidism, and even HIV. Often all these conditions may be considered before a physician diagnoses Lyme or the chronic form of the disease, Post-Treatment Lyme Disease Syndrome (PTLDS).

Second, Lyme disease is very difficult to diagnose definitively. For years, doctors believed that a "bull's eye" rash had to be present around the site of the tick bite to confirm diagnosis. We now know that such a rash is only present in about 20% of Lyme cases. Close to 80% of patients will exhibit some sort of rash, but most without the characteristic bull's eye shape. Unfortunately, not all doctors are aware of this updated information and continue to assume the absence of a circular rash rules out Lyme.

The blood test for Lyme disease (ELISA) is also notoriously inaccurate for several reasons. Unlike the bacteria that cause strep throat, for example, the bacteria that cause Lyme disease (*Borrelia burgdorferi*) are virtually impossible to culture in a laboratory to confirm their presence. The current Lyme test measures the total level of antibodies in the bloodstream, not the organism itself; the test is not sensitive enough to detect these antibodies within the first couple of weeks of infection, though, and the antibodies may not be present in sufficient quantity even up to six weeks later. This means that a patient may have the infection, but the test is unable to detect it and falsely yields a negative result.

## Pain and Lyme Disease

Active Lyme infection can be painful but usually resolves if treated with standard antibiotics: doxycycline for adults and amoxicillin for children less than 12 years of age. If the infection reaches the central nervous system, intravenous antibiotics are needed. Patients typically experience a rash and flu like symptoms in the form of headaches and muscle and joint aches.

These can be managed with nonsteroidal anti-inflammatory drugs (NSAIDs).

Unfortunately, 10%–20% of patients with acute Lyme disease develop Post-Treatment Lyme Disease Syndrome (PTLDS), which is pain and fatigue that persist months or even years after the active infection is gone and treatment has occurred. Often, patients experience a triad of symptoms that include fatigue, pain, and cognitive problems such as difficulty concentrating and focusing on tasks. Patients report musculoskeletal pain in the joints, ligaments, and tendons, as well as neuropathic pain affecting the large and small nerves of the body. The neuropathic pain can produce numbness, tingling, and pinprick sensations in the legs or arms. The pain can be so widespread that PTLDS mimics fibromyalgia.

Interestingly, the joint pain is more periarticular (surrounding the joint) than articular (inside the joint), so there isn't always joint swelling and inflammation that can be identified objectively on imaging studies. In fact, imaging studies may reveal normal joints and tissues despite the profound pain that they produce.

The impact of PTLDS can be devastating, comparable to congestive heart failure or other serious health problems according to one study. The combination of fatigue and pain prevents people from performing basic activities. Like other forms of chronic pain, PTLDS presents a diagnostic dilemma—the symptoms are real, but nothing really shows up on scans or blood tests. This has been a recipe for terrible frustration for patients. Many search for needed relief for years.

Sarah, an attorney, had several tick bites, but she was told by her doctor that she could not have contracted Lyme because she didn't exhibit the bull's eye rash. Her Lyme disease was left undiagnosed and she began to experience fatigue, memory loss, a spasm in her left eye, and extreme sensitivity to light and sound. She couldn't distinguish between the left side of the car and right side while driving, which left her housebound. Her body shook so badly that it looked like she had Parkinson's disease. MRIs of Sarah's brain were normal, but her symptoms progressed until she experienced extreme hair loss, searing burning pain, and seizures.

Sarah was hospitalized when she lost her ability to speak. Her memory had been so impaired that she couldn't remember to call her friends or family members anymore. Multiple Lyme tests came back negative, and she was told that she might be experiencing complications from menopause. Frustrated and in agony, she was bedridden for the better part of a year.

Finally, an infectious disease specialist gave Sarah one more Lyme test. Although she had tested negative just 11 days earlier, this test confirmed Sarah had an active Lyme infection. She was put on a course of antibiotics immediately and began to feel some relief from her symptoms.

Unfortunately, Sarah soon found herself in the crosshairs of a controversy within the medical community. The Infectious Diseases Society of America (IDSA) does not recommend prolonged re-treatment with antibiotics for PTLDS. When Sarah stopped her antibiotics after 28 days, her symptoms returned. The International Lyme and Associated Diseases Society (ILADS), on the other hand, believes in the value of longer courses of antibiotics for patients who continue to exhibit symptoms as Sarah did.

Sarah's first doctor was a member of the IDSA and, although he conceded to her privately that she was still sick, refused to continue to treat her. After an extensive and stressful search, Sarah found a doctor who was willing to treat her with an extended course of antibiotics, which she credits with finally putting her symptoms into remission and saving her life. She was able to return to her office and began working as an advocate for Lyme patients in her spare time. Sarah has 95% of her life back, but relapses occur with headaches and dull muscle aches.

## Causes of Post-Treatment Lyme Disease Syndrome

We are still not sure exactly what causes PTLDS, although there are three current theories. First, PTLDS may represent an ongoing immune response to the presence of the *Borrelia* bacteria in the body. Second, chronic symptoms may continue because the immune system has been abnormally activated, leading to an autoimmune inflammatory process. For instance, there is evidence that a overactive immune system is involved with chronic Lyme arthritis. Finally, the infection and related immune response may hyper-activate nerves in the brain and spinal cord causing changes in nerve synapses and neurotransmitters. These problems cause patients to experience central sensitization: hypersensitivity to light or sound, exaggerated pain from painful stimuli such as a pinprick, and pain in response to things that aren't usually painful (like a feather touching the skin).

It also seems that PTLDS falls within a category called the central sensitivity syndromes (CSS) that share similar clinical manifestations such as pain and central sensitization. Other conditions that are included under this CSS framework are fibromyalgia, chronic fatigue syndrome, migraine, and irritable bowel syndrome. There isn't evidence of persistent infection in these syndromes or in most patients with PTLDS, yet many Lyme patients do feel relief from continued antibiotics.

## Preventing and Treating Post-Treatment Lyme Disease Syndrome Pain

Like many other Lyme patients, Sarah benefited from a range of pain therapies including ridding her diet of gluten and other inflammatory foods, exercising regularly, and taking multiple dietary supplements. A gluten sensitivity test is important for PTLDS patients given that many of them experience both gastrointestinal intolerances and food sensitivities. Nutritionists can help patients steer away from foods that worsen symptoms. Sarah also used hyperbaric oxygen therapy (breathing pure oxygen in a pressurized room) and an infrared sauna (a sauna using infrared heaters rather than heated air to warm the body). Both of these therapies were very helpful. Sarah's tremors stopped and she began to retrieve her language skills.

Lyme patients benefit from acupuncture and cognitive behavioral therapy (CBT) as described in Part 3, Integrative Therapies for Pain. Aquatic therapy helps to maintain joint mobility and prevent deconditioning. Nonsteroidal anti-inflammatory drugs (NSAIDs) can help with muscle pain, as can muscle relaxants such as cyclobenzaprine (Flexeril) or tizanidine (Zanaflex) for muscle spasms. Several of the medications covered in Chapter 4, Neuropathic Pain, can be effective for patients with neuropathic pain (burning, shooting, stabbing, or tingling sensations), especially gabapentin (Neurontin) or pregabalin (Lyrica).

Anyone who spends time outdoors should take steps to prevent Lyme disease and the pain associated with it including performing regular tick checks after being outside. This can be easily done in the shower or bathtub. Make sure children are checked after playing outside, and don't restrict the inspection to the summer months. Special attention should be paid to areas behind the knees, in the armpits, and around the groin, since those are favorite hiding spots for ticks. These ticks are typically the size of a pinhead and can attach to the hairline, scalp, and back. Anybody who is outside can be bitten—hikers, landscapers, and children playing in fields or on playgrounds. Because deer ticks are tiny—some as small as the period at the end of a sentence—careful searching is essential. You should also take measures to protect your pets from ticks and to prevent them from bringing ticks into your home.

It is also incredibly important to correctly diagnose and treat a Lyme infection promptly. The best method of diagnosis is the correct identification of the rash because the immune system markers will not show up in blood work until weeks after the infection. Patients who catch the disease early have much better outcomes and a much smaller chance of developing PTLDS. If the diagnosis is delayed for months or years, the prognosis becomes more serious. Given problems with the available tests for Lyme disease, be aware of suspicious symptoms of Lyme disease that should prompt a visit with the doctor—brain fog, unusual fevers, migrating aches and pains, numbness or burning in your hands or feet, walking instability, or palpations.

Ally Hilfiger, daughter of fashion designer Tommy Hilfiger, was bitten by a tick when she was seven. Her mom found the tick, which rarely happens because it is so small, and had it examined for the Lyme bacteria. Tests were inconclusive.

Ally's joints began to hurt, and her muscles ached. Her legs burned, and she developed headaches and several strep throat infections. "It was like a terrible flu on top of a hangover, but I didn't look sick. I could function some days and not others. There were times when it felt like I had fiery spiders in my body and certain noises were intolerable," she said. The central nervous system can be a sanctuary for the bacteria that spread Lyme disease. They can evade the main immune system there, but activate the brains immune cells called microglia, triggering nerve inflammation along with neurological symptoms.

Ally never had the typical "bull's-eye" rash so no one considered Lyme disease. Instead, doctors diagnosed her with a host of other diseases that can mimic Lyme disease—mononucleosis, fibromyalgia, rheumatoid arthritis, and multiple sclerosis. None of the treatments for these diseases helped with her symptoms, though.

Middle and high school became impossible; blurred vision, fatigue, memory problems, and reading comprehension deficits all plagued Ally. Plus, odd behavioral changes took place. Rage began to surface from age eight until thirteen. Both the doctors and her family thought this was due to another diagnosis, Attention Deficit Hyperactivity Disorder and Attention Deficit Disorder. Nothing made Ally feel better and it became an all-encompassing battle—physical, mental, and spiritual.

Completely drained after over a decade of pain and confusion, Ally began having psychotic symptoms (writing on the walls and channeling Bob Marley), so her father made a decision that would change her life. He admitted her to a psychiatric hospital at age 18. One of the psychiatrists recognized that her symptoms reflected those of PTLDS and referred her to a specialist who confirmed the diagnosis. Ally had been tested three to four times since the onset of her symptoms but was told that the antibodies were not high enough to confirm the diagnosis. The Lyme disease expert felt that the Lyme bacteria were lying dormant and that she was co-infected with babesiosis, another tick-borne illness that mimics malaria.

After months of different antibiotics and an anti-malarial, Ally's symptoms finally improved. She credits NSAIDs, acupuncture, and especially a dietary detoxification program involving vitamins, enemas, and cleanses for helping her control the pain. According to her, what really freed Ally from the grip of the syndrome was harnessing the power of the mind. "I reset my subconscious mind into believing that I was healed and stronger," she said. "The more I took away the language of sickness, the more things started to change and the healthier I became." She reminds us to use tick repellant, wear long-sleeved shirts and pants, and tuck our pants into socks in order to protect ourselves. Today, Ally is a mother, successful producer, artist, and fashion designer.

As noted, the current blood test for Lyme may produce many false negatives, so patients who test negative but continue to have symptoms may want to have the test repeated several times. Researchers are hopeful that a more accurate Lyme test will be developed in the future, one that detects not just the antibody response but also uses a substance produced by the bacteria as a marker of infection. New combination antibiotic medications are also on the horizon. And with a variety of treatments (medications, good nutrition and sleep, gentle exercise, and mental health support), patients with Post-Treatment Lyme Disease Syndrome (PTLDS) can expect good relief of their pain.

## Hope for Disease-Related Pain Relief

To learn more about various self-care and pain treatment options and therapies, read the chapters in Part 1, Understanding and Treating Your Pain, and Part 2, Medical Therapies for Pain: Traditional and Innovative. There you will find more information and ideas for working with your physician and other healthcare providers to find ways to prevent, manage, and address your pain.

You can also learn more about disease-related pain by listening to the disease-related pain episodes of my weekly radio program, *Aches and Gains*. You can find the broadcasts on disease-related pain at the following URLs.

**Sickle Cell Pain—Prodigy**
http://paulchristomd.com/sickle-cell

**Lyme Disease—Ally Hilfiger**
http://paulchristomd.com/lyme-disease
http://paulchristomd.com/lyme-disease-2

**Lyme Disease**
http://paulchristomd.com/ticks
http://paulchristomd.com/ticks-2

# Suggested Further Reading

Cashel, Allie. *Suffering the Silence: Chronic Lyme Disease in an Age of Denial.* (n.p.) North Atlantic Books, 2015. This book aims to break the stigma and ignorance surrounding chronic Lyme disease. http://tinyurl.com/yanjfq3v

Harrod Buhner, Stephen. *Healing Lyme: Natural Healing of Lyme Borreliosis and the Coinfections Chlamydia and Spotted Fever Rickettsiosis.* (n.p.): Raven Press, 2015. This book examines the scientific research on Lyme infection and its tests and treatments, and outlines potent natural medicines. http://tinyurl.com/y7qt5bqn

Horowitz, Richard. *How Can I Get Better: An Action Plan for Treating Resistant Lyme & Chronic Disease.* (n.p.): St. Martin's Griffin, 2017. This book offers a direct, actionable step-by-step plan for dealing with Lyme Disease. http://tinyurl.com/ybn3t32o

McFadzean, Nicola. *The Lyme Diet: Nutritional Strategies for Healing from Lyme Disease.* (n.p.): BioMed Publishing Group, 2010. This book explores why dietary choices are critical for minimizing inflammation, optimizing immune function, promoting healthy digestion, balancing hormones, and detoxifying the body. http://tinyurl.com/ychmne9u

Platt, Allan F, and Sacerdote, Alan. *Hope and Destiny: A Patient's and Parent's Guide to Sickle Cell Disease and Sickle Cell Trait.* (n.p.): Hilton Publishing, 2006. A guide providing the facts patients, loved ones, and caregivers need to know in order to reduce symptoms, and relieve pain. http://tinyurl.com/ya79x9cg

Rawis, William. *Unlocking Lyme: Myths, Truths, and Practical Solutions for Chronic Lyme Disease.* (n.p.): Vital Plan, 2017. The book addresses common misconceptions about Lyme disease, how to obtain a diagnosis, limitations of antibiotics and how to strengthen your immune system through a healthier lifestyle. http://tinyurl.com/yb2f8f39

Strasheim, Connie. *New Paradigms in Lyme Disease Treatment: 10 Top Doctors Reveal Healing Strategies That Work.* (n.p.): BioMed Publishing Group, 2016. This book is based on interviews with ten leading Lyme doctors, and takes readers into their treatment programs. http://tinyurl.com/ybaeoz8a

Strasheim, Connie. *Beyond Lyme Disease: Healing the Underlying Causes of Chronic Illness in People with Borreliosis and Co-Infections.* (n.p.) BioMed Publishing Group, 2012. This book is based on interviews with 13 Lyme-Literate physicians discussing the underlying causes of disease. http://tinyurl.com/yd8ren64

## Other Resources to Explore

The American Lyme Disease Foundation's official website dedicated to the prevention, diagnosis and treatment of Lyme disease.

# 12

# Cancer Pain and Caregiving

"I think I might die."

Those were Carla's words as her husband drove her to the emergency room in the middle of the night. For a long time, Carla had struggled with bouts of stabbing upper gastric pain that radiated into her back. But tonight was different; the pain had woken her from sleep and taken a significant turn for the worse. As a nurse, Carla knew the situation was serious.

After some blood work, Carla was diagnosed with pancreatitis—inflammation of the pancreas. Things did improve after that first episode, but unfortunately after a few years of battling that condition, she became jaundiced and was diagnosed with pancreatic cancer.

Pancreatic cancer—the same cancer that afflicted Steve Jobs, co-founder and CEO of Apple, Inc.—is a terrifying diagnosis for anyone. But so far, Carla has beaten the odds. She is one of just 5% of patients who has survived for five years since her initial diagnosis. Although she's had a recurrence, chemotherapy has extended her life and I'm delighted to say that she's still living today. And like so many cancer patients, recovery has been about more than survival: it's been about fighting for her quality of life.

## Understanding Cancer Pain

More than 12 million Americans have cancer, and 90% of them experience pain as a result. Pain is among the most feared symptoms of cancer. Sadly, more than 30% endure severe chronic pain while undergoing therapy, and more than 70%

suffer greatly once the disease has become advanced. Family members of cancer patients report that almost 46% of dying patients don't have adequate control of their pain at death. Despite available medications, advancing pain research, and injection therapies and procedures, as many as 50% of cancer patients with pain may remain undertreated. A cancer diagnosis is never good news, but cancer pain can be better controlled. Importantly, cancer survival may even be linked to adequate pain control.

Cancer pain generally falls into one of three categories: pain from the tumor itself, metastatic pain, and pain from cancer treatments including surgery, chemotherapy, or radiation.

## Tumor Pain

Many common cancers—breast, lung, prostate, multiple myeloma, and others—can cause tumor pain. A tumor may begin to press against a vein, against a nerve, compress other tissues, or trigger an inflammatory response in the surrounding area. Bone cancer too, discussed in Chapter 8, Skeletal Pain, can be particularly painful. Cancerous tumors around nerves or those causing chemical abnormalities such as low calcium or high sodium can lead to muscle pain from cramps. Lung cancer tumors infiltrating ribs or the lung tissue can cause chest wall pain or shooting pain that patients feel across their chest.

Tumors can grow in or around organs too. For example, tumors obstructing the intestines from colorectal cancer cause pain from distension, decreased blood flow to the organ, or tension on the surrounding tissue. Patients describe terrible cramping and bloating or generalized abdominal pain. Cancers of the urinary or reproductive tracts or rectum can make patients experience bladder spasms or sharp, gnawing symptoms in the anal/rectal region or perineum, the region between the anus and the genitals.

Tumors can invade the spinal cord and nerves, compressing or inflaming them. When they do, neuropathic pain develops. About 40% of patients with chronic cancer pain have some kind of neuropathic pain. Tumors can also cause radicular pain (shooting pain in the distribution of a nerve) down the arm, leg, or chest along with more diffuse pain in an arm or leg.

## Metastatic Pain

Tumors can metastasize (spread) to other parts of the body causing pain. For example, multiple myeloma and prostate cancer can invade the bone or induce fractures causing both dull and sharp skeletal pain. Cancer spread to the hip causes groin, thigh, or knee pain, and if the cancer has travelled to the spine, it can cause back pain. Lung cancer can spread to the muscles of the chest wall, leading to substantial discomfort. Colorectal, uterine, and cervical cancer can all metastasize to the muscle, provoking spasms and sharp pain with movement.

Pain carries a particularly haunting quality for recovering cancer patients because they tend to worry that any pinch or ache is signaling the return of a tumor. After four years of remission, Carla began to feel pain in her lower abdominal area, always on the right side. Unfortunately, doctors determined that her cancer had metastasized to her liver. When tumors grow in organs or spread to organs such as the liver, intestine, or bladder, they frequently cause pressure-like sensations, internal squeezing, or cramps. It is often hard for patients to describe or even pinpoint the pain exactly, and many will also feel nauseated and sweaty. This type of pain, arising from tumor compression, infiltration, or distortion of an organ is called visceral pain.

## Treatment-Induced Pain

Cancer treatment—surgery, chemotherapy, and radiation—can also cause tremendous pain. Even though surgery can lead to pain, it may be critical for relieving symptoms of obstruction, nerve compression, or unstable bone caused by cancer. Carla had a Whipple procedure—named for the Columbia University surgeon who pioneered the technique—which removed the head of her pancreas, part of her small intestine, her gall bladder, and part of her common bile duct. Her surgical team then reconnected her digestive system.

The Whipple procedure was vital to Carla's survival, but it left her with significant pain at the site of her incision. Surgical pain related to cancer can occur from injury to nerves, inflammation, and from amputation of limbs (postamputation phantom pain). There's a growing appreciation in the medical community that surgery can cause significant long term pain complications. The risk of postsurgical pain is especially high for certain procedures such as modified radical mastectomy, thoracotomy, and limb amputation (all of which may be necessary to treat cancer). This is a major concern given that there are about 240 million surgeries performed across the world ever year.

Fortunately, we are making some progress in reducing postoperative pain. For example, hospitals now have guidelines for postoperative pain care and provide a pain team after surgery. Also more anesthesiologists are making available regional anesthesia (the technical term for epidurals, spinals, and nerve blocks) during surgery because the medical community is learning that regional anesthetic techniques are an effective way to prevent chronic pain from developing by blocking its transmission during and after surgery. You can read more about the benefits of regional vs. general anesthesia in Chapter 10, Postsurgical Pain.

Chemotherapy also causes certain patients tremendous pain and discomfort. It often affects the nerves of the feet and bottom of the legs as well as those of the hands and arms. Many chemotherapeutic drugs can cause pain. Several classes of these drugs such as the alkaloids, platinum-based compounds, and antimitotics can lead to burning, stinging pain in the feet or hands known as peripheral neuropathies. For instance, a platinum-based drug called oxaliplatin is used to treat colon cancer and carries an 8% risk of persistent neuropathic pain in the fingers and toes. Although tough to treat, this type of pain can respond to specific pain medications (discussed in Chapter 14, Pharmacological Therapies) and sometimes to acupuncture as well.

Unfortunately, Carla experienced neuropathic pain—like the kind we discussed in Chapter 4—after chemotherapy. Like many patients, after chemotherapy sessions Carla also experienced mouth sores, which prevented her from eating and drinking comfortably. She treated her sores with a pain-relieving mouthwash, which numbed the oral cavity until the sores subsided. She also found that once she knew they were coming and that they would eventually go away, she was able to mentally prepare for the sores, which made the episodes more bearable. Other side effects from chemotherapy include anemia, digestive problems, hair loss, and fatigue. Carla was able to continue working through her first round of chemotherapy, but after the cancer spread to her liver, she was unable to work.

Radiation therapy frequently causes acute muscle aches and stiffness, and it carries a risk of chronic pain from nerve injury, inflammation, or bone damage. Not as well-known by patients is that delayed pain from radiation therapy may occur several years after the treatment ends.

## Barriers to Cancer Pain Relief

A shocking number of cancer patients do not have satisfactory pain management during their treatment, and according to the American College of Clinical Oncologists, nearly half of all dying patients don't have adequate pain control at death. This is not usually because doctors lack the proper medicines and techniques; instead, it is often due to a lack of communication between the doctor and patient about the pain level the patient is experiencing. In short, patients are not telling their doctors about their pain soon enough or often enough.

Why do so many cancer patients stay silent about their suffering? Some are worried about bothering their doctors with their pain, while others think ignoring the pain will help them focus on getting better. Many are so stunned by their diagnoses that they aren't able to process what is happening to them. Regardless of the reason for not speaking up, patients should know that the earlier they alert their doctors—and get referred to a pain specialist, if necessary—the easier it is to get their pain under control. The longer the pain has gone on unchecked, the more difficult it is to manage effectively.

Both patients and healthcare providers may be concerned that cancer patients in pain may "become addicted" to opioids when used for pain control, and this has also contributed to undertreatment of pain in this population. Due to this excessive fear of addiction, some countries have even established laws and regulations that limit the availability of opioids for medical purposes.

Realistically, the evidence suggests that addiction and problematic opioid use occurs in 0%–7.7% of cancer patients, which is quite a low number.

Thankfully, because the pain of cancer can be identified by testing (MRI, CT, and blood tests, for example), most practitioners do not worry about prescribing opioids for the short term or long term in this group of patients. Additionally and unfortunately, cancer can also be a terminal condition and the opioid will no longer be needed in that case. Prescribers view these circumstances as providing support for the use of opioids in cancer pain and feel less worried about the risk of problematic use for cancer patients. This is in contrast to people with chronic, non-cancer pain, in which the pain is often not detected on images or tests, and opioid use can continue indefinitely. Typically, the expression "the opioid epidemic" is used to refer to this group of patients and not those using opioids for cancer pain. On the other hand, as cancer therapies improve the longevity of patients, their pain conditions will become longer lasting and therefore require proper monitoring to guard against opioid misuse, abuse, and addiction, especially if the condition leads to chronic pain.

Carla was able to handle the pain of her first round of cancer treatments with oxycodone combined with acetaminophen (Percocet), but her second round was bad enough that her doctor prescribed extended-release oxycodone (OxyContin). At first OxyContin made her very nauseated, but after about a week she was able to tolerate it much better.

## Treating Cancer Pain

Most cancer patients will have success treating their pain with medicines. These often include opioids—the mainstay of cancer pain control—coupled with anticonvulsants, corticosteroids, tricyclic antidepressants (TCAs), serotonin–norepinephrine reuptake inhibitors (SNRIs), or topical creams. Doctors and other healthcare providers use the World Health Organization (WHO) "ladder" for cancer pain relief. When applied in the sequence recommended by the WHO ladder, these medicines have a high percentage chance of decreasing pain. The stepwise approach first recommends nonsteroidal anti-inflammatory drugs (NSAIDs) and then progresses from weaker opioids to stronger opioids. Along the way, adjuvant drugs are provided. Adjuvants are drugs that are not typically used for pain but are helpful for pain management. They include antidepressants, anti-seizure medications, muscle relaxants, sedatives or anti-anxiety medications, and botulinum toxin (Botox).

Patients with cancer can have background pain and commonly experience breakthrough pain with a prevalence of 59%. This breakthrough pain comes on quickly and can last for minutes to hours. Traditional opioid pills don't always take effect fast enough, but newer formulations are available to control the pain more quickly. For instance, opioid formulations can be sprayed into the nose or mouth, placed under the tongue, attached to the inside of the cheek, or sucked like a lollipop.

A group of drugs called the bisphosphonates (pamidronate and clodronate, for example) can effectively reduce bone pain in patients with multiple myeloma and metastases from other cancers. Radiopharmaceutical drugs (Strontium-89 or Samarium (153Sm) lexidronam, for example) deposit radiation directly into the bone and can reduce pain for six months or more in up to 80% of patients with breast or prostate cancer that has spread to bone. Anticonvulsant drugs such as pregabalin (Lyrica) and gabapentin (Neurontin) can help neuropathic pain that results from nerve injury or nerve sprouting. Likewise, antidepressants can be effective for postsurgical neuropathic pain, chemotherapy-induced pain, and pain from radiation therapy.

## Biologic Therapies for Cancer Pain

Biologic therapies use substances derived from living organisms to treat disease. Monoclonal antibodies are laboratory-made proteins that attach to substances in the body such as cancer cells. One such biologic therapy, denosumab, is a monoclonal antibody that is able to block certain cells from breaking down bone when tumors spread to the skeleton, which can cause intense pain. A similar drug, tanezumab, is in clinical trials now. It blocks a neurotransmitter called nerve growth factor (NGF), which sensitizes nerve fibers to pain. Tanezumab has the potential to reduce bone pain from cancer too. Exciting work with biologic drugs that deactivate a protein called sclerostin may help pain due to cancers such as multiple myeloma. Sclerostin is found in bone cells called osteocytes and inhibits bone formation. There is great hope that drugs like these will improve pain and our ability to function when

affected by bone cancer, or skeletal pain in general.

## Interventional Pain-Relieving Therapies for Cancer Pain

About 5%–10% of cancer patients will need advanced procedures such as pain relievers delivered through epidurals, neurolysis (which involves injuring nerves or groups of nerves by chemical, thermal, surgical, or cryogenic freezing methods for the purpose of relieving pain), nerve blocks, and pain pumps. Some patients may need pain pump implantations, where a catheter is placed in the fluid-containing space that surrounds the spinal cord and is connected to an implanted battery-operated pump that delivers the medication. For these patients, advanced interventional procedures can be indispensable allies when the pain is unrelenting, doesn't respond to medicines, or those medications produce side effects that lead to needless suffering.

Neurolysis is an option for cancer patients, particularly those experiencing visceral pain in the abdomen or pelvis. In these cases, doctors first may perform a CT scan to ensure that the cancer has not metastasized to the lymph nodes in this area, which typically decreases the effectiveness of the block. Doctors can then inject neurolytic substances (such as alcohol or a drug called phenol) around nerves that are part of the sympathetic nervous system (these are the nerves which trigger the fight-or-flight response). This procedure is done to treat visceral pain that arises from organs such as pancreatic cancer, other abdominal cancers, or pelvic cancers. The procedure is safely performed under x-ray or CT guidance with needles, contrast dye, and local anesthetic. Neurolysis can provide needed relief and life-enhancing benefits. For example, one study noted that alcohol neurolysis provided significant analgesia for up to six months with improved survival in patients with inoperable abdominal pain from pancreatic cancer. Complications from these injections are minimal, and injections can be repeated for sustained relief. I've had patients who have undergone this procedure lower their intake of oral pain medications, allowing them to feel less sedated, more energetic, and better engaged in life.

Cancers that metastasize to the spine invade the bone, often causing fractures or instability. Patients have a hard time walking or carrying out daily activities such as dressing or bathing. Bed rest, bracing, and pain medications may not be enough, resulting in continued pain and progressive limitations. Surgery may help, but it's not often an option because of ill health. For spinal bones that have collapsed due to cancer or osteoporosis, vertebroplasty and kyphoplasty represent two minimally invasive options for patients with painful vertebral fractures. Kyphoplasty uses an inflatable balloon that's placed inside the bone to help re-expand it before the cement is injected. In both procedures, bone cement is injected into the broken bone by the physician under x-ray guidance to control pain and stabilize the spine. These procedures, which are also discussed in Chapter 8, Skeletal Pain, can be performed on an outpatient basis with light sedation. I've seen these procedures make a big difference in the right patients. A large evidence-based review concluded that both vertebroplasty and kyphoplasty safely reduce pain within two days, allow for lower opioid doses, and improve patients' ability to carry out everyday activities.

For patients who have difficulty tolerating oral medications or just don't get sufficient relief from them or nerve blocks, innovative devices called pain pumps (implantable drug delivery systems or intrathecal pumps) delivering tiny doses of medicines directly to the spinal cord can bring welcome relief. The device resembles a hockey puck, runs on a battery, and delivers drugs through a small tube called a catheter directly to the spinal fluid. Physicians implant the pump under the skin in the front of abdomen and tunnel the catheter across the flank to the spine. The medicine is contained inside a reservoir and is refilled through a port that is accessed by a needle inserted through the skin. Doctors control the continuous dose by an external, hand-held device in the office, and patients can self-administer a limited number of doses during the day with a special "remote control" device that they carry with them.

The main risks associated with pain pumps relate to problems with the catheter, but advances in catheter designs are decreasing this risk. The drugs used in the pump (opioids and local anesthetics, for example) all have potential side effects. For instance, opioids can lower hormone levels so patient testosterone, growth hormone, follicle-stimulating hormone, and luteinizing hormone levels should be monitored by a physician. Although rare (1.16% risk after six years of therapy), a collection of inflammatory cells located at the tip of the catheter called a granuloma can develop. If they increase in size, they can put pressure on the spinal cord leading to neurologic injury.

In my experience, patients with tumors that have invaded nerves, push on organs or spread to the bone, can benefit greatly from pain pumps. Several studies have shown the benefits of pain pumps in patients with cancer pain, highlighting better pain relief, less fatigue, fewer sleep disturbances, less nausea and fewer cognitive problems. A secondary outcome of one study indicated that cancer patients with pain pumps lived longer than those using traditional therapies for managing their pain. Pain pumps are also cost effective, with one study showing the greatest cost benefit between three and six months of therapy. You can read more about pain pumps in Chapter 15, Pain-Relieving Devices.

Because response to both pain medications and cancer treatments is so individual, it's very important to work closely with your oncologist to determine the right combination of medicines and well as the right dosage. Because of the complexities of cancer pain, interventional pain-relieving approaches should be explored to maximize patient care and comfort. Most doctors agree that if you've tried a treatment for one to two months without finding significant relief, it's time to try something else.

"I have probably tried every single alternative therapy out there," Carla said through laughter on my radio program. And she has tried quite a few: meditation, visualization, massage, music therapy, and Healing Touch. Carla has prayer partners who pray with her at the start of each day. She has found that every one of these alternative therapies has value for her, and if she is experiencing pain, each offers some relief. Prayer puts her in a different frame of mind for the entire day, while music—usually a soothing instrumental selection—calms her mind. Consider that the supportive mental health therapies including cognitive behavioral therapy (CBT), relaxation techniques, and education each reduce anxiety and help manage pain as well.

### Integrative Therapies for Cancer Pain

Tapping into the body-mind-spirit interface to access the subtle energy of the human body may offer a remarkable opportunity for healing. For instance, Jin Shin Jyutsu, (mentioned in Chapter 4, Neuropathic Pain, as an option for treating fibromyalgia and discussed in more detail in Chapter 22, Harnessing the Human Biofield) has shown benefits in breast cancer and multiple myeloma. Jin Shin Jyutsu practitioners also report their positive experience with breast cancer patients following surgery, improving range of arm motion, lymphedema, pain from radiation therapy, and fatigue. They have also reported success in reducing pain, increasing range of motion, facilitating swallowing, and improving saliva production in patients with head and neck cancers after surgery or radiation therapy.

There are many other integrative therapies for treating cancer pain, including the following, and these are discussed in more detail in Part 3, Integrative Therapies for Pain:

◆ Not only has hypnosis produced dramatic effects on controlling acute pain, but a number of studies have demonstrated its success in managing cancer pain and nausea from chemotherapy. See Chapter 19, Mind-Body Techniques for Pain Relief.

◆ Since ancient times, music has helped restore and sustain harmony in the body and soul. Indeed, music therapy can have remarkable success easing pain and suffering in those with cancer. See Chapter 21, Aromas, Music, and Pain Relief, for more on this topic.

- There is some research on the use of essential oils (aromatherapy) like rose and chamomile for cancer pain. For example, rose oil may favorably affect the bone when cancer has metastasized there. See Chapter 21, Aromas, Music, and Pain Relief.

- A form of energy healing that uses gentle hand techniques called Healing Touch has been shown to lower stress, pain, and fatigue in both adults and children with cancer.

See Chapter 22, Harnessing the Human Biofield.

- Pets can have a beneficial effect on pain by providing comfort, cheer, and stress reduction. Studies have shown that the stress hormone cortisol decreases and endorphins (the body's own painkillers) increase when we spend just five to 15 minutes with a dog. You can read more about animal therapy in Chapter 22, Harnessing the Human Biofield.

Perhaps the integrative therapy that is most challenging to entertain is the power of distance healing (covered in Chapter 22, Harnessing the Human Biofield ). This technique focuses on transmitting energy to a patient from afar (by telephone for example) in a way that heals pain. Edina, a guest on my show, shared a riveting story of how distance healing spared her from any pain related to radiation treatments for breast cancer and took away chemotherapy induced pain, nausea, headaches, and joint pain. She lives in Salt Lake City, Utah, and Kim, the distance healer, lives in Overland Park, Kansas. Edina also believes that distance healing has prolonged her life in conjunction with chemotherapy. Her remarkable story may not have a scientific explanation, but it should not be dismissed.

As we continue to find newer and better treatments for cancer, it becomes even more important to make sure that the pain associated with cancer is kept under control. Carla continues to enjoy her life, treasuring her time with her loved ones, and takes care to work with her doctors to ensure that her pain remains under control. Although cancer can be a terrifying ordeal for anyone, patients must stay in communication with their loved ones and their doctors to get the help and support they need.

# Caring for Those in Pain

Actor Patrick Swayze and his wife, Lisa, met as teenagers through their involvement in dance and theater. Shortly after, the two began dating. Lisa could have never imagined that the handsome, muscular young man in the peak of health would one day be depending on her to feed him, bathe him, and bring him his medications on a daily basis.

Caring for a loved one with chronic pain or illness is a life changing experience. It can be terrifying, frustrating, and draining, but it can also be deeply life-affirming. Lisa and I spoke about both the tremendous sacrifice she made as well as the hidden blessings she found as she cared for Patrick during the last 22 months of his life as he valiantly battled pancreatic cancer.

Lisa and Patrick Swayze married in 1976 when she was just 18 years old. They had met when Lisa's theatre group merged with the dance studio owned by Patrick's mother. Both continued to pursue their dancing and acting careers after they met, with Patrick receiving his breakout role as Johnny Castle in the 1987 hit film *Dirty Dancing*. Despite the inevitable ups and downs that accompany celebrity life, the two enjoyed one of Hollywood's most enduring marriages. Behind the scenes, Lisa said that Patrick was a "people person," who was unpredictable and surprising. At times, "I never knew what would come out of his mouth," laughed Lisa. He could be infuriating but quite charming, loving, and generous.

Patrick and Lisa had been married over three decades when he began having stomach problems that just wouldn't go away. He had always had indigestion, but this was more intense. He had a very high tolerance for pain and neglected to see a doctor for quite some time. One evening, however, Lisa noticed that his eyes were becoming yellow, indicating jaundice. They went to the doctor and learned the terrifying news that Patrick was suffering from Stage 4 pancreatic cancer, which had already spread to his liver.

On the outside, Patrick was calm and steady, but on the inside he was frightened, because the people he had known with pancreatic cancer had died. The doctor explained that it was an aggressive disease and urged him to get his affairs in order sooner rather than later. Lisa remembers experiencing the worst night of her life as she struggled to face the diagnosis.

About 75% of pancreatic cancer patients die within a year of diagnosis, and initially, Patrick was given just weeks to live. Yet he told his wife unequivocally that he wanted to fight and beat the disease. "I want to live," she recalls him saying with conviction. Both understood well what his diagnosis meant, but they were determined to meet it with hope. They believed that miracles happen.

Along with fear and uncertainty, pancreatic cancer brought crippling pain. The tumor itself caused sharp pains in the stomach and abdomen that radiated to the back, and chemotherapy and radiation left Patrick fatigued and lethargic. There were times when he was crippled by the pain or would fall to the floor from its intensity. Even simple activities like riding in the car caused pain, but Patrick chose, for the most part, to bear it silently. At times, he'd grimace when doing things around the house, but he never complained. Unlike others with cancer, Patrick didn't feel that the pain sapped him of his energy and motivation. He wasn't sure how much more pain there might be as the disease progressed, so he wanted to save his complaints for more serious problems.

Many patients with a terminal diagnosis choose to make the most of their remaining time by creating "bucket lists"—things they want to do before they die. Patrick simply wanted to go back to work as soon as possible, and he did. He starred in a television series *The Beast*, choosing to take very little pain medication so that he could perform. He scheduled his treatments around his filming. He worked 14 to 16 hours per day, five days a week while undergoing chemotherapy on the weekends. That's an unbelievable workload for somebody battling cancer. Lisa credits his incredible physical self-discipline and body-awareness—cultivated through years of dance—for his success in working through such a serious illness. She also felt that so many of Patrick's achievements during the last two years of his life were attributed to the forcefulness of "mind over matter."

Lisa completely supported Patrick's decision to continue to act, knowing that whatever kept his spirits up would likely prolong his life. Although his illness was equally painful and terrifying to her, she did her best not to cry in front of him or burden him with her own painful emotions as he fought for his life. She wrote in her 2012 book *Worth Fighting For*:

"There is a high price to be paid for the privilege of caring for your loved one when he's dying, but it's one I wouldn't have traded for anything. I always said that I'd have plenty of time to cry later."

Lisa says her mother, a nurse, taught her how to place her own emotional needs on the back burner while caring for Patrick. She wanted to support him completely and make the most of the time they had left together.

## The Role of the Caregiver

Caregivers play a vital role in the emotional support and day-to-day physical health of someone in pain, especially at the end of life and they face a very daunting task. Caregivers must often work with doctors and nurses to manage both treatments for the loved one's underlying disease or condition as well as pain control. Often, they are the ones who remember when medications need to be taken, including which ones need to be taken with food and which ones on an empty stomach. Caregivers also are often responsible for keeping everything clean and sterile to avoid exposing the patient to pathogens.

Depending on the patient's limitations, caregivers may have to prepare meals and give baths as well as help the patient dress and use the bathroom. They must learn to watch for signs of trouble, such as behavioral or emotional changes, or abnormal fluctuations in vital signs. Often, they transport their loved one to doctor's appointments and therapy visits as well as deal with the insurance companies and the daunting paperwork associated with claiming benefits. Many people suffering from chronic pain have good days and bad days, which can make the caregiver's life incredibly unpredictable.

Lisa Swayze worked around the clock for almost two years driving and even flying Patrick to cancer treatments, monitoring his medications, and staying in communication with his doctors. As his disease progressed, he was confined to his bed and completely lost his appetite. Patrick's doctors put him on total parenteral nutrition (TPN), which bypassed his gastrointestinal tract, and fed him intravenously with glucose, amino acids, and vitamins. This kept him nourished but meant that Lisa had to change his IV bags while she worked to keep his pain under control.

Both Patrick and Lisa became more spiritually engaged during his illness, and Patrick also practiced mindfulness to help control the pain. Lisa remarked that, "he was a master of mindfulness." This holistic approach to the illness brought them closer together and helped them cherish every moment together. "The connection was beyond words," said Lisa. "We lived in the moment."

## Hope and Support for the Caregiver

As devoted as Lisa was, she began to feel like she was hitting a wall as Patrick entered his second year of fighting his illness. Her energy reserves had virtually run out, and she felt drained physically and emotionally. As Patrick began to need more and more care, his brother Trevor moved in to the house to help Lisa, which provided a much-needed respite. Lisa began to take breaks when she could, taking the time to think about her own emotions and cry when she needed to. Even just going to the store for a couple of hours gave her a break from thinking about the illness, and she could come back with renewed determination and hope.

Caregivers who care for patients with prolonged illnesses or chronic pain may be looking after their loved ones for years. They can often stretch themselves too thin, leading to exhaustion or other illnesses. Caregivers must recognize their own limitations and be sure to find support and care for themselves as well. Many benefit from a support group, counseling, or someone to relieve their duties so they can take a day off.

If you know someone caring for a loved one in pain, calling to offer encouragement or even some time off can be a wonderful way to support his or her efforts. Be sure not to place demands on their time or energy, but make yourself available to serve in whatever way you can instead.

Lisa and Patrick also found it helpful to look at his illness as an opportunity to learn. They enjoyed asking the doctors questions and learning about new treatments and how they worked. Lisa joked with me that Patrick treated his illness as his own personal science project.

Caregiving changed the Swayzes' relationship, deepening their trust and connection with one another. The uncertainty of the illness forced them to live in the moment. They chose to see each of Patrick's days as a victory in and of itself and to make the most of their time together. Once a terminal illness is diagnosed (and continual pain can feel like a terminal illness), a lot of fear can push loved ones away from the patient. If that happens, try to do what Lisa and Patrick did: Set the fear aside, go through the journey together, and take each other's hand. You will be astonished by some amazing gifts and love that unfold during the process.

Even though the odds were stacked against them, Lisa and Patrick never gave up hope. Why shouldn't Patrick be the first person to beat a Stage 4 pancreatic cancer diagnosis? That was the question they chose to ask themselves each day. Whether a patient has received a terminal diagnosis or is living with chronic pain, continuing to hope that life can get better is a vital component of extending and making the most of life. "We were realistic optimists," said Lisa. "As long as Patrick was upright, talking, and breathing, there was hope."

## Pain Control When Life Ends

Palliative care provides the medical, emotional, and spiritual support for those with complicated or advanced diseases whose life expectancy is uncertain. Its goal is to improve the patient's quality of life and support his or her family. It can be given along with medical treatments whose aim is to treat the patient's disease or send it into remission. It is appropriate at any stage for serious illnesses such as cancer, congestive heart failure, Parkinson's disease, and Alzheimer's disease, among others.

Hospice care provides similar support for patients who are expected to live for six months or less. Care can be provided by visiting nurses or in a hospice center, and its goal is to keep the patient as comfortable and peaceful as possible. Both palliative and hospice care professionals work with caregivers to help them meet the patient's needs.

Switching to hospice care was a difficult choice for Patrick and Lisa, because, in some ways, it felt like they were giving up. But it is often helpful to look at hospice care simply as a shift in priorities—comfort over treatment—and a decision to make the most of the time the patient has left. Because they had fought so fiercely for Patrick to live, this transition was tough.

Like many terminally ill patients, Patrick benefited greatly from opioids for pain relief in the later stages of his disease. There is a harmful misconception that using and escalating the doses of opioids for terminally ill patients will hasten death. Research suggests that effective pain control during illness and even aggressive pain control at the end of life help patients stay encouraged, provide the positive attitude needed to engage the emotional and psychological aspects of dying, and can have the astonishing effect of actually prolonging life by reducing our body's exposure to uncontrolled pain.

Lisa put it this way, "Patrick was afraid to suffer, and nobody needs to suffer. Passing out of this world can be a special, delicate, and precious experience. If pain is out of control, it's heartbreaking for the patient and the family."

During the second year of his illness, Patrick was prescribed hydromorphone (Dilaudid) to control his pain. It was very important, providing needed relief and helping with his emotional pain and agitation, but it did cause mental fogginess, prompting him to joke with Lisa at times about having a "Dilaudid moment" when he forgot something.

As his condition worsened, Patrick began to need a Dilaudid shot in his IV every 30 to 45 minutes. After seeing how exhausting this was for Lisa and because Patrick wasn't a candidate for surgery or for a specific nerve block (neurolysis), he finally agreed to use a patient controlled analgesia (PCA) pain pump. This enabled him to have the pain medication automatically put into his IV with the touch of a button. Although convenient, it was a difficult decision because he wondered if he would ever come off of the pain pump.

As the body begins to shut down, patients experience new pain as well as anxiety and agitation. Caregivers should work with healthcare providers to ensure that their loved ones have effective medication in sufficient quantities to ensure their pain stays under control. For instance, opioids are central to effective pain relief at the end of life. Unfortunately, an estimated 46% of people do not have adequate pain treatment at death. One study reported that as many as 50% of patients with cancer pain may be undertreated. The World Health Organization has even declared that pain threatens to condemn one out of every ten of us alive today to die a painful death. This makes the experience even more heartbreaking and perhaps traumatizing for patients and loved ones alike. As one of my patients said to me, "Pain is all encompassing and can strip your life away. Without medicine and other therapies, it's a lot easier to think about dying."

Although opioids are the cornerstone of managing pain at the end of life, other pain medications, nerve blocks, pain pumps, and complementary and alternative medicine (CAM) such as spirituality and religion, music therapy, or pet therapy can all be effective and, in some cases, preferable to opioids. As a matter of fact, just simple touch and massage lead to meaningful differences in pain, distress, and quality of life according to one study. Integrative therapies are covered in more detail in Part 3, Integrative Therapies for Pain for Pain.

Interest in medical marijuana has experienced a resurgence in the palliative care and end-of-life communities as well. In general, the research shows that medical marijuana can reduce chronic pain by greater than 30% and can have two beneficial effects on those taking opioids: lowering the opioid doses and augmenting opioid effectiveness. In Europe and Canada, a marijuana oral spray is available to ease symptoms of cancer pain, neuropathic pain, and multiple sclerosis. Using a spray avoids the potential hazards and dosing uncertainties of inhaling forms of raw cannabis. A good many patients in pain at the end of life or in palliative care settings could potentially benefit from replacing opioids with marijuana or using lower doses of opioids in combination with marijuana. Read more about medical marijuana and opioids in Chapter 14, Pharmacological Therapies.

Thankfully, Patrick Swayze passed peacefully from this life, surrounded by loved ones and with Lisa holding his hand. She considered it an honor to be there, just as she felt honored to care for him in the last months of his life.

Death ends the patient's suffering but brings a flood of grief and loss to caregivers and other loved ones. Many feel blindsided by the emotional pain and feel unable to carry on with their daily lives for weeks or even months. Caregivers may feel a sense of relief that their duties have ended but, at the same time, may feel lost and unsure of what to do with themselves now that they have no one to care for.

Lisa Swayze described the grief of losing Patrick like being doused in gasoline and set on fire, but, in time, that feeling dissipated. Today, she continues to fight pancreatic cancer as a spokesperson for the Pancreatic Cancer Action Network and the Patrick Swayze Pancreatic Cancer Research Fund at Stanford University.

## Hope for Cancer Pain Relief

To learn more about various self-care and pain treatment options and therapies, read the chapters in Part 1, Understanding and Treating Your Pain, and Part 2, Medical Therapies for Pain: Traditional and Innovative. There you will find more information and ideas for working with your physician and other healthcare providers to find ways to prevent, manage, and address your pain.

You can also learn more about cancer-related pain and caregiving by listening to my weekly radio talk show, *Aches and Gains*. You can find the broadcasts on cancer-related pain at the following URLs.

**Cancer Pain**

http://paulchristomd.com/cancer-pain

**Suzanne Somers, Cancer Pain, and Phototherapy**

http://paulchristomd.com/breast-cancer

http://paulchristomd.com/breast-cancer-2

**Tommy Chong and Rectal Cancer**

http://paulchristomd.com/rectal-cancer

http://paulchristomd.com/rectal-cancer-2

**Colon Cancer**

http://paulchristomd.com/colon-cancer

Brittany Daniel and Non-Hodgkin's lymphoma

http://paulchristomd.com/non-hodgkins-lymphoma

http://paulchristomd.com/non-hodgkins-lymphoma-2

**Lisa Swayze and Caregiving**

http://paulchristomd.com/caregiving

http://paulchristomd.com/caregiving-2

# Suggested Further Reading

American Cancer Society. *American Cancer Society's Guide to Pain Control: Understanding and Managing Cancer Pain.* (n.p.): American Cancer Society, 2004. This book explains how to achieve acceptable pain control and how to understand the optimal balance between pain relief and the potential side effects of pain medications. http://tinyurl.com/y9kf43ok

De Conno, F. *Cancer Pain Relief: A Practical Manual.* (n.p.): Springer, 2012. A manual of useful information about treating pain from a pharmacological, surgical and psychosocial point of view. http://tinyurl.com/y9j3u6p3

Land, Susan S, and Patt, Richard B. *The Complete Guide to Relieving Cancer Pain and Suffering.* (n.p.): Oxford University Press, 2006. A handbook for cancer patients and their families to make informed decisions about their care. http://tinyurl.com/y79pj6xt

# Other Resources to Explore

Breastcancer.org is a nonprofit organization providing reliable information about breast cancer with a section on pain medications and other pain-reducing therapies.

Cancer.net is the official website for the American Society of Clinical Oncology (ASCO) with insights, tips, and inspirational posts on cancer, written by cancer physicians.

The American Cancer Society's official website, Cancer.org, includes a section on understanding and managing cancer pain.

Cancer Tutor is a project of the Cancer Research Foundation that lists types of cancer, causes, prevention, treatments, media, resources, survivor stories, forums, and articles on cancer pain.

Cancerwise is a blog run by The MD Anderson Cancer Center at the University of Texas featuring  real stories and  the latest news on cancer research, policy topics, and clinical trials.

The Cancer Treatment Centers of America blog offers details from the experts themselves, such as how doctors detect cancer and how to cope with a diagnosis.

Pain Control is a downloadable booklet by the National Cancer Institute. It includes causes of cancer pain, how to talk to your healthcare team, making a pain control plan, medicines and side effects.

Patient is an online health platform containing over 4000 health articles and thousands of discussion forums, named top health website by *The Times* newspaper. It includes articles on Pain control in palliative care.

SHARE Cancer Support blog was founded by survivors of breast cancer and ovarian cancer to offer personal stories, support groups, educational programs, and a hotline.

WebMD article on cancer pain management, including causes, symptoms, medicine and treatment.

# 13

# Autoimmune Pain: A Hidden Epidemic

"Oh God, I hurt!"

Few of Elvis Presley's millions of adoring fans would have believed that the undisputed "King of Rock and Roll" would ever say those words. On stage, even just months before his untimely death, his performances electrified his audience and brought many to tears. Yet Elvis's last years of his life were lived in a private agony of debilitating pain.

I had the privilege of speaking with Elvis's personal physician, Dr. George Nichopoulos, his life-long friend George Klein, and pain specialist and endocrinologist Dr. Forrest Tennant, all of whom offer profound insight into Elvis's life and complex medical history. During the 1970s, Elvis suffered from chronic pain that included headaches, low back pain, abdominal pain, as well as joint and muscle pain. He also suffered from related conditions such as chronic constipation, insomnia, isolation, irrational behavior, and likely depression. Many, if not most of these medical problems were probably triggered by an autoimmune response following several traumatic brain injuries sustained during Elvis's life.

Yet Elvis rarely complained. He continued to perform strenuous martial arts moves on stage despite his musculoskeletal pain, and he continued to eat an unhealthy diet despite terrible stomach, abdominal, and bowel problems. Elvis's private suffering highlights several important issues surrounding chronic pain in general and particularly autoimmune inflammatory disorders, which some doctors now believe were at the root of most of Elvis's health problems.

## Understanding Autoimmune Pain

Autoimmune diseases occur when autoantibodies in the bloodstream begin attacking healthy tissue instead of attacking pathogens like viruses and bacteria, which is their job in the body. The antibodies attack muscles, joints, organs, nerves, and bone and, left uncontrolled, can lead to complete debilitation and even death. Unfortunately, we still don't know much about why this happens to some people and not to others.

Many autoimmune diseases, such as Lupus and Crohn's disease, are acquired. Other autoimmune diseases are genetic. Acquisition seems to occur primarily from viral infection. For example, some patients experience fibromyalgia symptoms after mononucleosis infection or after Lyme disease. However, only about 5%–10% of people exposed to immune-stressors such as these infections ever develop fibromyalgia. This indicates that there may be a genetic component that predisposes patients to fibromyalgia as well as to other autoimmune disorders.

Autoimmune pain that goes unchecked can progress to central pain, which involves the brain and spinal cord. A more recent theory of central pain suggests that in people who experience central pain, an area of the brain becomes inflamed and painful, leading to a hyperarousal of the sympathetic nervous system and endocrine system. Severe pain stimulates the pituitary gland to release hormones such as cortisol, dehydroepiandrosterone (DHEA), testosterone, and progesterone to heal the painful area of the body. If the pain continues and the site doesn't heal, the hormones become depleted, leading to a decrease in appetite and sexual interest, insomnia, and even interference with the action of medications. Because many medications work by stimulating a hormonal response, this depletion can make such medicines ineffective. There is evidence that Elvis, for example, was experiencing central pain in the years leading up to his death.

## Elvis Presley and Autoimmune Pain

Many physicians believe that autoimmune diseases and the pain associated with them are becoming an epidemic in our society.

The impact of such diseases continues to be underappreciated and poorly understood, and we are really just learning how to treat them effectively. In addition to Elvis Presley, other iconic Americans including President John F. Kennedy and business magnate Howard Hughes suffered tremendous pain from what are now believed to be autoimmune diseases.

On the afternoon of August 16, 1977, Elvis Presley's girlfriend found him unresponsive on his bathroom floor. Attempts to revive him failed, and he was pronounced dead later at the local hospital in Memphis. The autopsy concluded that the cause of death was cardiac arrest and revealed the presence of several different drugs in his system.

His fans were understandably shocked and devastated, but the doctors who treated him had been worried about his health for some time. Elvis had been gravely ill the last three years of his life, requiring nearly round the clock care.

In addition to having ballooned up to 350 pounds, Elvis's known health problems in the three years preceding his death included severe headaches, hypertension, glaucoma, a protruding disc in his low back, anemia, prostatitis. and megacolon (the abnormal expansion of the colon and halting of peristalsis, the involuntary contractions which push food through the digestive system). The autopsy also revealed that his heart was nearly twice the size it should have been (cardiomegaly) and that he had terrible atherosclerosis (the buildup of fats and cholesterol in the arterial walls).

In light of the toxicology report, many would dismiss Elvis as an overindulgent celebrity who abused drugs for the fun of it and paid the price. Media outlets began speculating that Elvis had died of a drug overdose and that this was being covered up. It is true that the cardiac arrest Elvis experienced was not what we commonly call a heart attack (myocardial infarction), in which a coronary artery becomes blocked and heart tissue begins to die. According to the autopsy, Elvis experienced a fatal arrhythmia, a malfunction of the electrical impulses that cause the heart to beat. This is consistent with the idea that the combination of drugs in his system caused his heart to stop, but it does not mean that these same drugs would have stopped the heart of a healthy man.

Largely in response to the media speculation and public outcry, Elvis's personal physician Dr. Nichopoulos was brought up on manslaughter charges. "Dr. Nick," as he was known to his patients, was accused of overprescribing drugs to Elvis and negligently causing his death. A jury quickly cleared him of all wrongdoing at his trial, where they learned that only two of the 10 or more drugs in Elvis's blood had been prescribed by Dr. Nick. Unfortunately, Nichopoulos still lost his medical license and career and lived under the shadow of those accusations until his death.

Was Elvis simply a narcissistic drug addict enabled by an unethical doctor? On the contrary, his closest friends, like George Klein, remember Elvis as a deeply caring and religious man who suffered silently from constant pain at the end of his life. According to George, Elvis didn't like to talk about his pain and tried to fight through it. He really didn't complain much. Behind the scenes, Elvis was an avid reader, enjoying books on medicine, religion, and philosophy. He liked to ride horses, roller skate, play racquetball, and go to movies. George remembers Elvis as a great friend who was loveable and never wanted to hurt anybody's feelings. Doctors who understand chronic pain have concluded that Dr. Nick did indeed treat Elvis in good faith. And today, our knowledge of both autoimmune disorders and chronic pain sheds a very different light on the medical facts of Elvis's death.

Despite eating an unhealthy diet and abusing drugs like amphetamines recreationally, Elvis appeared to be quite healthy until about age 32. He was very physically fit during his military service and remained active afterwards through martial arts, horseback riding, and casual games of football. But something would happen in 1967 that would change that forever.

## Traumatic Brain Injury and Autoimmune Pain

In hindsight, it seems likely that Elvis's health troubles began with a serious concussion in March 1967. He tripped, hit his head on the bathtub, and was knocked unconscious. When he regained consciousness, he was unable to function normally for several days (possibly weeks) and hallucinated frequently. This was long before the days of strict concussion recovery protocols, so Elvis got back to his normal routine of performing and partying as soon as he felt he could.

It was after this incident that Elvis's unbearable headaches began. He had sustained three previous traumatic head injuries in the late 1960s prior to the most serious incident on the bathtub. After he sustained the head injuries, his health began rapidly declining, although the people managing his music career made sure the public never found out. In addition to weight gain and increasing pain all over his body, Elvis showed signs of mental impairment and irrational compulsive behavior. He gave luxurious gifts to complete strangers and took a spontaneous trip to Washington, DC, to meet with President Richard Nixon.

We now speculate that the kind of head trauma Elvis experienced (traumatic brain injury, or TBI) caused a small amount of brain tissue to leak into the blood stream, triggering an autoimmune response. In many autoimmune disorders, antibodies that form attack healthy tissue, leading to pain and multi-organ dysfunction. The antibodies begin randomly attacking normal tissue, such as the joints, nerves, and muscle, causing pain. Antibodies also may attack other organs such as the eye, heart, and liver. The autoimmune response involves the production of cytokines, small proteins released by cells. Cytokines trigger inflammation and activate nerves causing pain. A family of these cytokines (Interleukin-1) is associated with painful autoimmune disorders such as rheumatoid arthritis, multiple sclerosis, and inflammatory bowel disease (Crohn's and ulcerative colitis). Two of these conditions (rheumatoid arthritis and multiple sclerosis) are covered in Chapter 3, Arthritis Pain, and Chapter 4, Neuropathic Pain. Along with other physicians, I now believe an autoimmune disorder brought on by traumatic brain injury affected Elvis.

We hear quite a bit about traumatic brain injury in football players and boxers, but this phenomenon can occur from general repeated head trauma, not only from athletic injury. I see head trauma patients with a triad of symptoms: pain all over, insomnia, and headaches. They often complain of neck pain too. Like Elvis, patients experience constant pain, depression, and mental impairments, which can include irrational or obsessive-compulsive behavior. In addition to the organ problems already listed, additional information from Elvis's autopsy supports this hypothesis. Lymphocytes (white blood cells) had infiltrated his lungs, a symptom of emphysema or similar pulmonary disorders, although he was never known to smoke. Elvis's gamma globulin (proteins that include antibodies) levels were very low and his eosinophil (a type of white blood cell that elevates from conditions like asthma and autoimmune diseases) count was extremely high. These findings are consistent with a disorder of the body's immune system and most likely an autoimmune inflammatory disorder.

During the last years of his life, Elvis was in constant pain and unable to sleep without medication. Those who knew Elvis well, including his friend George Klein, saw that Elvis was putting Dr. Nick in an impossible situation. Dr. Nick knew Elvis was abusing drugs and tried desperately (and unsuccessfully) to get him to enter a treatment program. On the other hand, Dr. Nick knew Elvis's chronic pain was real and required treatment. Unbeknownst to Dr. Nick, Elvis was also getting prescription medications mailed to him by two doctors from other parts of the country.

To balance Elvis's need for treatment with his tendency to abuse drugs, Dr. Nick put together pill packets—small envelopes with several tablets or capsules. These were mostly to help him sleep and contained medicines like hydromorphone (Dilaudid), dextroamphetamine (Dexedrine), amobarbital (Amytal), and methaqualone (Quaalude). Because Elvis also suffered from depression, Dr. Nick recommended the more typical treatment for depression at that time—amphetamines. To prevent him from having control over his own dosing, Dr. Nick had a nurse move with her husband into a trailer on Elvis's property. She was under careful instructions from Dr. Nick regarding what medications to administer in response to particular symptoms. She cared for Elvis around the clock and when he was on the road.

An important key to Elvis's death lay in a probable genetic defect in a liver enzyme that controls the metabolism of certain drugs called cytochrome p450 2D6. Because of this condition, his body could not metabolize codeine properly, causing it instead to elevate to toxic levels in his blood. There are reports that Elvis had an allergic response to codeine. Unfortunately, the day before his death, Elvis mistakenly received codeine from a dentist who was putting a crown on one of his teeth.

The codeine Elvis received at the dentist, combined with the medications he was using to sleep (and other medications he obtained without Dr. Nick's knowledge), almost certainly caused his already diseased and enlarged heart to stop. That is, the toxic levels of codeine along with the other medications he was taking likely led to a lethal cardiac arrhythmia. Dr. Joseph Davis, the coroner retained for Elvis's second autopsy in 1994, explained the difference between dying of a typical drug overdose and what Elvis experienced:

"The position of Elvis Presley's body was such that he was about to sit down on the commode when the seizure occurred. He pitched forward onto the carpet, his rear in the air, and was dead by the time he hit the floor. If it had been a drug overdose, [Elvis Presley] would have slipped into an increasing state of slumber. He would have pulled up his pajama bottoms and crawled to the door to seek help. It takes hours to die from drugs."

Dr. Forest Tennant, a pain specialist, researcher, and editor emeritus of the *Practical Pain Management* journal, was called in 1979 by Dr. Nick's attorney. Dr. Tennant soon concluded that Dr. Nick had done his best to take care of Elvis in good faith and that it was not his fault that Elvis died, and he testified to that effect. The jury agreed with him, but much of the media continued to blame Dr. Nick for Elvis's death.

Elvis's story highlights how the issue of effective pain treatment can become intertwined with the issue of addiction. There is no question that Elvis abused drugs, but that was by and large a separate issue from his chronic pain. Elvis abused amphetamines recreationally from a young age, and he misused the medications prescribed to him by his doctors. His drive to obtain drugs later in life—legally and illegally—was more likely motivated by a frantic desire to treat his central, autoimmune-related pain, rather than by a dependence on a particular substance. In addition to grappling with pain throughout his body including headaches, low back pain, muscle and joint pain, and abdominal pain, Elvis also struggled with depression and insomnia, which he also sought to medicate.

## President John F. Kennedy and Autoimmune Pain

Elvis was not the only public figure to suffer silently from a poorly understood autoimmune disease. For his entire adult life, President John F. Kennedy was condemned to the same fate. Kennedy was the very picture of youthful vigor to the American public. We remember him playing touch football or standing next to his beautiful and stylish wife, Jacqueline. During his short time as president, he navigated some of the greatest challenges our nation ever faced, including the Berlin Crisis, civil rights challenges, the escalation of the Vietnam War, and the Cuban Missile Crisis, which was perhaps the closest our country has yet come to nuclear war.

Many knew that President Kennedy suffered from low back pain, which most assumed to be the result of injuries he incurred while serving in the Navy during World War II. But it was not until the release of his medical records in 2002 that the public became aware of his lifelong struggle with chronic pain. We know now that, even before he entered the Navy, he wore a brace to support his back and was already beginning to experience terrible pain in his joints. In 1944, he actually underwent back surgery—similar to what we would today call a discectomy—and was able to recover well.

President Kennedy's pain likely started during his teen years with severe spastic colitis, what we today call celiac disease. It is now believed that he was born with an autoimmune disease known as Schmidt's syndrome (autoimmune polyglandular syndrome type 2), which causes osteoporosis, nerve pain, arthritic pain, muscular pain, and many other disorders including colitis. In patients who suffer from Schmidt's syndrome, autoantibodies attack healthy tissues leading to

pain and deterioration. The syndrome also leads to adrenal insufficiency, thyroid disease, diabetes, and sometimes failure of the sexual organs. Even before serving in World War II, Kennedy suffered from joint pain in his lumbar spine and sacroiliac joint, most likely the result of autoantibodies attacking these areas. Doctors prescribed corticosteroids to treat Kennedy's colitis and those drugs likely saved his life. However, because the treatment was then relatively new, the dosages Kennedy received were very high by today's standards. High doses or long treatment duration with steroids decreases bone density causing osteoporosis and predisposing to fractures mainly in the spine and ribs. This almost certainly contributed to Kennedy's later development of osteoporosis and the subsequent collapse of his spine.

Surgical records noted that Kennedy's spine was osteoporotic. A trio of events might have caused this problem: autoantibodies attacking his bones, high cortisol levels induced by severe pain, and high doses of corticosteroids used to suppress his colitis. Kennedy was placing deoxycorticosterone acetate (DOCA) pellets under his skin with a knife and covering the area up with a Band-Aid. Elevated cortisol and continued use of steroids can both cause osteoporosis.

In 1954, Kennedy's spine had degenerated to the point where he required a second back surgery. He couldn't get out of bed at times and reportedly told his mother that he'd rather die than live in such pain. Surgeons attempted to fuse his vertebrae using a metal plate, but unfortunately the plate became infected and had to be removed. The ordeal was nearly fatal, yet while recovering, Kennedy wrote his Pulitzer Prize–winning book, *Profiles in Courage*.

Despite the incredible resilience and determination he showed throughout his life, Kennedy might never have lived to run for president had he not come under the care of Dr. Janet Travell, beginning in 1955. Kennedy's condition was deteriorating rapidly, and he was in such severe and constant pain that he felt hopeless. Dr. Travell immediately put him in the hospital and started him on several medications to bring his pain under control. When he was released, her multidimensional program of vigorous exercise, physical therapy, and a combination of medications (including methadone and codeine) kept him functioning at a very high level until his assassination.

During pain flare-ups, Dr. Travell also injected a local anesthetic called procaine into muscular trigger points of his low back two to three times a day. Some felt that this weakened his back, but Dr. Travell made sure Kennedy continued rehabilitation therapy. She thought that a vitamin B deficiency was causing nerve inflammation (neuritis) in his legs, so Dr. Travell also provided vitamin B and B12 supplements. Alternative therapies she utilized to control his pain included heel lifts to even out his legs, swimming, frequent hot showers, heating pads, and his famous rocking chair. Dr. Travell made sure Kennedy rocked and swam almost every day. The idea was to promote lymph drainage through movement. There is an intriguing theory about damaged nerves—that they are similar to damaged power lines. The sparks from damaged power lines are actually the release of electrons. When nerves are disrupted, they can elicit an inflammatory response that includes the accumulation of electrons or protons as well. Facilitating lymph flow can "release" these inflammatory molecules and electrically charged particles, removing them from the site of pain via a system of tiny channels in between cells. Activities such as rocking, swimming, massage, and walking all maintain lymph drainage, and Dr. Travell felt this type of movement was critical to Kennedy's treatment regimen and pain relief.

During his campaign and time in office, President Kennedy's health was a closely guarded secret. Robert Dallek, noted historian on Kennedy's life and guest on my radio show, said that the public had no idea Kennedy wore a back brace and he was never photographed using crutches or being assisted up and down staircases. In addition to him being the youngest president ever elected, Kennedy was the first Roman Catholic to run for the presidency of the United States. Dallek felt that Kennedy's advisors were certain that any other perceived problems by the public, such as his ailments, would hurt his chances as a candidate and his authority as president. Yet there is absolutely no evidence that his pain or the medications he took to treat it had any negative effect on his cognitive function. On the contrary, he seems to have maintained an incredible level of mental clarity throughout his career.

On November 22, 1963, President Kennedy was assassinated by sniper Lee Harvey Oswald as he rode in his motorcade through the streets of Dallas, Texas. Tragically, some have speculated that the secret back brace he had to wear contributed to his death by holding his body erect after Oswald's first shot passed through his neck. Had he slumped over, as he would have without the brace, Oswald's second shot might not have hit his head.

Although Kennedy suffered daily his entire adult life, he was able to win and serve in the highest office in the land. He led the country through some of its most perilous ordeals and rose to the demands of his office at all times. And although his ailment was not well understood at the time, he never stopped searching for the best possible treatment and never allowed his illness to limit his ambition or his commitment to his work.

## Hope for Autoimmune Pain Relief

The fact that a president of the United States and a man who many believe was one of the greatest performers to ever live both suffered from unrelenting autoimmune pain should inspire all of us not to allow physical ailments to limit what we hope to get out of life. They both experienced sorrow but accomplished a great deal in their lives. Their stories also remind us how much medicine has advanced in just a few decades, although we still have a long way to go.

> Dr. Nick believed that an operation to correct Elvis's toxic megacolon could have improved his health and extended his life. Unfortunately, the surgery in question was quite new at the time, and no one wanted to take the risk of operating on the King of Rock and Roll. Today, Elvis's severe 1967 concussion would have been considered an important piece of his medical history, and if treated early enough, he may have been spared much of his suffering. Modern genetic testing for the liver's ability to metabolize drugs could have explained why he had an allergic response to certain medicines like codeine or why they were not working for him, and today's doctors would have had a much greater range of medicines to choose from.
>
> President Kennedy suffered at a time when pain therapy wasn't even a recognized form of medicine. Yet he searched until he found a doctor who was able to treat his pain competently and holistically. Although his life was tragically cut short, his pain never defeated him. He took courageous and often drastic measures to maintain his health and performed perhaps the world's most difficult job until his death.

To learn more about various self-care and pain treatment options and therapies, read the chapters in Part 1, Understanding and Treating Your Pain, and Part 2, Medical Therapies for Pain: Traditional and Innovative. There you will find more information and ideas for working with your physician and other healthcare providers to find ways to prevent, manage, and address your pain.

> You can also learn more about autoimmune pain by listening to the autoimmune pain episodes of my weekly radio program, *Aches and Gains*. You can find the broadcasts on autoimmune pain at the following URLs:
>
> **Elvis Presley**
> http://paulchristomd.com/elvis-presley-1
> http://paulchristomd.com/elvis-presley-2

http://paulchristomd.com/elvis-presley-3

http://paulchristomd.com/elvis-presley-4

**John F. Kennedy**

http://paulchristomd.com/jfk

http://paulchristomd.com/jfk-2

## Suggested Further Reading

O'Bryan, Tom. *The Autoimmune Fix: How to Stop the Hidden Autoimmune Damage That Keeps You Sick, Fat, and Tired Before It Turns Into Disease.* (n.p.): Rodale, 2016. Two comprehensive 3-week plans to navigate conditions caused by autoimmune diseases, such as Alzheimer's, Multiple Sclerosis, Osteoporosis, Diabetes, and Lupus. http://tinyurl.com/yabwak75

Osborne, Peter. *No Grain, No Pain: A 30 Day Diet for Eliminating the Root Cause of Chronic Pain.* (n.p.): Touchstone, 2016. This book identifies grain as a leading cause of chronic suffering, while offering practical steps to find relief using a drug-free, easy-to-implement plan to eliminate all sources of gluten. http://tinyurl.com/y7n7cqf5

Myers, Amy. *The Autoimmune Solution: Prevent and Reverse the Full Spectrum of Inflammatory Symptoms and Diseases.* (n.p.): HarperOne, 2015. In this book Dr. Amy Myers offers her medically proven approach to prevent a wide range of inflammatory-related symptoms and diseases. http://tinyurl.com/ycto29f4

## Other Resources to Explore

The American Autoimmune Related Diseases Association's official websit including information and advocacy.

American Chronic Pain Association's articls on autoimmune diseases, with videos and patient resources.

Everydayhealth.com. Articles on autoimmune disorder of the joints, muscles, and nerves.

# Medical Therapies for Pain: Traditional and Innovative

# CHAPTER

# 14

# Pharmacological Therapies

When we think of treating pain, we often think of medicines. This is with good reason. For thousands of years, people have used various chemicals—from ple have used various chemicals—from alcohol to herbs—to relieve the pain of injury and illness. Today, pharmacological therapies make up an important facet of pain relief.

## Acetaminophen and NSAIDs

The most common over-the-counter pain relievers are acetaminophen (Tylenol) and various non-steroidal anti-inflammatory drugs (NSAIDs). Both acetaminophen and NSAIDs work by inhibiting the production of prostaglandins, molecules that cause pain, inflammation, and fever.

Acetaminophen is a weak anti-inflammatory medicine compared to NSAIDs, but is often a first-line medicine for mild pain. Acetaminophen has the advantage of being gentle on the stomach lining and doesn't inhibit platelet function, so bleeding isn't a concern. Kidney problems rarely occur with acetaminophen use as well.

Acetaminophen can cause liver damage in excessive quantities though, because the drug is metabolized in the liver. It should not be used by people with liver disease or a history of alcohol abuse. The maximum acetaminophen dose in adults is 4000 mg per day, but the FDA is considering lowering that dose to 3000 mg per day in order to protect patients from possible liver damage. One leading manufacturer of acetaminophen recommends 3000 mg per day. As a result, the FDA has limited the strength to 325 mg per tablet for prescription drugs, which includes combinations with other medicines such as short-acting opioids (for example, Percocet). When combined with NSAIDs, acetaminophen enhances the analgesic effect for patients with postoperative pain.

NSAIDs can be very effective for treating acute pain, osteoarthritis (OA), rheumatoid arthritis, headaches, metastatic bone cancer, and muscular pain. There are over 12 different NSAIDs on the market including aspirin, ibuprofen (Motrin, Advil), naproxen (Aleve), celecoxib (Celebrex) and diclofenac (Voltaren). No one NSAID is necessarily better than the others. If one doesn't produce much of an effect over 10 to 14 days, then another can be tried. Topical NSAIDs, such as diclofenac, can ease the pain of arthritic joints (Pennsaid solution or Voltaren gel) or acute discomfort from strains and sprains (Flector 1.3% patch).

NSAIDs are often better pain relievers than acetaminophen but may adversely affect the stomach mucosa, especially if taken for extended periods of time. This means that patients are at risk for ulcers or bleeding. In the quest to reduce potentially serious gastrointestinal side effects, a group of specialized NSAIDs called the COX-2 inhibitors were developed. These drugs confer a protective effect on the gastrointestinal tract and don't increase the risk of bleeding during surgery because they preserve the function of platelets in allowing blood to clot. Only one, celecoxib (Celebrex) is available in the United States. Two others, parecoxib and etoricoxib, are used outside the United

States for pain occurring at or around the time of surgery (perioperative pain) and musculoskeletal disorders, respectively. There are drugs that can also protect the stomach like the proton pump inhibitors (for example, esomeprosole (Nexium)) or H2 antagonists (for example, ranitidine (Zantac)) if patients require prolonged use of NSAIDS.

NDAIDs can also adversely affect the cardiovascular system. There is a "black box warning" for all NSAIDs indicating that they can increase the risk of serious cardiovascular events such as stroke or myocardial infarction (heart attack). These occur rarely, but it's important to be aware of the potential.

All NSAIDs—including aspirin—can reduce blood flow to the kidneys. This reduced blood flow typically causes a minimal effect in healthy people. But the risk of toxicity escalates when taken in high doses or taken by patients taking more than one NSAID, who have vascular disease, are of an advanced age, or who use NSAIDs chronically. For anyone taking NSAIDs who falls into these categories, a doctor can monitor kidney function with periodic blood tests if needed.

Patients who have a history of ulcers, kidney problems, or cardiovascular disease need to be careful with NSAIDs. In general, the rule of thumb is to use the lowest NSAID dose for the shortest period of time to prevent unwanted side effects. Many patients don't realize that NSAIDs can interfere with medicines they're taking to control their blood pressure (for example, diuretics) as well, so talk to your doctor if you're taking an over-the-counter NSAID regularly.

## Tricyclic Antidepressants and Serotonin–Norepinephrine Reuptake Inhibitors (SNRIs)

Tricyclic antidepressants (TCAs) have been used for several decades to treat depression as well as chronic pain. My patients often look at me in doubt when I recommend these medicines because they don't understand how antidepressants will treat their pain. Once I explain how they work, they usually feel comfortable trying one. Indeed, many have had good results from these medicines.

Amitriptyline (Elavil), nortriptyline (Pamelor), and desipramine (Norpramin) are commonly prescribed TCAs. They raise the levels of the chemical messengers (neurotransmitters) norepinephrine and serotonin in the blood by blocking their absorption (often referred to as "reuptake"). In turn, pain sensations are dampened. Both research and clinical experience show that these drugs can substantially reduce neuropathic pain conditions such as diabetic neuropathy and postherpetic neuralgia. In practice, these drugs can help treat many chronic pain syndromes such as migraine headaches, trigeminal neuralgia, radicular pain (shooting pain down the arm or leg), and facial pain. Studies also show a lowering of pain intensity for patients with chronic low back pain taking TCAs. For those with fibromyalgia, TCAs can help with pain, sleep, and fatigue, especially amitriptyline and a structurally similar drug called cyclobenzaprine (Flexeril).

Although most of their pain-relieving qualities are attributed to the increased levels of serotonin and norepinephrine, TCAs also interact with other receptors (including calcium, sodium, NMDA, and histamine), which may contribute to their analgesic affects. TCAs are gradually increased in dosage over time. Therefore, it can take several weeks before patients see an effect.

Patients with recent heart attack, epilepsy, hyperthyroidism, or urinary obstructions should not use TCAs because of possible complications. Frequent side effects include dry mouth and sedation; constipation, palpitations, blurred vision, drowsiness, lightheadedness and increased sweating can also occur. These drugs should be used cautiously in patients with cardiac rhythm problems. I've found that nortriptyline (Pamelor) combines good pain-relieving qualities with fewer side effects, especially in older adults. Pain often leads to sleep disturbances and anxiety, and I've seen these drugs help patients sleep at night and lessen their anxiety level. TCAs can lead to weight gain, so be sure to monitor this effect.

Another group of antidepressants used for pain control are the serotonin–norepinephrine reuptake inhibitors (SNRIs). Duloxetine (Cymbalta) is helpful for neuropathic pain conditions such as diabetic peripheral neuropathy (DPN) as well as musculoskeletal pain and fibromyalgia. I prescribe this drug for low back pain and neck pain too. Venlafaxine (Effexor) has evidence for treating DPN, and milnacipran (Savella) is used primarily for patients with fibromyalgia.

## Anticonvulsants

Also known as anti-epileptics, the anticonvulsant drugs (ACDs) are the most commonly used drugs for treating both epilepsy and neuropathic pain. There are dozens of anticonvulsants, but some of the more commonly prescribed for pain include gabapentin (Neurontin), topiramate (Topamax), carbamazepine (Tegretol), and pregabalin (Lyrica). Gabapentin and pregabalin are the two most often used for pain. These medicines block nerve hyperexcitability by modulating neurotransmitters such as GABA and glutamate, changing electrically activated channels inside cell membranes and influencing signals inside cells. Scientists believe the anticonvulsants are effective in treating neuropathic pain because its mechanism ("neuronal hyper-excitability") is similar to that of epilepsy. Because of their safety and good tolerability, many physicians turn to gabapentin or pregabalin as first choice medicines for any type of neuropathic pain.

Not only are ACDs effective in controlling neuropathic pain conditions such as postherpetic neuralgia (PHN), diabetic peripheral neuropathy (DPN), and spinal cord injury (SCI), they offer patients with migraine and fibromyalgia relief as well. Topiramate (Topamax) is specifically used for migraine prevention.

Like the TCAs, ACDs are gradually increased in dosage over time so it can take some time before patients see an effect. Don't give up if it's been a week or two and your pain hasn't changed. It may require two weeks or more before the drugs reach therapeutic levels in the blood.

Side effects of anticonvulsants vary depending on the specific medication and may include drowsiness, dizziness, weight gain, memory and concentration problems, and swelling in the feet. Once the medication is stopped, these problems resolve. In my experience, patients seem to experience fewer side effects with pregabalin, but patients can vary in their response to medications.

## Muscle Relaxants

Muscle relaxants, also known as antispasmodics, are typically used to treat acute pain associated with muscle tension and spasms. They can help ease musculoskeletal problems such as acute low back pain or muscle strain. In patients with spinal cord injury or multiple sclerosis, they can also be effective in controlling spasticity. Not many muscle relaxants are used for chronic pain; those that are include baclofen (Lioresal), cyclobenzaprine (Flexeril), tizanidine (Zanaflex), methocarbamol (Robaxin), metaxalone (Skelaxin), and carisoprodol (Soma).

A muscle spasm is an abrupt, involuntary muscle contraction. Muscle relaxants relieve pain by decreasing the frequency and intensity of muscle spasms. Although different muscle relaxants work in different ways, most seem to sedate patients, as opposed to acting directly on the muscles in question. Baclofen (Lioresal) is given orally and also administered into the spinal fluid through an implanted pump to treat spasticity from spinal cord injury, or multiple sclerosis. It can be quite effective in lowering muscle tone in people with these conditions, especially if there are limited results from taking the medication orally.

Tizanidine (Zanaflex) is also used for spasms due to spinal cord injury or multiple sclerosis. It inhibits motor nerves and decreases sympathetic nervous system activity, making it potentially helpful for neuropathic pain as well. Many of the other muscle relaxants work by inhibiting nerve activity in the spinal cord, but the exact mechanisms aren't clear. Unbeknownst to many patients and doctors, the muscle relaxant carisoprodol (Soma) is metabolized to meprobamate, a barbiturate, and therefore has abuse potential.

Muscle relaxants can work well in combination with other kinds of pain medications. For example, muscle spasms may accompany inflammation, so a nonsteroidal anti-inflammatory drug (NSAID) may bring added relief.

Common side effects of muscle relaxants include drowsiness, weakness, dizziness, dry mouth, and frequent urination.

# Opioids

Opioids are some of the oldest pain medications in use. We know that humans cultivated opium poppies as early as 3400 BCE In general, opioids mimic the activity of molecules called endorphins that we produce in our body. Endorphins bind to certain receptors in the brain, spinal cord, and even to nerves in other parts of the body, such as the knee, to reduce pain. Opioids also have the ability to dull our emotional response to pain.

There are many opioid medications available in the United States. Some, such as hydrocodone, last for relatively short periods of time whereas others are formulated to last for longer periods of time. The latter include medications such as extended-release oxycodone (Oxy-Contin), fentanyl (Duragesic) patch, or extended-release morphine (MS Contin). Most are available orally as pills, but certain opioids come in liquids, and now lozenges, sublingual sprays, sublingual tablets, nasal sprays, a film placed inside the lining of the cheek, or transdermal patches (fentanyl or buprenorphine [Butrans]). Across the world and especially in developing countries, only a few opioids are available and are primarily given for end-of-life care or cancer pain.

Opioids all work to relieve pain the same way, by acting on the opioid receptors. However, all patients do not experience the same level of pain relief from the same dose of opioid medication or from the same opioid, just as all patients do not experience identical levels of pain from the same disease or injury. As a result, doctors sometimes "rotate" from one opioid to another if a patient can't tolerate a particular drug due to side effects or if a specific opioid doesn't ease pain despite increasing the dose.

## Opioid Benefits and Harms

Opioids are the gold standard for reducing acute and postoperative pain. They also provide much-needed relief for patients with cancer pain as we discuss in detail in in Chapter 12, Cancer Pain and Caregiving. However, opioid use and benefit for treating chronic, non-cancer pain is controversial due to fears of abuse, addiction, and overdose deaths involving these medications.

Recently, the media and the government have highlighted the number of deaths related to opioid pain relievers. For example, the Center for Disease Control and Prevention (CDC) reported 18,893 opioid-related deaths in the United States in 2014. This is higher than the peak number of deaths reported in 2011, which was 16,917. These figures are very concerning and have led to a growing consensus that opioids are not appropriate for most patients with chronic, non-cancer pain. The primary concern of the CDC is the association between rising rates of opioid prescribing and escalating opioid-related side effects and deaths. Even though some of these opioid-related deaths also resulted from the combination of opioids plus other drugs such as benzodiazepines and alcohol, the non-medical use of prescription opioids is a major public health problem. Non-medical use means using opioids that are not prescribed for you or taking them to produce an experience other than pain relief (reduce anxiety, get to sleep, get "high").

In response to this public health problem, the CDC has issued guidelines for opioid prescribing in chronic pain. The guidelines include starting with immediate-release opioids instead of extended-release, providing patients with a three-day supply or less of opioids after surgery, and reassessing benefit and risks of 50 mg or more of equivalent daily morphine doses. Certain states are mandating adherence to the guidelines or creating their own stricter policies that limit opioid use.

Unfortunately, patients are feeling some harsh effects of these guidelines. As an example, a recent online survey of 3100 chronic pain patients shows that most believe the guidelines are negatively impacting them. They state that it is difficult to find doctors to treat their pain and that their pain is worsening because doses are lower. Forty percent of the online survey respondents state that they have considered suicide.

Pain is also a public health problem and in many cases it is clearly untreated or undertreated which was made clear by an Institute of Medicine Report in 2011. This report also indicates that prescription opioids may be an important element to treatment. Ultimately, our approach needs to balance both of these competing public health problems by decreasing non-medical opioid use and maintaining access to opioids when indicated.

Given the competing concerns and downward pressure on prescribing, a growing number of physicians and other healthcare professionals are viewing only a minority of patients with chronic, non-cancer pain as candidates for opioids. More practitioners will probably offer non-opioid and maybe non-drug therapy first to patients in chronic pain. Exercise, cognitive behavioral therapy (CBT), and weight loss are some of the first line therapies the CDC guideline recommends. It makes sense to consider opioids when pain is severe and unresponsive to other therapies (injection therapies, other medications, integrative strategies), negatively impacts function or quality of life, and will likely outweigh the potential harms.

Doctors are encouraged to do risk profiles before prescribing opioids long-term so that the medicines can be tailored to each patient according to level of risk. Opioid agreements, urine drug monitoring, and prescription monitoring programs offer methods of controlling risk that provide a higher level of safety for patients. The idea behind these risk-reduction strategies is to curb the use of opioids for non-medical purposes. Since 85% of addictions have expressed themselves by age 35, older patients with no prior history of addiction are typically much lower risk. And we cannot forget that people with an addictive or abuse

history who also suffer from unrelenting pain still need to have their pain treated.

## Opioid Addiction

Addiction is a complicated and individual phenomenon that is not widely understood. It is a chronic, neurological, and biological disease that has a strong genetic predisposition and is also influenced by environmental factors. Addiction takes hold when a drug with rewarding properties is introduced to vulnerable individuals at a vulnerable time in their lives. Risk factors include things such as a family or personal history of abuse, active psychiatric disorders, such as anxiety or depression, and being 45 years old and younger, as well as a lack of supportive family relationships.

Some patients do get into trouble for illegal use or non-medical use, but in my experience most chronic pain patients do not develop an addiction to opioids. Several experts estimate the risk of addiction in the general population to be about 10% and some researchers have concluded that abuse/addiction ranges from 3% to 19% in patients with chronic pain. The percentage may be even lower, though. One study indicates that addiction may be somewhere between 3% to 5% in patients who don't already have a history of substance abuse.

Some researchers and policymakers believe that a big rise in heroin use (147% increase since 2007) is due to the practices designed to curb non-medical opioid use. The thinking is that addicts are substituting heroin for opioids. The available evidence does not show this link, though. People have likely been driven to heroin because the cost is cheaper, it is more accessible, and has high purity.

## Opioid Risk Reduction Strategies

Safety precautions must be taken for all patients on chronic opioid therapy. Most pain specialists use opioid agreements, count pills during office visits for refills, check prescription monitoring programs, perform urine drug monitoring, check hormone levels intermittently, and assess a patient's potential for abuse with questionnaires. In my experience, patients may misuse an opioid medication by using it too often or for the wrong purpose (for example, as a sleep aid) and need to be reminded to take the medication as prescribed and for the intended effect (pain relief). If patients can't adhere to the treatment plan, divert the medication (sell it), forge signatures on prescriptions, or admit that they abuse the opioid to "get high," I discontinue the drug and may consult one of my colleagues specializing in substance abuse.

Addiction is a chronic disease that incorporates genetic, social, and neurobiological factors and leads patients down the path of losing control over drug use, compulsive use, continued use despite harmful consequences, and craving. On the few occasions that patients of mine develop the disease of addiction or abuse the medication, I refer them to addiction medicine specialists so proper treatment can begin.

Pharmaceutical companies with the support of the FDA have produced and continue to develop abuse deterrent opioids to help reduce the risk of non-medical misuse and abuse. Their focus is on decreasing the risk of abuse with extended-release opioids. Unfortunately, abusers can tamper with these tablets to release high doses of the drug by crushing or dissolving them. New technologies are designed to resist tampering by making it very hard to crush, chew, snort, or inject them intravenously.

Accidental ingestion by non-patients is also a public health concern that abuse deterrent formulations can address. For instance, children as young as one year of age have been known to put OxyContin tablets or other long-acting opioids in their mouths and chew them before swallowing which greatly increases the risk of serious side effects, especially death.

It's too early to know whether the abuse deterrent intervention will make a meaningful difference in the misuse, abuse, and overdose deaths related to opioids that are taken non-medically. However, early research on extended release oxycodone (OxyContin) provides some hope. Data have shown a substantially reduced interest in abusing it since the drug was reformulated as an abuse-deterrent opioid. Still, there is major need to address the underlying causes of substance abuse, such as despair and disengagement from society, depression, and anxiety. These fuel the desire for escapism and experimentation with legal and illegal drugs of abuse. Substance abuse and addiction are not due to the drug itself. It stems from the rewarding properties of the drug in a vulnerable person.

We discussed the biologic therapies in the context of osteoarthritis and rheumatoid arthritis in Chapters 3 and 4. Biologic therapies are vaccines, special enzymes, and monoclonal antibodies (special antibodies that bind to a molecule) used to treat diseases. These therapies offer similar promise for treating the abuse of opioids and stimulants, such as cocaine and nicotine. By preventing drugs of abuse from entering the central nervous system, these biologics can prevent and treat addiction. Because these biologic molecules don't travel to the brain, they instead bind or degrade the drug itself in the bloodstream, preventing it from achieving its effect. Several animal and some human studies show the exciting potential of these biologics in reducing overdose and curbing abuse.

## Using Opioids Wisely

When I counsel patients, I focus on making sure they take opioid medications as directed rather than as they "feel like" taking them. If patients of mine misuse or abuse opioids, they typically do so by swallowing too many tablets rather than altering them to snort or inject. Nevertheless, opioids can cause harm and any intervention that promotes safer use is important.

Keep in mind that opioids rarely provide 100% pain relief. Some studies mention that patients may only get as much as 35% relief and don't achieve higher levels of function or quality of life. Most of the research supports short-term use but lacks evidence for long-term improvement in pain or function for chronic, non-cancer pain. When patients aren't benefitting from opioids, they should be tapered gradually and stopped. On the other hand, while 35% relief may seem like limited reduction in pain, many of my patients would welcome an even 20%

improvement in their discomfort. For patients with cancer pain, opioids can be indispensable.

Opioids can be classified in many different ways, including abuse potential. Morphine (MSIR, MS Contin), oxycodone (Percocet, OxyContin), fentanyl (Duragesic), and methadone (Dolophine) are considered to have high abuse potential. Abuse potential with codeine (Tylenol #3) and buprenorphine (Butrans) is considered moderate and with tramadol (Ultram) is considered low.

As noted earlier, all patients using opioids long term should be carefully monitored for signs of misuse, abuse, or addiction, which are different from physical dependence and tolerance, both of which occur as a natural process of using opioids therapeutically. Physical dependence means that a patient will experience withdrawal when the opioid is stopped abruptly or if the dose is reduced quickly. It usually happens after two to 10 days of continual use of the drug. Tolerance means that larger doses of the drug are required to produce the same pain-relieving effect. Many patients confuse these words and tell me they're afraid of becoming "addicted" to an opioid that I may recommend as a therapy.

Opioids were believed not to produce a "ceiling effect"—the problem of increasing doses of medication with smaller incremental benefit. Animal and some human research have discovered that this might not be true. That is, larger doses and long-term treatment can lead to more pain, a problem known as opioid-induced hyperalgesia, the cause of which is unclear. These medications do have other side effects too, including drowsiness, dizziness, nausea, mental fogginess, respiratory depression, and constipation. Lesser-known side effects that patients should be aware of include fractures in older adults, hormonal effects, such as decreased cortisol and lower testosterone levels in men as well as menstrual changes in women, and opioid-induced hyperalgesia, when patients feel more pain rather than less pain from opioids. One useful strategy for opioid-induced hyperalgesia is to reduce the dose of the opioid analgesic or even stop it altogether which isn't easily accepted by patients.

Another lesser-known concern about opioids relates to possible immunosuppression. For instance, research findings in the laboratory and in animals have found a *possible* association between certain opioids (morphine, methadone, fentanyl) and the risk of infection. Another study in patients with rheumatoid arthritis revealed more hospitalizations from serious infections when opioids were started or continued compared to periods of nonuse. However, it's not yet clear how these immunosuppressive effects translate into a clinically meaningful risk of infection when opioids are used more broadly for patient care.

For women of childbearing age, exposure to opioids during pregnancy may be associated with a small increase in rare birth defects of the heart, intestines, and spinal cord. Many of these birth defects develop during the first few weeks of pregnancy, exactly when most pregnan-cies are not recognized. This means that all women who could become pregnant are at risk, and both doctors and female patients should make sure to discuss prescription opioid use before and during pregnancy. Certainly, opioids may be needed for pain, surgery, or infections while pregnant, but it's important to know about the risks of prenatal opioid exposure, including neonatal withdrawal, and to weigh the beneficial effects versus the adverse effects of these medications.

## Medical Marijuana: Uses and Controversy

One of the oldest documented medicines in history, marijuana has many therapeutic uses. It has been used by people over the ages to:

- manage pain, including the pain of childbirth
- relieve muscle spasms and the spasticity of multiple sclerosis
- reduce nausea
- ease irritable bowel syndrome
- stimulate the appetite
- control glaucoma

Unfortunately, marijuana is also the most commonly used illegal substance in the United States and the world. Because of this, its medicinal use is controversial, both in the eyes of the general public and in the medical community. Some believe that marijuana has no medicinal properties that cannot be obtained just as effectively with standard pharmacological therapies. Others believe that restricting or banning marijuana's use condemns countless individuals to needless and inhumane suffering. More recent studies highlight that medical marijuana does indeed have moderately good analgesic and antispasmodic effects and may help with sleep. Medical marijuana is already legal in several U.S. states and it may soon become a more common treatment option if it is ultimately approved by the FDA.

Cannabis is a flowering plant and a species of that plant, *Cannabis sativa*, contains chemical compounds called cannabinoids used for medical and recreational purposes. Cannabinoids are derived from plants (nabiximols), synthesized by pharmaceutical companies (dronabinol, nabilone), or produced inside the body (endocannabinoids). Pharmaceutical cannabinoids are cannabinoid-based medicines such as dronabinol (Marinol), nabilone (Cesamet), and nabiximol (Sativex). The popular term "medical marijuana" refers to using marijuana or cannabinoids as a medical treatment for diseases or alleviating symptoms from diseases. As a patient, this may mean receiving a medical marijuana certificate or recommendation in a state where it is legal to use. The specifics beyond its general approval for medical use are lacking—such as whether it should be smoked, vaporized, taken orally, in what dose and how often—because that would resemble a prescription, which doctors can't write.

Various forms of marijuana can be smoked, inhaled as a vapor, taken orally, absorbed topically, or given intravenously. There are differences in how the drugs act on the body (oral versus inhaled), contents of the active ingredients (tetrahydrocannabinol [THC] versus cannabidiol), and the source of the drug (plant-based versus synthetic). Dispensaries are not currently subject to federal government standardization, so the potency of the marijuana now being sold legally in certain states can vary greatly.

As a result of its historically limited legal use in medicine, very few studies exist examining appropriate dosing and levels of potency, or comparing the effectiveness of the form (oral, inhaled, or smoked, for example) in which marijuana is taken. Thus, patients have had to experiment to determine which methods and levels of treatment work best.

Patients with multiple sclerosis (MS), spinal cord injury, pain from HIV, fibromyalgia, and arthritis have all reported relief from using medical marijuana. The strongest scientific evidence for pain relief exists for cancer pain, but neuropathic pain from MS, HIV, and trauma also shows positive outcomes. Some studies indicate that medical marijuana can lessen chronic pain by 30% or more.

For Montel Williams, the Emmy award-winning host of *The Montel Williams Show*, marijuana can make the difference between sound sleep and a night filled with agony. He uses cannabis to control the pain and spasms that arise from his multiple sclerosis (MS). Williams has become a vocal advocate for the therapeutic benefits of marijuana and is pushing for full legalization.

After years of frustrating and baffling symptoms, Williams was officially diagnosed with MS in 1999. The pain was worst in his lower extremities and caused his left leg in particular to become weakened. He also developed agonizing trigeminal neuralgia on the right side of his face, producing lightning bolt-like pain that lasted as long as 25 or 30 minutes at a time. The pain woke him up at night, and for many years he got no more than four or five hours of continuous sleep. Sometimes these bursts of pain would even strike when he was on camera, and he would have to fight to keep his reaction under control.

Williams tried countless forms of pain management, including opioids and psychological treatments. In a letter advocating for medical marijuana, Williams explained:

"My doctors wrote me prescriptions for some of the strongest painkillers available. I took Percocet, Vicodin, and OxyContin on a regular basis—knowingly risking overdose just trying to make the pain bearable. But these powerful, expensive drugs brought me no relief. I couldn't sleep. I was agitated, my legs kicked involuntarily in bed, and the pain was so bad I found myself crying in the middle of the night.

All these heavy-duty narcotics made me almost incoherent. I couldn't take them when I had to work, because they turned me into a zombie. Worse, all of these drugs are highly addictive, and one thing I knew was that I didn't want to become a junkie. When someone suggested I try marijuana, I was skeptical—but desperate. To my amazement, it worked when these other legal drugs failed. Three puffs and within minutes the excruciating pain in my legs subsided. I had my first restful sleep in months."

For the past several years, Williams has found that marijuana offers him effective pain relief that allows him to work. Williams may smoke it or vaporize it for immediate relief of spasticity or consume it orally for help with pain that prevents him from sleeping well. He does not experience euphoria but rather an immediate cessation of twitching and a buffering of his pain.

## The Effects of Marijuana

There are several psychoactive cannabinoids in *Cannabis sativa*. The one responsible for many of the drug's effects is delta-9-tetrahydrocannabinol (THC). Others found in the plant include cannabidiol (CBD) and cannabinol (CBN). As noted earlier, all of these substances are derived from cannabis and are termed cannabinoids, which is any substance that acts on cannabinoid receptors.

In the 1990s, scientists discovered that our bodies actually produce chemicals—called endocannabinoids—which are cannabinoid substances very similar to THC. These chemicals bind to specific receptors in the body that are associated with sleep, appetite, memory, and pain regulation. More specifically, the body contains cannabinoid receptors called CB1 and CB2. CB1 receptors are located mainly in the brain, spinal cord, and nerves, whereas CB2 receptors are predominantly located in the immune system (spleen and tonsils, for example).

When the psychoactive components from cannabis—THC, CBD, CBN—or the endocannabinoids bind to CB1 receptors, they dampen excessive nerve activity and reduce pain. When CB2 receptors are turned on, they reduce inflammation and activity in the spinal cord, and can protect nerves from damage.

Recreational marijuana users treat the drug differently than medical users. They generally want to experience a euphoria ("a high") and a sense of relaxation. Along with those psychoactive effects, they also experience an increased heart rate (and other cardiovascular effects), dryness of mouth, and reddening of the eyes. Other acute effects of the drug (occurring within minutes of use and lasting for a couple of hours) include distractibility and impaired short-term memory. The inability to focus may lead in turn to slower reaction time to unexpected stimuli. Recreational marijuana users may also experience increased appetite and weight gain, a distorted sense of time, paranoia, anxiety, and depression. Men may notice lower testosterone levels, decreased sex drive, and lower sperm count and quality. It can disrupt the reproductive system of women as well.

Smoking marijuana is also known to irritate the lungs, and many studies show an increase in wheezing, coughing, and phlegm production in users. Other research notes a higher risk of bronchitis. Some patients worry about lung cancer, but the evidence is mixed and not particularly strong. Patients can avoid the toxic by-products of combustion by vaporizing (heating up the dried plant until the cannabis vaporizes on the surface) cannabis rather than smoking it. Much lower concentrations of carbon monoxide and other toxins are produced this way, which lessens the risk to the lungs.

Heavy or long-term marijuana use can lead to abuse and addiction, but at a lower rate than tobacco, alcohol, or cocaine, for instance. It's estimated that the lifetime risk of cannabis addiction is about 6%. Withdrawal can occur, but symptoms are less intense than withdrawal symptoms of other drugs. Demand for treatment for marijuana addiction has been growing rapidly worldwide. The potency (concentration of THC) of street marijuana has also been steadily increasing over the years (from 3% to 12%), which some speculate has led to greater rates of addiction. The standard treatment for marijuana abuse is outpatient counseling. Research is being done to investigate pharmacological therapies that would help with addiction and withdrawal symptoms.

## Marijuana Benefits and Concerns

Studies on the medical use of different forms of cannabis confirm Montel Williams' experience; many patients report significant pain-relieving effects and improvement in sleep, muscle stiffness, and spasticity. Many of the negative side

effects such as sedation, dizziness, dry mouth, nausea, or concentration problems were mild to moderate and did not last long. Cannabinoids also don't slow breathing down or lead to constipation.

Williams insists he has experienced very few negative side effects from using medical marijuana to treat his MS pain. He uses relatively little—just enough to take the edge off his symptoms and not nearly enough to experience euphoria. Williams says he has experienced no brain mass loss, no memory problems, no lethargy and confusion, or inhibited performance in his work.

Although there are risks, it seems that medical marijuana does indeed offer relief for some conditions that other drugs do not. Most patients don't report serious side effects either. Unfortunately, the political and medical controversy over use as well as its status as an illegal substance at the federal level has hampered research efforts and curbed drug development. Clearly, much more research needs to be done to investigate the benefits and side effects of medical therapy. Chronic pain is associated with the worst quality of life compared to other diseases such as chronic heart, lung, or kidney disease, and the risk of suicide is nearly doubled. Given the need for additional pain-relieving options, it's more than reasonable to consider medical marijuana as one of those choices for certain ongoing painful conditions.

Some groups, like the Canadian Family Physicians recommend that smoked cannabis only be used by patients after oral pharmaceutical cannabinoids such as nabiximol (Sativex) and nabilone (Cesamet) have failed. Unfortunately, there isn't much support from major medical societies for medical marijuana, nor is there direction from clinical studies on when to offer it as a therapy for pain. Some articles suggest waiting until previous evidence-based therapies fail. Federally, marijuana has no accepted medical use and a high potential for abuse even though it is legal in certain states. In addition, there are no standards for use at this point—what forms (smoked, oral), what cannabinoid (THC, CBD), at what dose, at what potency (% THC or other active ingredient), and what frequency should doctors incorporate medical marijuana into treatment for chronic pain? These knowledge gaps make many physicians uncomfortable recommending marijuana at this time. In the future, there is a strong interest in developing pharmaceutical cannabinoid medications derived from marijuana that maximize its pain and spasticity relief while minimizing the negative side effects.

You can learn more about pharmacological therapies by listening to the related episodes of my weekly radio program, *Aches and Gains*. You can find the broadcasts on pharmacological therapies at the following URLs.

**Pain and Addiction**

**Christopher Kennedy Lawford**

http://paulchristomd.com/addiction-pain

**Chris Herren**

http://paulchristomd.com/addiction-opioids-and-recovery

http://paulchristomd.com/addiction-opioids-and-recovery-2

**Opioids**

http://paulchristomd.com/war-on-opioids

http://paulchristomd.com/war-on-opioids-2

**Medical Marijuana with Montel Williams**
http://paulchristomd.com/medical-marijuana

## Suggested Further Reading

Backes, Michael. *Cannabis Pharmacy: The Practical Guide to Medical Marijuana*. (n.p.): Black Dog & Leventhal, 2014. Accessible book on the use and benefits of medical marijuana. http://tinyurl.com/y7tfsjef

Ballantyne, Jane, Tauben, David J. (eds). *Expert Decision Making on Opioid Treatment*. (n.p.): Oxford University Press, 2013. This book aims to provide expert opinion on how to manage common scenarios involving opioid management of chronic pain. http://tinyurl.com/y75ey2x2

Blesching, Uwe. *The Cannabis Health Index: Combining the Science of Medical Marijuana with Mindfulness Techniques To Heal 100 Chronic Symptoms and Diseases*. (n.p.): North Atlantic Books, 2015. This book presents evidence that cannabis is effective when used within the proper therapeutic window, especially compared with the risks of managing chronic symptoms with pharmaceuticals. http://tinyurl.com/yd5e5pyx

Casarett, David. *Stoned: A Doctor's Case for Medical Marijuana*. (n.p.): Current, 2015. In this book, palliative care physician, Dr. David Casarett, sets out to find evidence of marijuana's medical potential. http://tinyurl.com/y8quffan

Darnall, Beth. *Less Pain, Fewer Pills: Avoid the Dangers of Prescription Opioids and Gain Control Over Chronic Pain*. (n.p.): Bull Publishing Company, 2014. This book reveals the ramifications of using opioids and provides a low- or no-risk alternative. http://tinyurl.com/ybaabbdt

Darnall, Beth. *The Opioid-Free Pain Relief Kit: 10 Simple Steps to Ease Your Pain*. (n.p.): Bull Publishing Company, 2016. A self-help guide to reducing pain with less medication. http://tinyurl.com/y8lvtgj3

DeAngelo, Steve. *The Cannabis Manifesto: A New Paradigm for Wellness*. (n.p.): North Atlantic Books, 2015. This book is a case for cannabis as a wellness catalyst. http://tinyurl.com/ycace6w9

Federation of State Medical Boards. *Guidelines for the Chronic Use of Opioid Analgesics,* 2017. https://tinyurl.com/ycy8bcb8

Katz, Martin M. *Clinical Trials of Antidepressants: How Changing the Model Can Uncover New, More Effective Molecules.* (n.p.): Springer, 2016. This brief guide re-conceptualizes the clinical trial process with case studies and a review of salient depression scales. http://tinyurl.com/yack2595

Kramer, Peter D. *Ordinarily Well: The Case for Antidepressants.* (n.p.): Farrar, Strauss and Giroux, 2017. Peter D. Kramer addresses the growing mistrust of antidepressants among the medical establishment and the broader public. http://tinyurl.com/yc5chfu4

## Other Resources to Explore

Choosewisely.org is an initiative of the American Board of Internal Medicine with information about when opioids are needed to treat chronic pain.

Consumer Reports advice on treating chronic pain with opioids.

# 15

# Pain-Relieving Devices

Noah shattered his entire lower back in a tragic skydiving accident. Terry had a stroke that left him with burning pain all over the right side of his body. Lee had a spinal cord hemorrhage that led to constant stabbing pain from her chin to her feet. Stephen had three spinal surgeries to correct herniated discs and became a victim of failed back surgery syndrome. Kyla suffered from unrelenting fibromyalgia pain, and Colleen was miserable from idiopathic peripheral neuropathy.

All six of these individuals suffered from persistent pain that seemed immune to every treatment their doctors tried. Most of them became depressed and a few even contemplated suicide. Yet each found significant, and in some cases complete, relief from remarkable technologies that use electricity to stimulate the nervous system.

In this chapter, we discuss implanted devices that apply electricity to the nervous system—to the spinal cord, to the brain itself (the thalamus and the motor cortex), and to the vagus nerve. We also introduce other electrical devices—Transcutaneous electrical nerve stimulation (TENS) and Scrambler Therapy—that alter pain transmission by stimulating nerves on top of the skin, as well as an implantable pump that doesn't stimulate nerves, but instead delivers tiny amounts of pain medication directly into the spinal fluid.

These devices, with the exception of TENS and Scrambler Therapy, were typically considered treatments of last resort. Doctors turned to them only when everything else failed, because they involve surgery and some degree of risk.

But, in this chapter, we explore reasons why we may want to begin offering such treatments sooner and why they may actually be less risky and have fewer side effects than treatments like long-term opioid use.

These pain-relieving devices (neurostimulators) have evolved to the point where experts are recommending them earlier in the course of therapy for conditions such as complex regional pain syndrome (CRPS), certain neuropathic pain syndromes, and continual postoperative pain. Their growth has led to an estimated global market of $6.8 billion in 2017 and a predicted market value of approximately $4.6 billion in the United States alone by 2021.

The national concern over opioid use, abuse, and overdose for non-cancer pain has prompted the Centers for Disease Control and Prevention (CDC) to publish guidelines emphasizing non-drug therapies and non-opioid therapies for chronic pain. Among the list of these non-drug therapies recommended by the CDC are procedures like injections. Within the realm of procedures, it seems likely that more patients and physicians will turn to pain-relieving devices as an effective tool for easing chronic pain. In this chapter, we look at this tools in greater depth.

## Understanding the Nervous System and Chronic Pain

The nervous system is an electrical system. The central nervous system (the brain and spinal cord) and the rest of the body communicate through a series of electrical impulses. For example, the brain sends electrical impulses to the muscles to cause them to contract or relax, and the sensory nerves send electrical impulses back to the brain, which the brain interprets as tastes, smells, and other sensations. When you stub your toe, the sensory nerves in your foot send certain impulses to your spinal cord and brain, which the brain then interprets as painful.

In some chronic pain conditions, something goes wrong with these electrical impulses. The brain may misinterpret normal signals as pain, or damaged nerves may "misfire" and send abnormal pain signals to the brain—not unlike electrical wires shorting out.

It makes sense then to think of pain as partially an electrical problem within the body. Humans have known about the effectiveness of electricity for treating pain for thousands of years. For example, the ancient Egyptians, Greeks, and Romans applied electricity-generating fish (similar to electric eels) to painful areas of the body. The application of electrical impulses from a source outside the body seems to either intercept and block abnormal pain signals or change the way the brain interprets them. And today, new devices which function similarly to cardiac pacemakers, are able to modify or correct malfunctioning nerve impulses to relieve pain. Although the idea of a having an implanted machine generating electrical impulses can be scary, the voltage is extremely low and the devices are quite safe.

## Spinal Cord Stimulation (SCS)

Noah, a former member of the U.S. Army Golden Nights Parachute Team, hit the earth at 45 miles an hour when his parachute malfunctioned. Just before he crashed, Noah was able to tuck himself into a ball and take the impact to the side of the body. As the medevac unit rushed him to the hospital, the immediate threats to his life were his severed femoral artery and torn aorta. When he miraculously survived these injuries, Noah learned he had shattered his entire lower back from his fourth lumbar vertebra to his sacrum. When he recovered, he was left with constant stabbing pain in his low back and tailbone. Movement made it worse, forcing him to rely on a wheelchair most of the time.

Like Noah, Stephen was injured during his military service. After three back surgeries, he still felt electrical pains shooting down his legs—a classic symptom of failed back surgery syndrome. Dependent on opioids to make it through the day, Stephen began experimenting with chiropractic treatments and physical therapy to try to reduce his dosage.

Despite love and support from friends and family, both Noah and Stephen began to lose hope. Their rescue came from a spinal cord stimulator.

A spinal cord stimulator is a device consisting of a battery known as an implantable pulse generator (IPG) connected to thin wire leads placed on top of the spinal cord. Multiple circulator metallic electrodes, called contacts, are placed at the end of the leads. They deliver tiny "doses" of electrical current. The pulse generator—a thin 1 × 2 inch unit that's 0.4 inches thick—has a rechargeable battery and can be programed and charged remotely.

Spinal cord stimulation (SCS) began with experiments conducted in 1965, which revealed that small doses of electricity applied to the spinal cord could block pain signals within the cord itself. Although the mechanism by which this happens is still not completely understood, animal research suggests that the electricity may help prevent or reverse "central sensitization." Central sensitization refers to changes that occur in the spinal cord—due to injury or a chronic pain condition—that cause pain signals to be amplified. The stimulator device is thought to inhibit pain signals before they reach the brain. Interestingly, animal research also suggests that stimulating the spinal cord may also activate a region in the brain itself that contributes to suppressing pain.

Patients who are candidates for spinal cord stimulation undergo a trial period, during which a lead or leads are placed on the spinal cord through a needle and are left to protrude through the skin and connect to an external pulse generator. The stimulator remains in place for several days. Patients use it at home or at work. Once the test period ends, the leads are removed in the doctor's office. If the stimulator made a significant impact on pain or helped improve function, or sleep, or limited the need for pain medications, a permanent implantable pulse generator (IPG) device (battery) and the leads are implanted in the patient in the operating room.

The implantable pulse generator (IPG) is typically placed surgically in the upper buttock, and the leads are run under the skin to the spinal cord. With traditional "tonic" stimulation, patients feel a tingling sensation in the area of pain when the device is activated. This tingling sensation replaces the painful sensation. Newer modes of stimulation, referred to as "burst" or "high frequency," cause little or no sensations at all. The implant surgery takes place in the operating room usually over a two-hour period. Most patients return home the same day.

Unlike a cardiac pacemaker, which pulses only as needed to keep the heart rhythm regular, the spinal cord stimulator emits electricity constantly, and the strength can be adjusted by remote control. Some patients find they may need to adjust the current for certain body positions—standing, sitting, or lying down. Newer stimulators can even adjust their output automatically, based on the pattern of adjustments the patient makes over a period of time.

There are now six different companies that sell spinal stimulator devices in the

United States: Medtronic, Boston Scientific, St. Jude Medical, Nevro, Stimwave, and Nuvectra. Each one offers something unique. These innovations include the following:

♦ More contacts on the leads

♦ The ability to obtain an MRI of any part of the body after the device is implanted

♦ The ability to sense the body's position and automatically adjust the stimulation

♦ Software programming advantages that move current in a number of different patterns along the leads

♦ Special leads that can modify pain in a nerve bundle near the spinal cord called the dorsal root ganglion (a nerve bundle which is sort of like the grand central station for painful impulses traveling from the body to the spinal cord)

♦ High frequency stimulation that doesn't produce the typical tingling sensation in the body and can be especially beneficial for low back pain

♦ A wireless stimulator device that doesn't require an IPG (battery); and stretchable leads that offer better body compliance

## Choosing Spinal Cord Stimulation

Patients with unrelenting low back pain or leg pain may not be sure how to choose between a spinal cord stimulator and corrective back surgeries, such as laminectomies or vertebral fusions. Most doctors agree that surgery is probably the best option for isolated herniated discs that are pushing on nerves or when the back itself is physically unstable and compromising the spinal cord or spinal nerves, while pain caused by malfunctioning nerves will be better treated by spinal cord stimulation. Keep in mind that repairing or cutting injured nerves surgically often does not control neuropathic pain, and spine surgery for improving low back pain has yielded disappointing results, not to mention a new pain diagnosis known as failed back surgery syndrome. However, spine surgery is key if you're experiencing neurologic changes such as progressive weakness or bowel or bladder changes from spinal cord compression.

Some patients are worried that the pain relief from spinal cord stimulation will mask the worsening of an underlying condition, but doctors agree that spinal cord stimulation only "corrects" or modifies malfunctioning nerves; it does not mask the physical signs of bone, nerve, or tissue degeneration. Spinal cord stimulation has been most successful in treating neuro-pathic pain (covered in Chapter 4), including the typical burning pain and allodynia (extreme sensitivity to touch).

Approval for using SCS devices for pain or other conditions varies by country. In the United States, the FDA has approved SCS devices for chronic painful conditions of the trunk and/or limbs such as failed back surgery syndrome, complex regional pain syndrome, and radiculopathy (shooting pain down the arm, across the chest, or down the legs). In my experience, they can also help with other conditions such as nerve pain following hernia repair, post-herpetic neuralgia, and sometimes visceral pain of the abdomen or pelvis.

## Spinal Cord Stimulation and Pain Relief

Patients want to know how much re-lief SCS devices will give them. I tell them that the majority of patients experience about 50% or more relief. What's underappreciated is that there is a critical time period for offering this device after the chronic pain syndrome develops. That is, research shows that there is an 85% success rate if the stimulator is implanted less than two years after the beginning of specific chronic pain syndromes, compared to a mere 8% success rate if placed after 15 years or more of having pain. That's a big difference and highlights the need for a timely and accurate diagnosis, as well as greater awareness of pain-relieving devices.

It's important to know that pain relief from the device may be less effective over time. For instance, a patient may experience 70% relief during the first two years of therapy, and then notice that it drops to 50% in the third year. Disease progression, or spinal cord plasticity (adaptation of the nervous system) may account for this change. The most frequent complication relates to lead migration or connection failure with loss of pain relief, and then pain at the IPG site.

Both Noah and Stephen felt significant relief during their trial periods and had spinal cord stimulation devices implanted permanently. Both were fortunate that their doctors did not allow their pain to linger for years before offering spinal cord stimulation, since the longer pain goes without successful treatment, the less treatable it becomes. They were able to wean off their medications and return to normal physical activity, including rehabilitation exercises. They returned to work and school, and Noah even began sky diving again.

In the future, patients can look forward to all neurostimulation devices becoming smaller and the batteries longer-lasting. We may see the use of something called optogenetic neuro-modulation too. It's a fascinating technique that uses viruses to introduce genes into a nerve. That nerve then produces a protein which can turn the nerve off or on by using different wavelengths of light. The switching off or on may help to reduce pain. It is being tested on animals and in the early stages of development.

## Deep Brain Stimulation

Electrical stimulation of areas deep inside the brain—deep brain stimulation (DBS)—is used to treat severe tremors and movement disorders caused by conditions such as Parkinson's disease and other dystonias. Dystonias are neurological disorders that cause continual muscle contractions, twisting, or abnormal postures. When we talk about the "deep brain," we're referring to special regions called the thalamus as well as the periventricular gray and periaqueductal gray.

The DBS device used is nearly identical to the spinal cord stimulator, but the electrodes are placed in the thalamus, two walnut shaped masses located very close to the center of the brain, and in the periventricular and periaqueductal gray regions. The thalamus acts like a switchboard for sensory information such as pain and relays both sensory and motor signals from the body to higher brain areas. The DBS implantable pulse generator (IPG) is typically placed under the collarbone.

Before a DBS trial, the doctor orders a magnetic resonance imaging (MRI) or a computed tomography (CT) scan of the brain. These allow the neurosurgeon to develop a "map" of the various regions of the brain, and have a clear picture of where to implant the electrodes. The patient is sedated, and the shaved head is placed in a halo-like brace (stereotactic frame) to prevent it from moving. The scalp is opened, burr holes are drilled in the skull, and the electrodes are placed. Once the electrodes are placed, patients are awakened so they can respond to the surgeon's questions about whether the painful area is being covered and whether there are any side effects. Once the placement is confirmed, the lead wires are secured and the holes in the skull are plugged. After the DBS device is turned on, patients will not typically feel anything except—if the device works for them—pain relief.

Although not approved by the FDA for pain control, DBS has been used for over 40 years to treat certain kinds of unrelenting pain, but only rarely. It seems to work best for nerves that have been torn away under the arm (brachial plexus avulsion), facial neuropathic pain syndromes, post-stroke pain, cluster headaches, and in some cases, failed back surgery syndrome, particularly the leg pain component.

Unlike other forms of nerve stimulation, DBS involves penetrating the surface of the brain. It's invasive and reserved for those who don't respond to medicines, injections, or alternative therapies. Because DBS isn't approved for chronic pain control by the FDA, reimbursement from insurers is unlikely and funding for clinical research is tight. The risks of DBS include intracranial hemorrhage leading to stroke, headache, neurological injury, and infection, for example. Although not widely used, DBS has had remarkable success in individual patients.

Terry suffered a stroke that left him with the sensation that someone was constantly pouring scalding water over the right side of his body. He had to take sponge baths and wear loose fitting clothes. When lying down, he placed a pillow in between his feet so that his right leg wouldn't touch his left. Confined to his house, Terry spent each day moving from the bed to the recliner. That's it. After his stroke, Terry was unable to work, hunt, fish, or care for his land. Pain medicines brought little relief and left him feeling like a zombie. Unable to leave the house or get a good night's sleep, Terry actually considered suicide.

During Terry's DBS trial, he felt a small electrical shock, but then the pain started to melt away. He did experience some flashes in his right eye, but these went away with time. Although some patients may experience 40%–50% pain relief from DBS, Terry found his pain entirely gone. "It was like I was reborn," he said. Today, he gets about 90% relief and has stopped all of his pain medicines. Similar to other patients with DBS devices, he can exercise and work. Most importantly, he can visit with his grandchildren, work on his land, fish and hunt, and do all the things he loves to do. The physical limitations he does have are due to his stroke, not his DBS.

Although DBS involves brain surgery, it shows great promise for a small group of patients who would otherwise suffer tremendously. There's renewed interest for DBS as a pain therapy because it's been so successful in treating movement disorders. Research is also underway to test its efficacy in treating Alzheimer's disease, depression, stroke, and Tourette's syndrome.

## Motor Cortex Stimulation

Like DBS, motor cortex stimulation (MCS) also simulates the brain, but on the surface. Also like deep brain stimulation (DBS), MCS is not approved by the Food and Drug Administration for pain control. However MCS is particularly promising for central pain (pain following a stroke, for example), spinal cord injury pain, and the chronic neuropathic facial pain called trigeminal neuralgia. (This term refers to stabbing, burning, and unpleasant sensations along the nerves of the face, or along certain branches of the trigeminal nerve which supply sensation to either side of the face; it is discussed in more detail in Chapter 4, Neuropathic Pain). Patients with neuropathic pain that is burning and constant are the best candidates for MCS if all other treatments have failed.

The motor cortex is part of the brain involved with the planning and execution of voluntary movement. It is located in the back of the frontal lobe and sends electrical impulses to the spinal cord in order to move parts of the body. It's surprising that stimulating a part of the brain focused on movement can reduce pain, a sensory disturbance. Quite astonishingly, it can, but the mechanism isn't fully understood. A working theory is that exciting the motor cortex leads to a blockade of the pain-sensing nerves located in the main sensory area of the brain called the primary somatosensory cortex. MCS probably affects the thalamus (the switchboard area for pain processing) and other structures of the brain as well.

As with deep brain stimulation, patients having an MCS device implanted get an MRI to map the brain. They are then either awake or asleep for the placement of the electrodes on the brain. Doctors deliberately contract certain muscle groups to confirm the electrodes are placed correctly over the motor cortex. They are looking for the painful region of the body such as the face or arm to contract because this corresponds to the best analgesic effect. If patients are weak or paralyzed or lack sensation in the painful region they are not good candidates for MCS, unfortunately.

Once placement is confirmed, permanent electrodes are sewn into the dura (the membrane surrounding the brain) and the small opening in the skull is closed. Like DBS, the IPG is placed under the collarbone and the leads travel from the battery under the skin all the way to the brain. There is a mini plate that secures the lead to the outside of the skull. As with DBS and high frequency spinal cord stimulation, patients do not sense the stimulator when it's turned on. They just feel better.

Motor cortex stimulation is safer than deep brain stimulation, since the neurosurgeon doesn't actually penetrate the surface of the brain. Most studies report no side effects, but there are risks similar to those associated with DBS. The one difference is that MCS can cause a postoperative seizure. Patients aren't limited in what they can do after implantation either. For example, they can exercise, swim, play golf, or go bowling. One patient even went zip-lining.

Choosing between MCS and DBS for controlling chronic, unyielding pain can be tricky. Sometimes, either technique will help. In general, DBS seems to have a wider coverage of relief, and MCS is probably more effective at reducing pain in a specific area of the body, such as the face or arm, rather than the broadly defined area of the low back, for instance. We don't have any studies that compare these two for treating similar pain syndromes, which hampers our ability to guide patients. An analysis of MCS studies on patients with central neuropathic pain (pain from injury to the brain or spinal cord) found that 64% described significant pain relief. The best results seem to be in patients with neuropathic facial pain. Unfortunately, up to 40% of patients may lose the benefit over a year. This could result from neuroplastic changes in the brain or scar build up around the electrodes.

Along with other pain specialists, I believe that we should offer neurostimulation earlier in a patient's quest for pain relief. I have two reasons for this opinion. First, the longer chronic pain has persisted, the more difficult it is to treat. Second, there is growing evidence that most forms of nerve stimulation are safer and more cost effective than a lifetime of pain medications, which can lead to multiple side effects of their own. For example, studies show that SCS is cost effective when compared to conventional medical management (medicines, imaging, physical therapy, massage, and hospital admissions, for example) and that the higher costs of surgical implantation are recouped after about two years.

Unfortunately, because neither MCS nor DBS is FDA-approved for pain control, patients who find relief must often pay over $100,000 for a device, its implantation, and the associated hospital costs. Given that DBS and MCS may only help a small number of patients with chronic central pain (500 to 1000 a year,

for example), it is particularly challenging to find the tens of millions of dollars needed to conduct the large scale, randomized controlled clinical trials that the FDA requires for approval and widespread acceptance. Yet the delay leaves hundreds of patients each year who cannot afford the surgery living in perpetual agony. It is my hope that the FDA will approve both DBS and MCS for pain control based on humanitarian reasons and allow physicians to provide relief to patients who can benefit from them.

Lee experienced a spinal cord hemorrhage in her neck due to a surgical error that left her with extremely painful symptoms that mimicked those of post-stroke pain. Faced with burning and stabbing pain from her chin to her foot on the right side of her body, she had to give up practicing law and was barely able to care for her four young children. Lee dragged her right leg, had right arm weakness, and endured tremors on her right side. She had low quality of life. She missed family vacations. Just walking around the mall was a major endeavor.

Feeling completely robbed of her life, Lee became depressed, lost hope, and contemplated suicide. When she learned about neurostimulation, she wanted to try it. After spinal cord stimulation didn't work, she heard about motor cortex stimulation by accident. Because she did not fit the typical profile of a candidate for MCS, she had to search for quite a while until she found a doctor who was willing to consider this treatment.

Lee came home four days after her procedure feeling like a new person. "It's like a light switch was turned on," she said. The MCS device has stopped her tremors and produces substantial relief. It's dramatically changed her life. "I can chase my three-year-old now. I'd be in a nursing home taking medications all day otherwise," said Lee. She uses her stimulator 24 hours a day seven days a week and has done so for years. If she turns it off, within 10 minutes she develops a bad headache and the pain returns. Lee also uses pregabalin (Lyrica), hydromorphone (Dilaudid), fentanyl (Duragesic) patch, and oxycodone (Percocet), but she credits the motor cortex stimulator for giving her a new lease on life. "Don't be afraid to try MCS because it requires brain surgery. Don't let that limit you. The benefits can be much bigger."

## Vagus Nerve Stimulation

Vagus nerve stimulation (VNS) places electrodes of a nerve stimulator on the vagus nerve. The vagus nerve sits between a large artery and a vein in the neck. There are associations between the vagus nerve and many different brain functions related to the perception of pain. Interestingly, studies in animals have shown that VNS inhibits painful impulses traveling through the spinal cord. VNS involves a pacemaker-like generator implanted in the chest wall that is programmed to stimulate the vagus nerve in the neck. VNS is approved by the FDA for drug-resistant epilepsy and chronic depression and has been studied for its efficacy in treating chronic pain disorders such as migraines and cluster headaches.

The vagus nerve is the tenth cranial nerve. It starts in the brain, runs down the neck, behind the ear, and then splits into smaller nerves that extend throughout the body, branching to the heart, blood vessels, the gut, uterus, and every smooth muscle. This means that the vagus nerve and its branches are involved in all our involuntary movements including heart rate, breathing, sweating, and peristalsis (the contraction of the digestive tract). It also branches into the skeletal muscles of the larynx, so its stimulation affects speech. The vagus nerve has sensory fibers on the inside of the ear called the auricular branch too.

VNS began in 1997 to treat drug-resistant epilepsy. Not only was it extremely effective in controlling epileptic seizures, but it was also much less invasive than previous treatments, which involved disconnecting or removing parts of the brain. In 2005, VNS was approved for chronic or recurrent depression.

Kyla experienced widespread body pain from fibromyalgia that developed during her second pregnancy. In addition to nerve, muscle, and joint pain, she experienced irritable bowel syndrome, and general mental fogginess that robbed her of two years of memories, and disrupted sleep. Soon she had to give up working and began to rely on her mother and mother-in-law to help take care of her infant and toddler. Her husband couldn't touch her because pressure against her skin was so uncomfortable. She found the most relief from pregabalin (Lyrica), and tramadol (Ultram), while nonsteroidal anti-inflammatory drugs (NSAIDs) helped a bit and tai chi kept her calm. But she still spent about 80% of her day in bed. "I spent a lot time crying in bed and endured six years of hopelessness and pain," Kyla shared.

Kyla kept hope alive for the sake of her children and, after six years of suffering, she was invited to enroll in a vagus nerve stimulation (VNS) study on fibromyalgia at a nearby medical school. She agreed and went to the hospital to have an electrode wrapped around her left vagus nerve and a pulse generator placed under her collarbone. The neurosurgeon spent four hours implanting the device. It took her about four weeks to recover from the surgery, but the VNS was turned on after a week.

Like other forms of nerve stimulation, VNS is generally felt by the patient, especially at first. Kyla knew right away that hers was on, because her neck and throat tightened up. Unlike brain and spinal cord stimulators, which deliver a constant current, the VNS pulse generator sent electrical impulses to the vagus nerve in her neck for 30 seconds every five minutes, which initially triggered an uncontrollable cough for Kyla. Today, she has it set so the stimulator goes on every 10 minutes for 30 seconds. To sleep at night, she had to put a magnet over the stimulator to turn it off. She also noticed that her voice changed during the stimulation and that sometimes she couldn't speak at all from shortness of breath. Fatigue following the surgery took a while to improve too.

Other possible side effects of VNS include dry mouth, headache, facial pain, and bradycardia (slow heart rate). Kyla experienced some minor heartburn as well. Yet despite these challenges, Kyla found that within several months, her intense nerve pain and radiating joint pain faded away. Soon she could get out of bed without assistance, hug her husband and children, and do other activities that had seemed impossible before. The side effects continued to dissipate and she began to leave the stimulator on 24 hours a day. By the time the first year of the trial was over, she reported feeling "reborn." Seven years later, she's 80% better and feels that VNS has, "given me back who I am."

The results of the pilot study that Kyla was part of were very positive. Five of the patients saw their symptoms of fibromyalgia completely disappear, and others were able to cut back on their pain medications. A few experienced side effects that removed them from the study. Kyla is not completely pain free, but VNS has been a life-changing therapy for her. She still takes medications, but takes about 75 mg of pregabalin (Lyrica) per day instead of 350 mg, and two tramadol (Ultram) pills instead of 16 per day. Most importantly, she can go about her daily life and care for her children without assistance. She no longer worries about her short-term memory. The "brain fog" has lifted and her husband can hug her like he once did. She has returned to work and even earned her master's degree.

VNS may work by tuning down central sensitization or by affecting levels of pain neurotransmitters in the brain and spinal cord. Animal studies show increased levels of the neurotransmitters, serotonin and norepinephrine in the blood of those receiving stimulation. This is similar to the action of serotonin–norepinephrine reuptake inhibitor (SNRI) drugs, such as duloxetine (Cymbalta) and milnacipran (Savella), that are prescribed for fibromyalgia and other pain conditions. New evidence suggests that VNS may have great potential for inhibiting inflammation by suppressing the production of inflammatory molecules called cytokines, specifically tumor necrosis factor (TNF). This is exciting because it's prompted an interest in studying VNS for arthritis, colitis, and myocardial infarction (MI; heart attack).

European researchers have developed transcutaneous (placed over the skin instead of implanted) VNS devices. One of these, gammaCore, has been shown to reduce the symptoms of acute migraine attacks and may decrease the frequency of future attacks. It's approved in Europe for both migraine and cluster headaches. GammaCore is handheld and battery operated. Patients position it on one side of their neck and push a button to adjust the current delivery to the vagus nerve in the neck for about 90 seconds, three to four times a day. GammaCore is FDA approved for episodic cluster headaches in the United States. Another transcutaneous VNS device, NEMOS, stimulates the branch of the vagus nerve on the inside of the ear through an earpiece. It is used in Europe for treating epilepsy and preliminary studies show that it can reduce chronic pelvic pain.

VNS may help treat gastrointestinal pain, asthma, pain after stroke, and heart failure. Unfortunately, because VNS is not FDA-approved for pain relief and not covered by insurance, Kyla may lose her stimulator when the battery dies if she cannot find a neurosurgeon to replace it. Though the current pain market is small for VNS, we are just beginning to explore the science and application of this technology. It holds promise as a future therapy for several chronic pain conditions.

## Transcutaneous Electrical Nerve Stimulation

Transcutaneous electrical nerve stimulation (TENS) involves a device that applies electrical currents to the skin for pain relief. It's very safe and noninvasive. Patients place skin electrodes (like EKG pads) over the area of pain and turn on a small battery-driven device. Most of these units can be set to deliver high or low frequencies. Pulse duration can be controlled and they can be set to deliver burst stimulation or continuous stimulation. Usually,

patients feel a pins and needles sensation in the area under the electrodes. Research on this device has found variable results for managing chronic pain. For instance, several studies have shown benefit for musculoskeletal pain, but others have not. I find that a TENS unit helps some patients with low back pain or neck pain and others with neuropathic pain. The degree of relief seems mild to moderate in patients of mine who use it.

## Scrambler Therapy

Like transcutaneous vagus nerve stimulation (t-VNS), Scrambler Therapy (ST) is a new form of noninvasive electrical

stimulation. Some people confuse it with transcutaneous electrical nerve stimulation (TENS), because nerves are stimulated by placing electrodes over the skin. The difference is the type of nerves that are activated. Scrambler Therapy (ST) is believed to target nerves that sense pain, called C fibers whereas TENS activates nerves that conduct touch and pressure information, called A-beta fibers.

In 2014, ST was FDA-cleared for the treatment of neuropathic pain and cancer pain. Several studies of varying quality demonstrate dramatic pain relief without side effects for patients using ST. Patients included in these studies had intense hand and foot pain after chemotherapy (chemotherapy-induced peripheral neuropathy); visceral pain from pancreatic, colon, or gastric cancer; failed back surgery syndrome; complex regional pain syndrome (CRPS); post-herpetic neuralgia (chronic shingles pain); or chronic low back pain.

Doctors treating a patient with Scrambler Therapy gather as much information as possible about the original injury or problem to determine where to place the electrodes. The electrodes (similar to EKG pads) are placed above and below the painful area within a single dermatome, (an area of skin supplied by a single spinal nerve). The inventor, an Italian biophysicist, Giuseppe Marineo, believes that ST replaces painful signals with synthetic "non-pain" or "healthy" signals. It's like retraining the brain to believe that the pain is no longer there.

The device transmits a low-frequency electrical stimulation. As soon as the patient feels the vibration in the first pad, the doctor raises the stimulation intensity until the patient feels it in the second pad. Five sets of electrodes can be used. Electrodes are placed above and below the area of pain and the device usually runs for 30-45 minute sessions, during which patients report a tingling or humming sensation. Some patients feel tired afterwards. Typically, if the therapy is going to be effective, patients will experience relief with the first treatment.

Patients can receive only one ST treatment per day. Most doctors schedule new patients for five sessions a week for two weeks, a total of 10 treatments. Patients typically feel significant relief the first week, which increases the second week with many reporting a substantial drop in pain after completing the entire treatment protocol. Some patients have even achieved complete pain relief, and others find that the pain does not return at all. Generally, the beneficial effects last several weeks to months, but patients can get a "booster" Scrambler session that re-establishes the therapeutic effect for months or longer. Patients who treat their returning symptoms promptly may find that they can go longer without a booster session in the future.

Since the therapy is noninvasive and side effects are minimal, there aren't many disadvantages to trying ST. However, it can't be used on pregnant women, patients with epilepsy, or on anyone with cardiac stents or a pacemaker. It can be used on patients with implanted spinal cord stimulators and deep brain or motor cortex stimulators, but the stimulators must be turned off during ST. ST appears to be less effective when patients are already taking anticonvulsant pain medications, most likely because they interfere with the way ST modifies pain processing. As a result, patients on these drugs must stop taking them before beginning the therapy.

Colleen suffered from idiopathic peripheral neuropathy, which began as clumsiness and progressed to spasms in her legs and constant burning pain, especially in her feet. "It was like walking on a bed of hot coals," she said. In addition, it was hard to hold objects and she felt sad and just humiliated at times. She tried various drug therapies and did find some relief with the fentanyl (Duragesic) patch, diazepam (Valium), meditation, and guided imagery. But Scrambler Therapy (ST) changed her life.

During her first ST treatment, Colleen initially felt small vibrations from the electrodes against her skin. It was uncomfortable until the doctor reduced the magnitude of the stimulation. When she got up after treatment, she immediately felt like she had better balance. Soon, she discovered that 80%–90% of her pain was gone. "I was aware that my feet were no longer on fire, and I didn't have to grab anything to keep myself upright," she remarked.

By the end of Colleen's tenth session, the burning in her feet was completely gone, her balanced was restored, and she found she didn't need a booster session for a full year. Her relief was long-lasting until "I suddenly noticed that I was standing on hot pebbles," and that's when she knew she needed a booster. Her numbness didn't completely go away with ST, and she experiences occasional muscle spasms. Still, she's now free to travel and drive without worrying, and she is highly functional.

Although it has been used for about 20 years in Europe, there are unfortunately very few U.S. physicians certified in ST. As of this writing, the cost is approximately $2500 for 10 ST treatments, but it is increasingly covered by insurance and worker's compensation plans because patients have been able to return to work post-treatment. Good results rely on practitioner skill, so make sure if you pursue this option, you locate a doctor specifically trained in this therapy.

## Pain Pumps

Pain pumps, also known as intrathecal drug delivery systems (IDDS) work differently from all the other devices discussed in this chapter. Instead of stimulating the nervous system with electrical impulses, they deliver tiny, controlled doses of pain medicine directly to the spinal cord. They have been used successfully since the 1980s, yet pain pumps remain a little-known alternative to standard medical management of pain from cancer or non-cancerous conditions.

Patients receiving a pain pump have a small battery-operated pump the size of a hockey puck surgically implanted under the skin in the abdomen. The pump is filled with pain medicine and connected to a small tube known as a catheter that delivers tiny amounts of that medicine into the spinal fluid. Because the medication goes directly to the spinal cord, very small doses can be quite effective. This allows for a faster and more effective response, smaller doses, and fewer side effects. It also offers doctors the ability to target a variety of pain receptors with drugs that can be uniquely administered through the spinal fluid (intrathecally). Most medications are several hundred times more potent delivered this way, compared to taking them orally.

There is good evidence that pain pumps can reduce pain, limit medication side effects, improve function, enhance quality of life, and probably improve survival in patients with cancer pain. This is welcome news for the more than 1.6 million new patients diagnosed with cancer each year in the United States alone. For patients with spasticity from spinal cord injury or even post traumatic brain injury, a medicine known as baclofen (Lioresal) can provide much needed muscle relaxation from excessive tone when given directly into the spinal fluid, and the data support its use. For chronic, non-cancer pain (failed back surgery syndrome or diabetic nerve pain, for instance), the potential value also exists, but the evidence is less strong.

In my experience, patients with abdominal pain from pancreatic cancer, cancerous tumors pressing on nerves, or cancer that is metastatic to the bone, for instance, particularly benefit from pain pumps. Some patients with persistent back pain and/or shooting leg pain (failed back surgery syndrome) are candidates as well, but interventional pain specialists are implanting fewer pumps due to declining reimbursement. The FDA has approved two programmable pumps: SynchroMed II (Medtronic) and Prometra II (Flowonix). Many times, oncologists don't refer patients for pumps because they aren't aware of their effectiveness or they believe the cost is too high. On the contrary, research shows that pain pumps are cost effective for cancer pain and non-cancer pain alike when compared to conventional medical management.

Non-cancer patients are only offered pain pumps when they haven't responded to anything else. Maybe that paradigm should shift toward an earlier consideration for pump therapy in appropriate patients rather than positioning it as a "last ditch effort" when controlling pain becomes tougher. We are learning that treating pain sooner can be more effective. For example, we already know

that patients have a much better chance of success with spinal cord stimulation when implanted less than two years after developing chronic pain. And there is growing evidence that cancer patients can not only enjoy a better quality of life earlier, but that adequate pain control can prolong their lives even with a terminal diagnosis.

Drugs used in pain pumps include opioids such as morphine and hydromorphone (Dilaudid), the antispasmodic called baclofen (Lioresal, Gablofen), and a synthetic form of the venom of marine snail called ziconotide (Prialt). Baclofen is particularly helpful for spasticity from multiple sclerosis, spinal cord injury, or post-traumatic brain injury. Doctors have also successfully used local anesthetics such as bupivacaine (Marcaine) and another drug called clonidine (Catapres). Clonidine can lower pain when placed in the spinal fluid but is used to treat hypertension when taken orally. While these and other drugs can be used alone, they are often combined to better address pain. This happens because each drug binds to a different pain receptor in the spinal cord. Prescribing morphine with bupivacaine, for instance, targets two pain generating signals compared to just one. Many patients report better pain relief with more than one drug too.

There can be side effects of pain pumps and the most common relate to bad reactions to the drugs. This can be corrected by lowering the dose, adding another drug, or just removing the drug from the pump altogether. It's critical to make sure you find a pain doctor who knows how to adjust pump medications and manage the many variables of pump therapy. It's delicate and much more precise than taking medicines by mouth. Other side effects are caused by the catheter or pump. Unlike the leads of spinal cord stimulators, we deliberately place the catheter of a pain pump into the spinal fluid and this can cause a continuous leak in as many as 20% of patients. Unfortunately, a spinal headache can result, but it usually resolves by itself.

Be aware that opioids given into the spinal fluid can decrease female and male hormones or growth hormones leading to sexual dysfunction, reduced libido, or fatigue. It's a good idea to talk to your pain doctor about monitoring these hormones and treating any deficiencies. Rarely, granulomas (a benign growth that forms at the tip of catheter) can form.

As of this writing, the average life of a pain pump is about 7 to 10 years. The pump then must be removed surgically and replaced with a new one. Newer external remotes allow the patient to self-administer a little extra dose of pain medicine during the day, and innovative catheters now better resist kinking or occlusion. Ongoing research into non-opioid drugs with different mechanisms for inhibiting pain will broaden our therapeutic options as well.

---

Graciela was plagued by extreme pain from multiple sources. She suffered from chronic pancreatitis and endometriosis, which led to a hysterectomy, and she had two vertebrae fused in her back following an injury (failed back surgery syndrome). Because she missed too many work days, she was fired from her job as a high school teacher. The pain robbed her of her dreams, hopes, and aspirations, and her husband said that she wasn't the person he married. That person was gone. After 12 years of pain patches and all sorts of pain pills in ever-increasing doses, along with physical therapy, nutritionists, and weight loss, she decided to try an implanted pain pump. A friend of hers had one and didn't do well, so Graciela was petrified. Yet, "I can't tell you how it saved my life," she said.

During her trial, or screening test, a catheter was inserted into the intrathecal space (the fluid containing space surrounding the spinal cord), and Dilaudid, an opioid, was delivered from an external pump. Graciela immediately felt better, although she had a mild spinal headache, which can be a normal side effect.

After she had the pump permanently implanted in her abdomen, Graciela felt her quality of life improve immediately. Her depression disappeared, her pancreatitis pain improved 50%, and her low back pain improved 90%. She no longer wakes up in pain or worries about running out of her medicines. She's been able to stop the antidepressants and the fentanyl (Duragesic) patch, but does need oral Dilaudid for breakthrough pain—spikes of intense pain occurring during the day. Graciela particularly benefited from having the opioid medication bypass her digestive system, which eased many of her gastrointestinal side effects, such as constipation.

After Graciela lost weight, the pump flipped around inside the surgical pocket, requiring a revision surgery to reposition it. Other than that, she has had no complications. Every two to three months, the pump medication runs out, so Graciela has it refilled. A thin needle goes through the skin to access the reservoir at which point any remaining solution is withdrawn before the new medication is injected. She can no longer sit in a hot tub (heating pads or hot tubs can increase the dose of medicine) and the pump protrudes a bit, but she can exercise, bend and twist carefully, and just started practicing yoga. The overall improvement in quality of life is well worth some of the limitations.

You can learn more about pain-relieving devices by listening to the related episodes of my weekly radio program, *Aches and Gains*. You can find the broadcasts on pain-relieving devices at the following URLs.

### Spinal Cord Stimulation

http://paulchristomd.com/pain-pacemakers

http://paulchristomd.com/innovations

**Deep Brain Stimulation**

http://paulchristomd.com/brain-stimulation

**Motor Cortex Stimulation**

http://paulchristomd.com/cortex-stimulation

http://paulchristomd.com/cortex-stimulation-2

**Vagus Nerve Stimulation**

http://paulchristomd.com/vagus-nerve-stimulation

http://paulchristomd.com/vagus-nerve-stimulation-2

**Pain Pumps**

http://paulchristomd.com/pain-pumps

# Suggested Further Reading

Chou, Kelvin L, Grube, Susan, Patil, Parag. *Deep Brain Stimulation: A New Life for People with Parkinson's, Dystonia, and Essential Tremor.* (n.p.): Demos Health, 2011. A case for no longer using DBS as a last resort treatment option, but rather using it earlier to improve quality of life for patients. http://tinyurl.com/y8gzvdy8

Deer, Timothy R, and Pope, Jason E. (eds). *Atlas of Implantable Therapies for Pain Management.* (n.p.): Springer, 2016. An essential guide to the treatment of pain using neuromodulation. http://tinyurl.com/y6w34nm5

Fishman, Scott, and Kreis, Paul. *Spinal Cord Stimulation Implantation: Percutaneous Implantation Techniques.* (n.p.): Oxford University Press, 2009. This book describes how spinal cord stimulators (SCS) are used to treat chronic pain of neurologic origin, such as sciatica, intractable back pain, and diabetes. http://tinyurl.com/y76r3w3h

Montgomery Jr., Erwin B. *Deep Brain Stimulation Programming: Mechanisms, Principles and Practice.* (n.p.): Oxford University Press, 2016. This book explores new techniques of deep brain stimulation programming. http://tinyurl.com/y7pjymto

Rosenberg, Stanley. *Accessing the Healing Power of the Vagus Nerve: Self-Help Exercises for Anxiety, Depression, Trauma and Autism.* (n.p.): North Atlantic Books, 2017. A practical guide to understanding the cranial nerves as the key to our psychological and physical wellbeing. http://tinyurl.com/ycbexqlb

## Other Resources to Explore

Painscience.com article about Central Sensitization in chronic pain.

UCLA Medical Center's online resources about motor cortex stimulation pain management through oral medications, injections and nerve blocks.

# 16

# Regenerative Biomedicine

Our bodies are home to many automatic processes that heal and regenerate damaged tissue. In most of us, minor cuts, scrapes, and bruises all heal relatively quickly if we are healthy. Of course, more serious injuries, such as bone breaks or ruptured tendons, take longer to heal, and if the process takes too long, we are at risk for experiencing continued pain.

Today, researchers are making exciting advancements in enhancing our bodies' own healing mechanisms, an area of medicine we call regenerative medicine. Doctors are beginning to apply these advancements as injection therapies for treating painful conditions, such

as bone and cartilage defects, osteoarthritis, tendon and ligament injuries, and perhaps even nerve damage. You may have already seen a number of clinics or centers offering regenerative medicine. These techniques are evolving rapidly and have become increasingly popular in the United States and internationally.

In this chapter, we talk about three kinds of therapeutic injections that encourage the healing of damaged tissue as well as exciting developments in nerve regeneration. All these techniques have tremendous implications for treating injury and chronic pain.

## Prolotherapy

Trenton was born with tendons and ligaments in his shoulders that were looser than they should have been, leading to subluxation—a condition that caused his shoulder to partially dislocate easily. From the age of nine, Trenton experienced multiple shoulder dislocations, which forced him to wear a brace during physical activities to help keep his arm in the socket. Trenton was so prone to dislocations, he would sometimes even wake up in the middle of the night with searing pain from a shoulder dislocation.

As an adult, Trenton's constant shoulder pain left him unable to lift his right arm above his head, prevented him from doing most upper body exercises, and interfered with his sleep. Eventually, x-rays revealed that the cartilage in his shoulder joint had deteriorated to the point where bone was rubbing against bone, and his doctor recommended shoulder replacement surgery.

Because Trenton was a young 48 years of age, the orthopedic surgeon recommended he postpone surgery as long as possible. However, no one offered him any options for pain control outside of the normal medications. Medicines, physical therapy, shoulder injections, massage therapy, and herbals did little to strengthen the joint or reduce the pain. Fortunately, Trenton's wife had friends who had benefited from prolotherapy and urged Trenton to give it a try.

Tendons, ligaments, and fascia are tough connective tissues that join muscle to bone, bone to bone, and muscle to muscle, respectively. Muscles contain connective tissue as well. Prolotherapy helps stimulate the healing of chronically injured ligaments, tendons, or joints thereby reducing pain and regenerating new tissue. Legend has it that the practice of prolotherapy originated with Hippocrates himself, the father of Western medicine, in the days of ancient Greece. The story goes that Hippocrates would treat dislocated shoulders in soldiers by inserting hot silver wires in and around the joints, creating scar tissue and preventing the shoulders from dislocating again.

Modern prolotherapy involves the injection of various substances into affected tissues. These injections generate a controlled inflammatory response that mimics the body's natural healing process. In the 1930s, doctors injected strong irritants during prolotherapy to stimulate inflammation, but today the injections typically consist of a hypertonic dextrose solution (a kind of sugar water) or sodium morrhuate (cod liver oil). Dextrose is the most common substance that is injected. Other chemicals may be added to the injections such as lidocaine, glycerin, or phenol. These injections stimulate the production of healthy collagen fibers.

## Understanding Prolotherapy

Collagen is a protein that provides structure and elasticity to many parts of our body, including ligaments, tendons, cartilage, and bone. Healthy collagen fibers lie parallel to one another and properly transmit forces from muscle to bone and bone to bone. In an injured joint, collagen fibers become jumbled, transmitting forces abnormally, destabilizing the tissue, and activating nearby nerves.

How do prolotherapy injections stimulating the production of healthy collagen fibers help with healing and pain relief? Prolotherapy injections are thought to stimulate an inflammatory reaction around injured tissue. This promotes the release of substances necessary for new growth and tissue repair. The injections trigger the body to send fibroblasts—cells that produce collagen—to the site of injury. These fibroblasts lay down new collagen in a parallel structure. The entire cascade of events heals the tissue, strengthens a joint, restores normal function, and reduces pain.

In many cases, the pain from certain conditions is not due to chronic inflammation but rather a failure to heal properly. Prolotherapy stimulates the body's natural resources in an effort to speed the healing. Ultrasound images even suggest that prolotherapy can encourage the regeneration of tissue when injected into areas such as the meniscus and the medial collateral ligament in the knee.

## Choosing Prolotherapy

The best candidates for prolotherapy are patients with chronic musculoskeletal conditions, such as knee osteoarthritis or finger osteoarthritis. Others that may benefit are patients with Achilles tendon problems, tennis elbow (lateral epicondylosis), plantar fascia problems, rotator cuff tendon problems, and sacroiliac joint pain. It's not clear yet whether prolotherapy is beneficial for patients with low back pain. Prolotherapy is an option only if more conservative treatments have failed. In certain circumstances, prolotherapy may be a good alternative. For example, patients may not be able to get a joint replacement for medical reasons, or, like Trenton, they may want to postpone the replacement as long as possible. Prolotherapy is suited for chronic pain (lasting more than three to six months), not acute pain.

Patients receiving prolotherapy must go through an initial examination, during which the doctor determines exactly where the tissue is damaged. Many physicians initially identify injured tissue by palpation (touch) and confirm with ultrasound or x-ray. During the prolotherapy treatment, the doctor numbs the skin and inserts a needle into all the areas where the damaged tendons and ligaments connect to bone and muscle, in a process that has been compared to "spot welding." A larger volume of solution may be injected into the joint itself.

Most courses of prolotherapy treatment involve a minimum of three sets of injections, spaced four to six weeks apart. There are several injections and they can be painful, so a patient may be offered acetaminophen (Tylenol) or even a short-acting opioid before or after the procedure. Temporary soreness and stiffness after the treatments can be expected. Many patients experience convincing relief after the third session but begin to feel some difference from the underlying pain even after the first one. Similar to other injections, patients may need "booster" sessions for continued benefit. Insurance does not typically cover prolotherapy, and the cost (as of this writing) ranges between $200 and $600 per session.

Trenton had his doubts, but after some research he learned that there was clinical evidence supporting the effectiveness of prolotherapy. He agreed to try a few sessions on his right shoulder to see if it helped. After his first session, he was sore for about a day and half, but he found that sleeping was already much more comfortable and that he had an increased range of motion of his arm. After the third series of injections, he was convinced that it was working; he experienced good pain relief, was able to reach above his head, and was moving his arm in new ways. He's had about six treatments so far, each requiring 20 injections per session, lasting 30 minutes, and costing him $200 per session. When I last spoke to him, he was planning to have his left shoulder treated as well.

We do not yet have evidence that the ligaments and tendons treated with prolotherapy become stronger than the original undamaged tissue. However, prolotherapy patients like Trenton consistently report that their joints feel less painful and more stable. As the prevalence of musculoskeletal conditions leading to pain increases, both insurers and physicians are discovering that non-surgical approaches such as prolotherapy can be viable solutions—so much so that I wonder whether this and other regenerative therapies might even be used as a form of strength enhancement for athletes in the future.

# Platelet Rich Plasma Therapy

Platelet rich plasma (PRP) initiates an inflammatory response in the area of injury. In this way, it is similar to prolotherapy. PRP therapy also involves injections into or around damaged connective tissues of the knee joint, tendons, plantar fascia, or ligaments, for instance. In platelet rich plasma therapy, however, the substance injected is not dextrose solution but is cellular material from the patient's own blood. Platelets are colorless blood cells in our plasma (the colorless fluid part of the blood) that contain over 1100 biologically active proteins. Because it involves injecting cells from our bodies, PRP therapy is a biologic therapy. (Biologic therapy uses living organisms, substances from living organisms, or versions of these substances made in the laboratory to treat disease. Vaccines and antibodies are examples of biologic therapies. Another biologic therapy you may have heard of is stem cell therapy.)

Platelets are important in blood clotting and wound healing, and they promote tissue regeneration. Platelet rich plasma contains many growth factors that specifically stimulate the production of muscle cells, cartilage, bone, and blood vessels. Studies in animals have shown that PRP therapy speeds up healing in muscle, ligament, joint, and tendon injuries by leveraging the remarkable ability of platelets to deliver growth factors directly to the site of injury.

Beginning in the 1950s, dentists used PRP to enhance wound healing in cancer patients with jaw reconstruction. Since the 1990s, orthopedic surgery, plastic surgery, dentistry, and spine surgery have applied it to surgical sites to enhance wound healing. Professional football player Hines Ward tore one of the major ligaments of the knee called the medial collateral ligament two weeks prior to the Super Bowl in 2008. PRP injections are credited with accelerating his healing process and allowing him to play the game. Furthermore, the International Olympic Committee expert group has suggested that PRP may be a good option for treating athletic sports injuries but recommends proceeding with caution due to the need for more scientific evidence.

Physicians are using PRP in the United States and other countries. However, many insurers consider it experimental and don't cover the cost. Doctors currently use PRP injections to treat tennis elbow (lateral epicondylitis), plantar fasciitis, ankle sprains, ligament tears of the anterior cruciate (inside the knee joint) and medial collateral ligament (outside the knee joint), tendon injury to the Achilles and patella (knee cap), and acute muscle tears. There is exciting work on humans and animals showing nerve regeneration in the spinal cord and peripheral nerves too. We may be able to use PRP for treating spinal cord injury or nerve injuries in the future. Not only that, but early animal research shows that PRP can slow down intervertebral disc degeneration that can lead to chronic back pain and nerve compression.

## Choosing Platelet Rich Plasma Therapy

During a PRP therapy session, the patient's blood is drawn and spun in a centrifuge for a few minutes. This separates the blood into three layers. The blood is often spun again. This process increases the concentration of the patient's own platelets and growth factors in the blood sample to between three and five times the normal concentration found in the blood. How much blood is needed? It depends on the area being treated, but about 20 cc of blood produces 3 cc of PRP for injection into the tendon around the elbow (tennis elbow), for example.

Platelet rich plasma can be stored for eight hours or more, but most doctors inject it back into the patient within the first 20 to 40 minutes. There are a variety of commercial techniques that create PRP, and the final PRP end product often differs according to patient age, diseases, and circulation. There is no standard PRP content of platelets or growth factors either. Some PRP samples contain white blood cells, which may be helpful or harmful to tissue healing, according to scientific research.

When rest, anti-inflammatory medications, and physical therapy have failed to resolve an injury, PRP therapy can be a good option. For Jerome, who suffered for 15 years with pain and physical limitations from a partially ruptured Achilles tendon, PRP therapy was a less invasive short-term alternative to surgery that wouldn't prevent him from getting surgery in the future if it was needed. Prior to PRP therapy, Jerome had suffered repeated injuries to the tendon, rehabilitation was lasting longer for each subsequent injury, and pain relief was poor. It became hard to wear shoes, and the pain was limiting his time with his children since he was no longer able to run and play with them.

After each of Jerome's three sets of injections, which were made directly into the tear, Jerome wore a boot to immobilize his foot and walked with crutches. After the injections, he began a regimen of stretching and physical therapy (PT) to strengthen the area. PT and education are critical to recuperation, but not all parts of the body require immobilization.

After the treatment was complete, the swelling in Jerome's heel was completely gone, and his pain was substantially reduced. Jerome felt the biggest improvement about a month into PRP therapy. He has had no noticeable side effects and is now able to lead an active life and play sports without the constant fear of re-injury that plagued him before treatment. "I can play with my kids without worrying that my next step may be my last," he said.

Like other biologic therapies for managing pain, researchers are trying to develop standard, safe methods for the correct application of PRP therapy — optimal dose, platelet processing, volume injected, number of injections, and rehabilitation protocol after injections. Accurate diagnosis is absolutely vital, and patients must inform their doctors of any previous injections to the affected area, such as steroid shots. Steroids and nonsteroidal anti-inflammatory drugs (NSAIDs) can interfere with the healing properties of PRP.

Because we are not sure how local anesthetics affect PRP injections, they are usually avoided as well. Jerome mentioned that the injections were painful, but not for very long. It's normal for patients to have pain at the injection site for one to two days. Today, doctors use ultrasound guidance to make sure they are placing the injections in exactly the right locations. Imaging such as MRI or ultrasound can track tissue healing following PRP therapy, and establish the baseline condition before the treatment begins. Injections can be performed directly into or around the injured tissue (a tendon, for example) just one time or many times in a "spot welding" or "peppering" manner.

## Platelet Rich Plasma Therapy and Pain Relief

Mild tendonitis may resolve with one PRP treatment, whereas a partial tear like Jerome's may require two or three sessions with four to seven days between sessions. Some patients experience enough healing and relief from PRP therapy that they are able to avoid surgery, although a complete tear of a ligament or tendon will still require surgical reconstruction. For instance, PRP will not re-attach a full tear of a rotator cuff tendon. Similarly, severe degenerative osteoarthritis (grade 4) won't likely respond to PRP. These patients need joint replacement.

If you're considering PRP, the evidence base that exists suggests improvements in lateral epicondylitis (tennis elbow), knee osteoarthritis, plantar fasciitis, rotator cuff tendinitis, and patellar tendinitis (jumper's knee). Other chronic tendinopathies (disease of a tendon causing pain, swelling, or inflammation, for example) like Jerome's may benefit as well.

Right now, doctors prefer to use a patient's own blood (as opposed to the blood of a donor), to prevent problems with infection or the immune system rejecting the PRP.

PRP therapy is relatively expensive, costing between $300 and $2000 per injection. However, this expensive treatment may ultimately be cost effective. For example, the total cost for tennis elbow surgery may exceed $15,000, so PRP injections for tennis elbow are a cost-effective measure if they prevent further medical interventions. The potential for healing damaged tissue looks bright, and there are no reported complications from PRP, but remember that the science still lags behind clinical practice and uncertainties do remain.

## Stem Cell Therapy

The clinical application of stem cells for replacing injured or diseased tissue began after World War II. Since the 1960s, stem cell therapy has been used in the form of bone marrow transplants to treat conditions such as leukemia. More recently, stem cell therapies are a topic of great interest for health, disease, and biomedical research into regenerative medicine. Concurrently, a growing number of stem cell clinics are marketing the benefits of stem cells for pain conditions such as arthritis as well as other diseases such as Parkinson's disease and multiple sclerosis (MS).

New applications show exciting promise for treating painful conditions such as bone and cartilage defects, osteoarthritis, tendon and ligament injuries, and even nerve damage. There is concern, however, about safety, effectiveness, and compliance with federal regulatory standards. A core question relates to whether the stem cell products produced by clinics are considered biological drugs and if so, are they subject to regulation by the FDA.

## Understanding Stem Cell Therapy

Stem cells are special cells that have the capacity of regeneration; they can divide and become replicates of themselves. Stem cells can also become or differentiate into specialized cells of the body (nerve cells, bone cells, tendon cells, for example). Stem cells are able to change the behavior of other cells around them too. There are two main categories of human stem cells: embryonic stem cells and adult stem cells (which are found in fat, skin, and muscle, for example). A third type of stem cell (called induced pluripotent stem cells, or iPSCs) can be created by reprogramming an adult stem cell.

You may have heard about certain populations of stem cells in the news media. For example, the bone marrow contains hematopoietic stem cells (HSCs) that can differentiate into all the cells in the blood. HSCs are the basis of a well-established treatment for leukemia/lymphoma and bone marrow injury from radiation. Another population of cells, bone marrow stromal cells (BMSCs) can become bone cells, cartilage cells, and fat cells, for instance. BMSCs are classified as mesenchymal stem cells (MSCs). MSCs are being increasingly studied for their therapeutic potential. There are many sources of MCSs including adipose tissue, bone marrow, amniotic fluid, the placenta, and the umbilical cord. It appears that bone marrow MCSs and adipose-derived stem cells represent the most available sources of MSCs for tissue regeneration.

There is early but groundbreaking research on creating patient neurons from stem cells taken from the patient's own skin. These adult stem cells are genetically reprogrammed to become neurons that retain the genetic identify of the patient. Studies on these neurons formed outside the living body are helping researchers analyze pain mechanisms in the nerve and potential drugs that treat the disease. The process of removing adult cells from the skin, reprogramming them, and then producing a specific cell type like a neuron is called induced pluripotent stem cell (iPSC) formation.

When Derrick tore his anterior cruciate ligament (ACL), medial collateral ligament (MCL), and meniscus in his knee, he feared his days of skiing were over. He was a healthy 57-year-old who loved to ski and ski jump. His orthopedist told him he would need immediate arthroscopic surgery, but he didn't want to pursue that option when he was told there was only about a 14% chance that he could resume his former athleticism on the ski slopes after a high-grade tear of his ACL.

Limited to going to work and sitting around the house, Derrick felt helpless and discouraged. NSAIDs and RICE (Rest, Ice, Compression, and Elevation) made a difference, but not enough. Derrick went to physical therapy just once. He couldn't exercise, wore a knee brace, and used crutches. He lived in fear that he'd worsen his injury with movement.

Derrick's own research on his injury led him to a clinic that performed stem cell therapy in conjunction with the platelet rich plasma (PRP) treatments described in the previous section of this chapter. One month had lapsed since his knee injury. After meeting with the physician and reading a book about stem cell therapy and results, Derrick felt comfortable undergoing the treatment. He also felt that surgery would still be an option if the therapy wasn't successful.

Although cautiously concerned about the novel nature of stem cell therapy, Derrick liked the non-surgical regenerative injection approach to his knee injury. He was hopeful that the therapy would re-grow his torn ACL to its original size and strength, and heal his torn meniscus. Many clinics don't restrict the procedure based on age, weight, previous arthroscopy, or other types of surgery.

Derrick's entire procedure took less than a month and was performed in three steps. First, about 60 cc of blood was removed from Derrick's arm and processed in the clinic's lab. That same day, PRP was injected under ultrasound and x-ray guidance into his knee. Next, a fairly large needle was inserted into his upper hip bone to remove some bone marrow containing the stem cells. A couple of holes were made into the bone, which hurt briefly. Derrick's bone marrow was then processed in the clinic's lab.

About 10 days later, Derrick returned to have the stem cells injected under x-ray guidance into his ACL. This injection was uncomfortable. The doctor injected more PRP along with the stem cells during this session. Finally, 10 days following the stem cell injection, more of Derrick's blood was removed and processed, and PRP was injected under ultrasound guidance in the region of the ACL, MCL, and meniscus.

The doctor informed Derrick that he typically injects about 5–10 ccs of bone marrow concentrate into the area of need. That volume of bone marrow concentrate included PRP as well. The doctor removed 100 cc of bone marrow and spun it down to about 3–5 cc. In preparation for the therapy, Derrick took a proprietary supplement containing glucosamine, resveratrol, vitamin D, and vitamin C. He also cut out sugar, stopped lifting heavy weights, lost 12 pounds, and strengthened his body.

The bone marrow extracted from Derrick's hip contained stem cells: HSCs and MSCs. HSCs can differentiate into red and white blood cells as well as platelets, and MSCs can become bone, fat, connective tissue, or cartilage. Both types of stem cells are concentrated in a centrifuge, a proprietary formula is added, and then they are injected into the area of injury.

Although studies have been conducted on implanting MSCs into degenerated intervertebral discs or arthritic knee joints, researchers still are trying to determine exactly how MSCs function. Do they differentiate into cells that replace injured ones or produce growth factors that stimulate repair, for example? Figuring out how MSCs function may lead to further options for MSCs in pain treatment. They may even have the potential to modify diseases such as osteoarthritis (OA) by inhibiting molecules that destroy cartilage and by suppressing harmful effects of the immune system.

Because MSCs have a lower risk of rejection by the immune system compared to other stem cells, they might be used as a regenerative therapy for the broader community. In other words, most stem cells are harvested from a patient's own body and then given back to that same patient, a process called *autologous* stem cell therapy. Placing stem cells into a patient that were removed from a different person who acts as a donor, can potentially offer greater accessibility provided we don't have to worry about rejection by the immune system. Using donor cells is the key to this procedure, which is called *allogeneic* stem cell therapy. Allogeneic stem cell therapy may soon become more available due to the "hypoallergenic" nature of MSCs.

We don't understand exactly why stem cells used in this way are successful and why the cells do not differentiate incorrectly—by becoming bone instead of cartilage, for example. If the stem cells were to differentiate incorrectly, it would pose the risk of harmful growth of an unwanted tissue. And as a matter of fact, in some studies, leakage of MSCs injected into the intervertebral disc of animals has caused undesirable bone to form on the sides of the discs. Consequently, it may be important to add technologies to avoid the migration of stem cells out of the target region. Another question that arises is whether or not the stem cells might overgrow, causing a tumor. Avoiding this complication is critical. Thankfully clinical observation from practitioners suggests that this has not occurred.

### Stem Cell Therapy and Pain Relief

Although research is in the early stages, several human studies in knee osteoarthritis have shown pain relief and better functional status after stem cell therapy with MSCs. A few other studies have noted improvement in articular cartilage quality. Limited studies in humans with degenerative disc disease causing low back pain have demonstrated pain and functional improvement after MSC treatment, and work in animals suggests that

stem cells stop the disc degeneration process while promoting regeneration.

In Derrick's case, stem cell therapy in conjunction with PRP was performed with the assumption that the PRP growth factors would activate the stem cells to replace the damaged ligament and meniscus, or that the PRP would trigger substances around the injured tissue to begin the healing process. The belief is that the therapy re-grows the damaged tissues of the knee itself in either case. Interestingly, PRP added to stem cell therapy in animal and test tube studies has enhanced the healing process.

The role of stem cells in treating tendon injuries—Achilles tendon, patellar tendon, rotator cuff tear, and lateral epicondylar tendon (tennis elbow)—is weak. Tendon disorders (tendinopathy) are increasing as more people take part in exercise but, unfortunately, stem cell treatment has only shown minor benefit in human studies. In fact, the Australasian College of Sports Physicians has recently written in a position statement that there is a lack of evidence for MSCs in treating tendinopathy.

Research suggests that stem cells may confer a pain-relieving effect that's separate from their regenerative effect. It may do this by changing how nerve cells interact with each other or reducing inflammatory molecules called cytokines that lead to the development of neuropathic pain.

Neuropathic pain, affecting up to 8% of the population is one of the most challenging chronic pain conditions to control. Recall some examples of neuropathic pain discussed in Chapter 4, Neuropathic Pain, in Part 1, Understanding and Treating Your Pain. These include diabetic peripheral neuropathy, postherpetic neuralgia (PHN), spinal cord injury, and multiple sclerosis. Neuropathic pain continues until the damage is healed or pathways of pain reduction are amplified. Medicines, nerve blocks, spinal cord stimulation, and cognitive behavioral therapy (CBT) are strategies that we use for amplifying pain-reducing pathways.

In order to more effectively treat neuropathic pain, scientists are exploring ways to repair damaged nerve cells by transplanting stem cells at the site of injury such as spinal cord injury. Researchers have seen certain kinds of stem cells differentiate into nerve cells when transplanting them into animals with spinal cord injury, providing hope that this can be done safely and effectively in humans.

Other animal studies have shown positive effects of stem cell therapy on nerve pain from diabetes and spinal cord injury. Preliminary experiments in humans have reported pain reduction when stem cells were injected around the trigeminal nerve in patients with facial pain (trigeminal neuropathic pain), and there has been early work on studying stem cells for treating amyotrophic lateral sclerosis (ALS) and multiple sclerosis as well.

Fascinating investigations on transplanting genetically engineered stem cells into an injured spinal nerve of animals has revealed therapeutic benefits for neuropathic pain. These stem cells have been programmed to produce an analgesic protein inside the injured nerve, acting somewhat like a pain-relieving mini pump. Advances like this may offer patients with poorly controlled peripheral nerve pain (sciatica or carpal tunnel, for example) a means of restoring normal sensation and function.

For those patients with bladder pain syndromes, such as interstitial cystitis (IC) or pelvic pain, sleep disturbance, sexual dysfunction, and chronic stress, can all be overwhelming. Current conventional treatments can help, including sacral neurostimulation (similar to spinal cord stimulation, but the lead is placed along the nerves in the sacrum) but as Deede, one of my own patients said, "some therapies help my ability to urinate, others may ease the constant burning, but none really makes me feel whole again." Fortunately, MSC therapy injected into the bladder of animals with IC symptoms has substantially improved most of the damage caused by this syndrome. These early studies in animals are providing the foundation for therapeutic trials in humans. Stem cell therapy may indeed become a standard therapeutic approach for bladder disorders in the future—a great hope for this group of patients.

There are also early investigations into MSC therapy for temporomandibular joint repair and regeneration, mostly in animals and the test tube. This is an innovative approach to treating a major cause of non-dental orofacial pain collectively known as temporomandibular disorder.

Derrick's results from the mesenchymal stem cell (MSC) therapy were dramatic. His doctor told him to expect symptom improvement anywhere from right after the therapy to three months later. He also mentioned that it may be nine to 12 months before Derrick saw long term tissue healing of the meniscus or ACL. Within 12 weeks of Derrick's treatment, he was back to normal activities, running, jumping, and golfing with no problems. Within a year, he was back to skiing regularly. An MRI of Derrick's knee performed nine months after the treatment confirmed that his damaged tissues had completely healed.

When arthritis began in Derrick's other knee, he had it treated with platelet rich plasma (PRP) therapy and the symptoms have not returned. "My knees feel like they are 25 years old. I can run with my son and my knees feel loose and lubricated," he said. Derrick told me it was like discovering the fountain of youth for his joints.

It cost Derrick about $7000 for the three-step therapy, which was not covered by insurance. As you might imagine, stem cell therapy costs more than PRP, ranging from $6000 to more than $30,000 per procedure.

## Stem Cell Therapy and the Future

The promise of restoring normal structure and function to damaged tissues without surgery is very exciting for those with injuries like Derrick's and for the millions who suffer from degenerative arthritis, disc disease, neuropathic pain, and bladder pain syndromes. Today, artificial "bionic" implants represent the standard of care for severe joint disease, but progress in tissue engineering with stem cells may one day allow us to offer "biologic" replacements instead (a completely regrown meniscus or a regenerated nerve, for example).

Regenerative therapy offers radical results and its allure can be irresistible. However, there are still many gaps in our understanding about safety, efficacy, therapeutic mechanism, route of administration, dose of cells, frequency of administration, processing, stage of disease, and source of stem cells. Still, stem cell rejuvenation offers doctors the opportunity to move pain medicine from merely managing symptoms to complete healing of the disease process—a phenomenal possibility.

## On the Horizon: Nerve Restoration

Medical conditions such as diabetes, HIV, cancer, or traumatic injury can damage the peripheral nerves and lead to burning pain, numbness, or even paralysis. The peripheral nervous system is made up of all the nerves outside the central nervous system. (The central nervous system consists of the brain and spinal cord.) The peripheral nervous system is the major connection between the brain, spinal cord, and the rest of the body, joining it to the muscles, limbs, and other organs, and it is responsible for all movement and sensation as well as autonomic functions like heartbeat, breathing, and sweating. Peripheral nerves range in size from the tiny nerves in our skin to large nerves like the sciatic nerve, which stretches all the way down the leg. Damage to even our smallest nerves can cause intense pain, and nerves that do not heal or reconnect properly after injury are much more likely to cause chronic pain.

For many years, physicians and researchers assumed that damaged peripheral nerves were not capable of significant healing or regeneration the way skin, bone, and muscle tissues are. But, today, neuroscientists have determined that nerve cells can actually regrow and reconnect. However, the process is limited and very slow. For instance, peripheral nerves regrow at a rate of one inch per month at best. Researchers are currently working on ways to stimulate nerve regrowth in an effort to restore sensory and motor function to damaged areas of the body and to ease pain. This has exciting implications for patients suffering from nerve damage due to trauma or disease—bone fractures, knife wounds, diabetic peripheral neuropathy, chemotherapy-induced peripheral neuropathy, and carpal tunnel syndrome to name just a few.

## Understanding Nerve Cells

Nerve cells, known as neurons, are made up of a cell body (like a flat tree stump), dendrites (tree branches), and a long "tail" called an axon. The axon is like a wire that conducts electrical impulses to and from other neurons, muscles, and organs, and to the central nervous system. Often, but not always, the axon is surrounded by a sheath of myelin, which acts like insulation for the "wire." Myelin allows impulses to travel more quickly.

Nerves can become damaged in any number of ways. Trauma caused by accidents, and bullet or knife wounds can crush or even sever (transect) one or many nerves. Tumors may compress nearby nerves, and the environment around the tumor may also inflame them. Diseases such as diabetes cause nerves to degenerate, as do certain chemicals such as the medicines used in chemotherapy. In many instances, the result is burning pain or tingling, sensitivity to touch, or numbness.

## Nerve Damage and Pain

There is a link between the improper re-growth of nerves and pain. Once damaged, nerve endings are unfortunately stubborn and don't want to grow back together. For instance, only 10% of axons ever reconnect to their targets after they are cut. In addition, the environment around the nerve doesn't support rapid regeneration.

Scientific investigations are looking at ways to make the environment more suitable for re-growth or to change the nerve's point of view so that it's able to grow despite the barriers. The goal is making the axon re-connect with itself or with its target. This would help restore lost sensation or motor function, and decrease pain.

Once a nerve becomes damaged, a complicated and fascinating cascade of events begins. First, the ends of the nerve separate by as much as several millimeters, creating a nerve gap. Expert surgeons can sometimes micro-suture the ends together, but most of the time such reconnection is impossible. (Imagine cutting a piece of rope and trying to reconnect each fiber exactly as it was.) The longer the nerves remain disconnected, the less likely they will re-connect too.

Surgeons can also graft a portion of another nerve into the gap, but the longer the ends have been separated, the more difficult it is for the nerve to function properly after a graft or surgical reconnection. Crush injuries generally regenerate easier than transections, since the nerve fibers don't need to reconnect, just heal. Similarly, nerves that are malfunctioning because of disorders of the myelin can recover fairly well. In these cases, the "wiring" (axon) is still intact; it just needs to reform the myelin, and function usually returns. In contrast, if the wire (axon) is severed, the nerve has to re-grow from its stump and that is what's so difficult. Neuropathic pain develops when the nerves are damaged, but if they can heal, then there is a greater chance of suppressing those painful sensations.

Barring immediate surgical intervention, the "distal stump"—the part of the damaged axon farther away from the cell body—begins to deteriorate rapidly in a process known as Wallerian-like degeneration. Then the proximal portion of the nerve, the part closer to the cell body, begins to upregulate, or change the genetic program to increase the expression of molecules known as regeneration-associated genes (RAGs). This prepares the nerve to regrow.

In response to the RAGs, axon sprouts begin to form, and ideally these sprouts reconnect with the distal portion of the injured nerve. Then new myelin often needs to form around the axon for proper function to be restored.

Peripheral nerves damaged in the outermost layer of the skin (from a paper cut or sunburn, for example) regenerate rather quickly. We lose skin cells every day, and the nerve supply replenishes without a problem. This is astonishing given that everywhere else in the peripheral and central nervous system the process of nerve regeneration is very slow and incomplete. Even when sprouts form, it is very difficult for the axons to reconnect with each other or with the appropriate part of the body such as a muscle or organ.

## Protein Inhibitors and Nerve Restoration

Nerve restoration encompasses a number of strategies that researchers are developing to help the axon (wire) heal properly and reconnect more quickly with the appropriate part of the body. Nerve restoration involves overcoming the body's chemical inhibitions to nerve growth and then directing that growth to the area of need. You wouldn't imagine that the body produces blockers of nerve growth, especially after injury. But growth can't continue unchecked, so our bodies produce molecules that put the brakes on the process. And as we saw in Chapter 4, Neuropathic Pain, and Chapter 8, Skeletal Pain, nerves that sprout in areas where they don't belong can lead to pain. However, when these "growth-inhibiting" molecules do their job too soon, beneficial growth is stopped.

Researchers are therefore working on techniques to temporarily block these inhibitory molecules in situations where nerves are damaged and need to regrow. One such growth-inhibiting protein molecule is the retinoblastoma (Rb) protein, which is present in adult nerves and appears to act as a brake to slow or stop nerve growth. Researchers have successfully inactivated the Rb protein in animals for a brief period of time to entice nerves to grow faster.

Another growth-inhibiting molecule is a protein called phosphatase and tensin homolog deleted on chromosome 10 that is known as PTEN. PTEN is a protein that puts the brakes on nerve regeneration after injury. PTEN exists in nerve cells and normally prevents unwanted growth. (PTEN is found in tumors as well, but the PTEN in tumors is thought to have a mutation that causes abnormal cell growth). Researchers have found that temporarily suppressing PTEN production in animals causes nerves to grow much more robustly. The challenge is to inhibit PTEN very locally and temporarily to avoid increasing a patient's risk for cell overgrowth and cancer.

Interestingly, diabetics show abnormally high levels of PTEN. This leads some researchers to think that PTEN may contribute to the nerve damage (or failure to regrow nerves properly) that is associated with abnormal blood sugars and insulin levels in diabetes. It's estimated that more than 20% of diabetics have bad nerve pain (discussed in more detail in Chapter 4, Neuropathic Pain), and we don't have therapies to halt or reverse the damage caused by diabetes yet. This is particularly disappointing because diabetic peripheral neuropathy ranks as the most common form of peripheral neuropathy.

In examining methods of regenerating damaged nerves, investigations have also identified a protein called RhoA in peripheral nerves and the central nervous system. Like Rb and PTEN, RhoA stops nerve growth. This leads to growth retraction during peripheral nerve injury. Blocking RhoA in animal studies also increases sprouting and growth of nerves after injury without necessarily increasing the risk of cancer. Researchers are working on creative ways to combine proteins such as RhoA and PTEN to facilitate the effects of RAGs and allow for even better nerve regeneration.

## Nerve Growth Factor and Nerve Restoration

Instead of blocking protein inhibitors such as Rb, PTEN, and RhoA, another nerve regeneration alternative is to apply a protein stimulant called nerve growth factor (NGF). The body produces NGF, which attaches to a nerve and triggers growth. NGF has been shown to stimulate nerve growth and protection, although it can also encourage nerves to sprout in regions of the bone where they don't belong, sensitizing nerves and leading to bone pain. In peripheral nerves, however, it appears that nerves signaled by NGF or even insulin (which is also a growth factor and like NGF binds to nerves and signals growth) activate a regenerative mode that makes the nerve more resistant to damage, disease,

or death. NGF has been used to regrow nerves in clinical trials with mixed results. There is some promise that NGF will be helpful in treating HIV neuropathy.

## Nerve Restoration in the Future

Innovative and ongoing research for nerve regrowth involves genetic manipulation—transferring genes that block PTEN production—and electrical stimulation.

Electrical stimulation has been shown to encourage healthy nerve reconnection in conjunction with surgery. Studies have shown that if a nerve is stimulated after injury, it recovers more effectively than if nothing at all is done to it, or if it is sutured together. There has also been some work in carpal tunnel surgery showing better outcomes with direct stimulation around the nerve. Electrical stimulation doesn't have to be directly on the nerve. Stimulation can occur transcutaneously (across the skin) as well. The theory is that electrical stimulation may trigger the regeneration-associated genes (RAGs), which in turn, accelerate nerve growth.

## Hope for Damaged Nerves and Pain Relief

Although several of these nerve regeneration therapies are still a few years away from rigorous clinical trials in diabetic peripheral neuropathy or traumatic nerve injury, for instance, they offer tremendous hope for people suffering from peripheral nerve damage and neuropathic pain.

You can learn more about regeneration therapies by listening to the related episodes of my weekly radio program, *Aches and Gains*. You can find the broadcasts on regeneration therapies at the following URLs.

**Prolotherapy**
http://paulchristomd.com/prolotherapy

**Platelet Rich Plasma**
http://paulchristomd.com/regenerative-biomedicine

**Stem Cell Therapy**
http://paulchristomd.com/stem-cell-rejuvenation
http://paulchristomd.com/stem-cell-rejuvenation-2

**Nerve Restoration**
http://paulchristomd.com/nerve-restoration
http://paulchristomd.com/nerve-restoration-2

# Suggested Further Reading

Baldelomar, Raquel, and Jacoby Richard. *Sugar Crush: How to Reduce Inflammation, Reverse Nerve Damage, and Reclaim Good Health.* (n.p.): Harper Wave, 2016. This book helps readers assess their nerve damage, offers practical dietary advice, and includes the latest thinking on ways to prevent and reverse neuropathy. https://tinyurl.com/ycdfulme

Boomer Hauser, Marion A., and Hauser, Ross A. *Prolo Your Pain Away: Curing Chronic Pain with Prolotherapy.* (n.p.): Sorridi Business Consulting, 2017. This book describes how Prolotherapy can treat chronic pain, osteoarthritis and sports injuries. https://tinyurl.com/ybdcvk8x

Darrow, Marc. *Prolotherapy: Living Pain Free.* (n.p.): Protex Press, 2004. An introduction to Prolotherapy covering history and medical research to success stories. https://tinyurl.com/y89d4p22

El-Badri, Nagwa. (ed.) *Advances in Stem Cell Therapy: Bench to Bedside.* (n.p.) Humana Press, 2016. The book reviews the main approaches for generation of differentiated cells from various types of stem cells. https://tinyurl.com/y7zemfjw

Soliman, Dina. *Pain Management by Prolotherapy and Perineural Injection Therapy: Non-Surgical Interventional Regenerative Orthopedic Medicine.* (n.p.): Lap Lambert Academic Publishing, 2016. This book discusses Prolotherapy as a way to repair connective tissue in patients suffering from chronic pain. https://tinyurl.com/yblxvec6

Weekes, Cheryl. *Taming Nerve Damage: Pain Relief Without Drugs.* (n.p.): PurposelyPositive, 2015. This book is designed to help readers control their own health care and lower pain levels without drugs. https://tinyurl.com/yadkjopg

## Other Resources to Explore

The Conversation is a source of news hosted by Boston University's College of Communication published a beginner's guide to understanding stem cells.

Nerve injury articles published on the Johns Hopkins Medicine website.

OnHealth.com, a publication owned and operated by WebMD, including article about nerve pain symptoms, causes and treatment options.

# Integrative Therapies for Pain

# 17

# Weight Control, Exercise, and Diet

Pain can often make us feel helpless. So often a disease or an injury seems to snatch away someone's ability to enjoy life. But there are many lifestyle choices that can make pain worse or make it better. These factors are within our control, so they offer us hope both to improve existing pain as well as to prevent pain from occurring or reoccurring.

Most of us have heard the conventional wisdom about diet and exercise: Eat plenty of fruits and vegetables and stay active. But this is often easier said than done. So how do we motivate ourselves to make lasting lifestyle changes? I have found that when my patients are able to connect their food and exercise choices to the way they feel, they are much more likely to continue with a program of healthy eating and regular physical activity.

This chapter outlines the role that diet and exercise play in increasing or decreasing pain and discomfort. It turns out that relationship may be far more intricate and complex than previously thought.

## Understanding Obesity, Pain, and Weight Control

Americans are becoming overweight and obese at unprecedented rates. According to the Centers for Disease Control and Prevention (CDC), 34.9% of Americans (nearly 79 million) are obese. More than two-thirds (68.8%) of Americans are overweight. There are many reasons cited for these alarming numbers. The typical American diet is full of processed foods, sodas, animal fats, and refined carbohydrates. Most Americans lead sedentary lives; more than 80% fail to get a recommended amount (30 minutes, five days a week) of exercise each week. Obesity affects people globally too; 50% of adults are projected to be obese by 2030.

Obesity puts us at greater risk for many diseases, including (but not limited to) heart disease, stroke, high blood pressure, diabetes, osteoarthritis (OA), gout, and even some cancers. Obesity also makes us more prone to injuries such as fractures and sprains. Many of these conditions cause pain, of course, but the relationship between obesity and pain is even more multifaceted than previously thought. In addition to causing diseases which in turn cause pain, many scientists now believe that obesity itself causes and increases pain as well. The available evidence points toward an elevated response by obese people to molecules in the body that produce pain.

Clinical research shows that excess body fat stimulates the secretion of cytokines, proteins that cause inflammation and pain. Scientists believe cytokines play an important role in coordinating the hormonal and immune response to stressors like disease and injury. Immune cells produce cytokines during periods of inflammation and, in turn, these substances make nerves in the body more sensitive to pain signals. These cytokines—molecules such as tumor necrosis factor and Interleukin-1—can cause pain in the joints, the muscles and even the organs (visceral pain). Rheumatoid arthritis (RA) is an example of a painful, destructive, and inflammatory reaction caused by cytokines going haywire.

Many effective pain medications for RA target cytokines to inhibit their production. Thus, losing the excess body fat that stimulates the secretion of cytokines and maintaining a healthy weight can reduce or prevent pain.

Fortunately, you don't have to look like a fitness model to see the benefits of weight loss. Overweight individuals who lose as little as 5%–10% of their body weight greatly reduce their risk of heart disease and other illnesses. Many osteoarthritis patients also see improvements in their pain when they lose weight. On the surface, this makes sense: Less body weight means less wear and tear on the weight-bearing joints in the knees, ankles, back, and hips. But many patients have reported that their hand and wrist pain also improves as they lost weight. This would seem to affirm the theory that the relationship between excess body fat and pain is not merely related to the work of carrying around extra pounds. In other words, it is not just mechanical overload on the joints. Obesity seems to promote a body-wide state of inflammation that triggers pain in specific parts of the body (arms and neck, for example) and painful conditions such as headache, shoulder pain, and fibromyalgia

No one wants to be overweight, but it can be difficult to stay motivated to lose that excess fat. Yet the more individuals understand how maintaining a healthy weight can decrease their chances of experiencing chronic pain, the more likely they are to find the strength and determination to keep trying.

## Understanding Exercise and Pain

Regular, moderate exercise is a vital part of wellness and pain prevention. We all have heard that exercise helps us lose extra fat, decreasing the chance of obesity and the pain caused by it. But exercise does more than that. Even before any pounds are shed, increased movement helps relieve and prevent pain. Individuals who are not overweight also need to exercise. Regular exercise increases blood circulation, releases endorphins (the body's natural painkillers), increases energy, and improves the quality of sleep and sex.

Pain and lack of mobility often become a vicious cycle: People in pain are reluctant to move, but lack of movement makes their pain worse. It can and often does hurt to move, but the less you move, the greater the likelihood of muscular deconditioning. Once this occurs, it's even more painful to move and exercise. For many people of all shapes and sizes, stiffness and immobility can become chronic. That's why working to stay flexible and in good cardiovascular condition—particularly as you age—is one of the best things you can do to minimize and prevent pain. Studies tell us that losing weight lowers levels of inflammatory molecules, such as cytokines, and even modest weight loss improves pain and the consequences of having pain such as sleep problems, fatigue, depression, and mechanical overload. More remarkable is that physical activity raises our pain threshold and lowers pain perception.

Consider low back pain. For many years, doctors recommended bedrest for alleviating the pain. Today, it's the opposite. High-quality scientific evidence has shown that staying in bed actually worsens low back pain. Surprisingly, regular movement and exercise not only lower chronic low back pain, but they also enhance mobility and facilitate function even into older adulthood. Research shows that exercises in the form of strength training, stretching, lumbar stabilization, and aquatic therapy can all help improve low back pain.

Katherine was an obese woman suffering from arthritis, diabetes, and high blood pressure. She also had arthritis in her knees, tendonitis in her legs, and heel spurs in her feet. For years, Katherine felt that her pain controlled her life. She couldn't sleep well, and her pain was so debilitating that she was unable to leave her house or play with her grandchildren. She tried multiple over-the-counter and prescription medications but found little relief.

At her doctor's urging, Katherine had tried to exercise, but she felt discouraged by the pain and gave up. Then Jeanette DePatie, a certified fitness instructor who was also a member of her church, told her about exercise classes she offered that were specifically designed for overweight individuals. Jeanette herself weighed 200 pounds but had become a professional fitness instructor, a marathoner, and a triathlete.

Katherine began attending Jeanette's classes. At first, her pain was so severe that she had to exercise while sitting in a chair. She started by moving her legs, pointing her toes and flexing her feet for just five minutes a day. Gradually, she built up to stretching more, trying yoga, tai chi and other types of therapeutic movement. She stuck with Jeannette's program for four years, and, today, Katherine exercises for an hour a day, three days a week. Other gentle exercises that plus-size people find useful when beginning to exercise include walking around the block and marching in place.

Although Katherine is not yet pain-free, she is much more active than she used to be. She is able to travel, take care of her grandchildren, and do many other things she hadn't been able to do for years. Her sleep has improved tremendously, and she is no longer depressed. The exercise helps her to control her pain and sometimes even forget about it. Katherine still needs to lose weight, and she is working on it, but her quality of life is so much better that it's undeniable that the exercise has proven extremely beneficial.

Obese individuals are more prone to injuries while working out, but this risk can be greatly reduced by selecting the right kind of exercise. In addition to simple movements, like the ones Katherine started with, riding a stationary bike or exercising in the water can be very good options for overweight individuals. It is often beneficial if they can start exercising under the supervision of a professional fitness instructor who is trained to work with plus-size individuals. Obviously, some pain during exercise is normal—muscle soreness or even mild cramps, but any chest tightness or sudden sharp pains should be evaluated immediately by a doctor or nurse.

Jeanette reminds her students that they can accomplish amazing things if they start small and increase incrementally. Starting an exercise too suddenly leads to injury and discouragement. Jeanette's students increase their training only about 10% a week. This may not sound like a lot, but over time, most see results like Katherine did, or even better. Tailoring the exercise program to the needs and abilities of the individual person improves compliance and encourages people to engage in low-impact activities gradually. Jeanette encourages her students to gain a sense of accomplishment from their progress, and to continue working at it consistently.

Katherine credits her successful exercise—which shocked her family—to Jeanette's patience and encouragement. She never felt pushed or pressured and was allowed to progress at her own pace. It took Katherine two full years of working out regularly before she was able to reap significant pain relief from it, so anyone trying to gain benefits from exercise should not give up. Don't feel as though you need to lose weight before beginning an exercise program. Focus on a regular fitness program at your current weight with professional guidance.

If moderate, low-impact exercise can improve the lives of those suffering from multiple health disorders, think what it can do for those who are relatively healthy. Making the time for regular exercise goes a long way toward relieving and preventing ongoing pain.

## Understanding Diet, Food, and Pain

The food we eat—or don't eat—can make a huge difference in the way we feel. Obviously, diet plays an important role in losing weight or maintaining a healthy weight. But a growing body of research suggests that some foods actually promote pain while others tend to relieve it. We also know that pain and inflammation are interconnected. Thus, a healthy, anti-inflammatory diet is another important element of treating and preventing pain.

When we're young, most of us feel like we can eat almost anything we want without noticing any negative consequences. As we age, these habits can catch up with us, sometimes sooner than we expect.

Many doctors now believe that certain foods stimulate the production of cytokines—the inflammation-stimulating proteins mentioned earlier in the chapter and throughout this book—while others inhibit them. Unfortunately, much of what we call "fast food" falls into the pro-inflammation category. Foods fried in oils at high temperatures and foods that are high in animal fats are among the worst offenders.

Anti-inflammatory foods, such as salmon, tuna and halibut; dark cherries, blueberries, kale, and green beans; cinnamon, ginger and rosemary; walnuts; green tea; and avocado oil can provide real benefits. For instance, vegetarian diets can have an impact on fibromyalgia symptoms, and higher quantities of fruits and vegetables lead to some protection against gout. There are several versions of the anti-inflammatory diet. Most versions eliminate or greatly reduce fatty meats and fried, processed foods. They also increase fresh fruits and vegetables and lean proteins including plant proteins, turkey, chicken, and fish. A higher fiber diet reduces cholesterol and belly fat, lowers blood pressure, and reduces the risk of many different diseases. There is also a growing consensus that when it comes to overall wellness, pain prevention, and even weight loss, quality of food is even more important than total calories consumed.

There is a tremendous variety of healthy dishes that can be prepared in accordance with anti-inflammatory diet guidelines. Hundreds of dishes from virtually any ethnic tradition can offer good nutrition and be part of a pain-reducing lifestyle. Herbs and other beneficial substances found in anti-inflammatory foods can also be taken as supplements, including bromelain (from pineapple), ginger, cinnamon, and turmeric. Even foods associated with indulgence, such as dark chocolate and red wine, can offer anti-inflammatory benefits when consumed in moderation.

Tami was a single mother with young children who developed both osteoarthritis and rheumatoid arthritis in her thirties. She suffered pain in her knees, ankles, and shoulders, accompanied by debilitating fatigue. Despite trying several medications, herbals, and a knee injection, her pain soon became bad enough that she couldn't play with her children or even leave the house very often. Tami also struggled to find the energy to cook, turning to carryout food and prepackaged meals that were often highly processed and full of fat and preservatives. Before she knew it, Tami was 50 pounds overweight.

Tami's breakthrough didn't come from a new medication or a typical therapy. It came from a change in diet suggested by her doctor. Initially the thought of changing the way she ate terrified her. Comfort foods, after all, were one of her few sources of pleasure in life. But she was experiencing so much pain that she was willing to try anything.

Tami's dietary changes were not primarily designed to help her lose weight, although that was a welcomed side effect. Her diet was instead geared toward reducing inflammation. Tami stopped eating red meat and prepared, canned, and processed foods, and she was surprised at how much she enjoyed the new foods that were rarely part of her diet before. She became more mobile, more motivated, and less sluggish. When she stopped drinking soda, she noticed less achiness and fatigue. She started eating fresh blueberries, blackberries, cherries, and a variety of fresh vegetables. She added grilled fish, russet potatoes, and artichokes and started drinking green tea.

Within a few weeks, Tami found the pain from her arthritis significantly improved. She lost about 50 pounds, so she is back to her ideal weight. She was able to eliminate her opioid pain medication and now only occasionally takes nonsteroidal anti-inflammatory drugs (NSAIDs). More importantly, she was able to begin living a more active life again. Tami knows the diet works because if she gets off track with her eating, she will find the pain returning. For example, when she started eating red meat again, her pain returned.

Tami also discovered she can eat a wide variety of foods as long as they are prepared correctly. She was shocked at how much her children enjoy the new foods she prepares. She is delighted that they are starting their lives with healthy eating habits that will reduce their risk of experiencing chronic pain in the future.

## Other Sources of Information about Weight Control, Exercise, and Diet

Many dietary and exercise changes seem so basic that it is easy to underestimate how much of a difference they can make in our overall well-being. It sometimes feels easier to try an expensive new medication with the hope that it can radically change how we feel. It can be a little more challenging to make consistent, incremental changes in the way we eat and move, but the improvement in our health and wellness can be tremendous.

You can learn more about weight control, diet, and exercise by listening to the related episodes of my weekly radio program, *Aches and Gains*. You can find the broadcasts on weight control, diet, and exercise at the following URLs.

**Plus-sized and in Pain:**
http://paulchristomd.com/plus-sized

**Foods and Pain Relief:**
http://paulchristomd.com/foods-that-fight-pain
http://paulchristomd.com/appetite
http://paulchristomd.com/appetite-2

**Exercise and Pain Relief:**

**Gunnar Peterson – Beverly Hills-based Personal Trainer**
http://paulchristomd.com/gunnar-peterson
http://paulchristomd.com/gunnar-peterson-2

**Mark Sisson – Fitness Expert**
http://paulchristomd.com/mark-sisson
http://paulchristomd.com/mark-sisson-2

## Suggested Further Reading

Amen, Daniel G., and Amen, Tana. *The Brain Warrior's Way: Ignite Your Energy and Focus, Attack Illness and Aging, Transform Pain into Purpose.* (n.p.): Berkley, 2016. A guide to improving overall health, focus, memory, energy, mood stability and more. https://tinyurl.com/yaodycdm

Neal D., Barnard. *Foods That Fight Pain: Proven Dietary Solutions for Maximum Pain Relief Without Drugs.* (n.p.): Rodale Press, 2008. This book offers a wealth of new research from prestigious medical centers around the world that shows how food can counteract pain. https://tinyurl.com/y7pc8yxa

Rawlings, Deirdre. *Foods that Fight Fibromyalgia: Nutrient-Packed Meals That Increase Energy, Ease Pain, and Move You Towards Recovery.* (n.p.): Fair Winds Press, 2012. This book includes new information on the link between food allergies and fibromyalgia, how to use nutrition to balance neurotransmitters for less pain and depression. https://tinyurl.com/ybxau9q9

## Other Resources to Explore

Fibromyalgia News Today article on the link between chronic pain and obesity.

Future Medicine, a UK based imprint of Future Science Group, addresses information needs in clinical and translational medicine and the biosciences including articles on obesity and chronic pain.

Health Essentials' article on an anti-inflammatory diet to relieve pain. Health Essentials is an intitative of Cleveland Clinic, a nonprofit multispecialty academic medical center.

A LiveScience article discussing whether obesity causes more pain in people.

Clinical news and information portal, MD Magazine's, article on understanding the relationship between chronic pain and obesity.

Practical Pain Management's high-protein-intake diet for patients with chronic pain.

CHAPTER

# 18

# Sleep, Stress, and Emotional Health

We think of pain as a physical phenomenon, but it has emotional, mental, and even spiritual components. Keeping ourselves emotionally, mentally, and spiritually healthy is incredibly important for preventing pain as well as in recovering from injury and illness.

For many years, most doctors dismissed the emotional aspects of pain as unimportant or even as simply imagined by their patients. As a result, they ignored these aspects of pain or referred patients for psychotherapy rather than recognizing and then treating the multidimensional aspects of pain in each person. Today, we are learning much more about how our mental state affects the way our brains process pain. New neuroimaging studies reveal that anticipating pain, imagining pain, or even empathizing with someone else in pain activates the same regions of the brain that process a physically painful event like burning a finger or stubbing a toe.

To lower our risk of chronic pain, we need to safeguard our emotional, mental, and spiritual health. This includes getting enough sleep, reducing stress, and maintaining healthy, supportive relationships. We must also be sure to treat any mental illnesses such as depression as promptly as possible. These steps might seem like common sense, but they are easy to neglect when life gets busy or circumstances seem to spin out of control.

## Understanding Sleep and Pain

A 2013 Gallup poll found that nearly half of American adults surveyed do not get the recommended seven or more hours of sleep a night. Seventy million Americans suffer from some sort of sleep disturbance, whether it is sleep apnea, narcolepsy, or insomnia. And almost 70% of those suffering from pain complain of sleep problems. This often becomes a vicious cycle: Pain disrupts sleep, and lack of sleep worsens pain. Sleep disturbances are linked to worsening pain after surgery, in fibromyalgia and rheumatoid arthritis, among patients with migraine and tension type headaches, and for patients with cancer pain.

Sleep is made up of two major phases: non-rapid eye movement (NREM) and rapid eye movement (REM). NREM sleep is composed of four stages. During stage 1, we experience light sleep. During stage 2 our body temperature drops. Stages 3 and 4 (also referred to as slow wave sleep) are characterized by slower breathing, lower blood pressure, and muscle relaxation. Various hormones are released into our bloodstream during these stages, regulating growth, appetite and healing. About 90 minutes after we fall asleep, we enter the REM phase, which is when we dream. Our body is completely relaxed during this time and our eyes dart back and forth under our eyelids. REM sleep recurs about every 90 minutes through the night.

Sleep problems such as sleep apnea do not necessarily reduce the total number of hours a person sleeps but instead disrupt REM sleep. These disruptions continually bring the individual back to stage 1 of NREM sleep, resulting in restless, poor-quality sleep. There are three major types of sleep apnea: Central apnea, where the brain signals to breathe are absent; obstructive apnea (the most common type), where the anatomy of the throat, sometimes coupled with excessive weight, prevent the individual from breathing easily; and mixed apnea, which is a combination of the two. Sleep apnea puts tremendous strain on the heart and should be treated promptly.

In the past, many doctors tended to overlook the importance of sleep. Today, however, there is growing evidence that many significant medical problems can develop in the absence of the right quantity and quality of sleep. Typical symptoms of sleep deprivation include irritability and weight gain, and we now know these can extend to problems like depression, hypertension, heart disease, and diabetes.

Getting a sufficient amount of quality sleep is vital to our health and well-being. Our daily activities drain both our physical and mental resources, and sleep restores both. The lower metabolic rate we experience during sleep facilitates the production of protective antioxidants and allows for restorative processes like memory encoding and tissue repair. Sleep deprivation also increases levels of the inflammatory substances called cytokines, such as

TNF-alpha, and Interleukin-1. These substances can excite nerves and amplify pain signals, leading to a chronic pain cycle. Cytokines also play a role in diseases such as rheumatoid arthritis (RA) and fibromyalgia (FM). Sleep helps to restore cytokines to normal levels.

We tend to sleep more when we're sick because our bodies need it. Animal studies demonstrate that increased sleep can speed recuperation. Sleep deprivation can aggravate chronic inflammatory conditions such as RA and make symptoms of FM worse. If your sleep has been disturbed, you might have experienced another consequence of sleep loss—muscle aches and pains.

People suffering from chronic pain often find themselves in the seemingly impossible position of having their pain disrupt their sleep, while lack of sleep makes their pain worse. Sleep deprivation itself lowers our threshold for pain, aggravates inflammatory conditions, and can lead to chronic pain even in the absence of other problems. Some studies have found that lengthening our slow wave sleep (deepest level of sleep) offers more effective pain relief than even a large dose of ibuprofen (Motrin). And, if deprived of slow wave sleep, people experience the reverse. For instance, studies show that when sleep is limited, people develop muscle aches and their pain threshold lowers. It's fascinating to note that functional neuroimaging scans reveal that when we sleep, the pain and arousal systems are turned off. This prompts the question: Can chronic pain prevent us from getting the sleep we need by fueling a state of perpetual arousal? It certainly seems possible.

Fatima was a typical, healthy mother of two until one afternoon when her car was rear-ended while she was stopped at an intersection. Initially diagnosed with whiplash, Fatima began to experience increased pain radiating all over her body, which eventually lead to diagnoses of fibromyalgia, migraines, and temporomandibular joint disorder (TMJ). Many of the pain medicines she was prescribed caused her to break out in hives, leading not only to daily misery, but also to a 17-year struggle with insomnia.

Like many people suffering from chronic pain, Fatima struggled both to fall asleep and to stay asleep. She could often drift off to sleep with the help of medication but would find herself waking from pain within four hours. Today, she has been able to manage her insomnia reasonably well using a combination of melatonin and trazodone (Desyrel) (both help her to fall asleep), while utilizing cognitive behavioral therapy (CBT) techniques and meditation to help her fall back to sleep if she wakes up.

## Treating Sleep Problems

For people struggling to fall asleep, melatonin supplements can be a good option. Melatonin is a substance produced naturally by the pineal gland, and it facilitates sleep without causing a hypnotic state. Antiepileptic drugs such as gabapentin (Neurontin) and pregabalin (Lyrica) improve sleep quality in some people as well.

Opioids can be useful in treating pain for certain patients, but they have mixed results when sleep disorders are involved. In short, their pain-relieving qualities help some patients sleep, but they may also increase the risk of central sleep apnea, reducing the quality of a patient's sleep. To complicate the issue even more, opioids can suppress REM sleep and thereby decrease the pain threshold. However, if they improve pain control, sleep may improve overall. Affected individuals using opioid medications should be closely monitored by their doctors.

Other sleep medications have mixed results as well. Tricyclic antidepressants (TCAs) are useful for both pain control and improving sleep quality, but some such as amitriptyline (Elavil) can reduce REM sleep. Diazepam (Valium), alprazolam (Xanax), and other benzodiazepines are not only anxiolytics but also muscle relaxants, so they can aggravate obstructive sleep apnea by relaxing the muscles of the throat. Insomnia drugs such as zolpidem (Ambien) and temazepam (Restoril) have been associated with increased mortality rates and even cancer. This does not mean that these drugs should not be used or that they cause death or cancer, but patients must be aware of the risks.

Such side effects are good reason to make non-drug approaches like cognitive behavioral therapy (CBT) and the other therapies covered in Chapter 19, Mind-Body Techniques for Pain Relief, the first line of defense. For example, several studies report a significant benefit on sleep quality and hygiene from CBT, and you can achieve longer term correction of insomnia through CBT compared to other strategies. More alternative therapies, discussed in the other chapters in Part 3, Integrative Therapies for Pain, are also good to investigate. Some patients swear by acupuncture or herbals, for instance. Others find massage therapy good for relaxation and getting to sleep. In addition to CBT and meditation, Fatima has benefited from acupuncture and is seeing an herbalist specializing in Chinese medicine. You can read more about these in Chapter 20, Alternative Medicine and Pain Relief.

## Practicing Good Sleep Hygiene

Practicing good sleep hygiene can also help improve sleep tremendously. This includes doing your best to establish a consistent routine by going to sleep and waking up at the same time each day. Have a wind-down period each day before you actually get into bed at night when you do enjoyable and relaxing activities. Turn off your cell phone and your computer and avoid screens a few hours before bedtime. Keep lights low in the evening, and maximize the bright light you are exposed to during the morning and midday.

If you find your mind racing before you sleep, write down your concerns on a piece of paper and turn the list face down. This helps to direct your mind away from your problems. If you do not fall asleep within 15 to 20 minutes of trying, get out of bed, do something boring (do not turn on your computer and check your email!) and go back to bed when you are tired. Try not to work, argue, or do anything negative in the bedroom; use it only for sleep and sex. The goal is to keep all associations with the bedroom positive and relaxing.

Although exercise is very important and helpful in regulating sleep and improving its quality, be sure to finish your exercise four to five hours before you plan to go to sleep. This facilitates sleep onset and sleep maintenance. Exercising too close to bedtime raises levels of norepinephrine and promotes a state of arousal. Also, avoid alcohol and tobacco use close to bedtime. All of these habits can help you safeguard the quality of your sleep, heal from illness and injury, and prevent the worsening or development of chronic pain.

# Understanding Stress and Pain

Stress can trigger pain and make existing pain worse. Both reducing stress and improving how we deal with it are vital to healing and pain prevention. A stressor is a thought, word, or action that our brains perceive as a threat. Illness, infection, and injury are physical stressors, while relationship problems, financial strain, and overloaded schedules are examples of psychological stressors. Traumatic events, such as accidents, the death or serious illness of a loved one, or the loss of a job, can produce huge amounts of stress. For some, even seemingly harmless situations like social events or public speaking opportunities can act as significant stressors.

Stressors activate our general defense system. The response to an actual event or even just the anticipation of a threat triggers our nervous system to arm our muscles to escape or to fight. Stress arouses the endocrine system to maximize our survival by mounting the fight-or-flight response. (During the fight-or-flight response, the sympathetic nervous system sends messages to the endocrine system to release adrenaline and other excitatory substances.) Stress also alerts the immune system to set up an inflammatory reaction that protects against the threat and promotes wound healing. Our endocrine, nervous, and immune systems are all involved. Various glands release a range of hormones including adrenaline and cortisol into the blood stream, while some of our nerves become more sensitized to molecules that promote pain. Our pupils dilate, our vision sharpens, and we become hyper-aware of our surroundings.

For millennia, this stress response played a vital role in our ancestors' survival. The extra energy supplied by the stress hormones would be burned off when they fought a predator or ran from danger. Even today, stress can enable us to optimize our performance in sports, on stage, or in work-related situations. But our stress response is supposed to be a temporary state, not a constantly recurring feature of our lives. Furthermore, in the modern world, psychological stressors frequently pose no physical threat, so individuals find themselves full of stress hormones with no natural activity to flush them out of the bloodstream.

The bad pain of a kidney stone, migraine, or heart attack threatens the body and acts like a stressor that causes all three systems (the endocrine, nervous, and immune systems) to mobilize.

Extended periods of stress can predispose us to developing and even maintaining a chronic pain state. Chronic pain may develop from a stressor such as surgery, an infection, or an emotionally traumatic event that alters the normal function of these three systems. Both stress and pain affect our health, functional abilities, and sense of well-being.

The two most common types of chronic pain associated with stress are low back pain (often in men) and headaches (frequently in women). Some research demonstrates that chronic stressors in the workplace lead to neck pain, especially in the trapezius muscle.

Extended periods of stress can make us more sensitive to pain and may have several other harmful effects on the body. These detrimental effects include hypertension, obesity, heart disease, skin disorders, digestive problems (heartburn and irritable bowel syndrome), and depression. Stressful lifestyles are also associated with early death. A study in the journal *Psychosomatic Medicine* found that stress-induced conditions in teenagers raised blood levels of C-reactive protein—a marker for inflammation—and increased their chances of developing cardiovascular problems later in life.

## Resilience, Catastrophizing, and Stress

No one is immune to stress. People from all socioeconomic, racial, and cultural backgrounds are affected by it, although obviously economic insecurity can be a stressor on its own. People caught in poverty, abusive relationships, dysfunctional families, or high-pressure work environments may feel trapped and find that stress in one area overflows into all aspects of their lives. Work stress can bleed into relationships, and vice versa. Many of us overlook the impact of psychosocial stress on our bodies.

It is also clear, however, that some people are able to handle stress more effectively than others. The ability to deal with stress productively is frequently referred to as resilience. Resilience results from a combination of family environment, motivation, and genetic makeup. Many doctors believe that some aspects of resilience may be genetically inherited. Other aspects of resilience are shaped by factors such as the security of relationships in childhood and how well the adults in a child's life handle stress. Children living in a safe, stable environment with loving relationships and parents who handle stress well are better able to cope with the unpredictable aspects of life than children who lack these social factors in their formative years.

In the absence of resilience, patients in pain induce stress through catastrophizing—assuming a minor pain is a sign of a serious illness or otherwise focusing on the worst-case scenario when confronted with a challenge—and this process, in turn, perpetuates or even worsens their level of discomfort. Several aspects of modern life make some individuals prone to catastrophizing. The internet and the 24/7 news cycle have allowed us access to all kinds of medical information, even about very rare conditions we are very unlikely to have as well as informing us of every natural disaster and tragedy as it unfolds. Individuals prone to anxiety may do well to avoid excessive exposure to such information. We're realizing that thoughts can have destructive physiological consequences. Anticipating or remembering a stressful event mobilizes the stress response even when there is no physical trauma.

## Managing Stress

Resilience can be learned. Cognitive behavioral therapy (CBT), discussed in Chapter 19, Mind-Body Techniques for Pain Relief, helps many sufferers improve their response to stressors. This technique opens up our awareness of our thoughts, feelings, and behaviors related to daily life. Patients can also learn resilience by observing others who are able to handle stress better than they do. The world is full of very successful people who are able to convert stress into productive energy. Surrounding oneself with inspiring, supportive people is an important part of managing stress effectively.

Biofeedback, also discussed in Chapter 19, Mind-Body Techniques for Pain Relief, helps individuals gain awareness of the relationship between their thoughts and their physiological responses. Biofeedback offers a wonderful way of reducing stress and pain by decreasing muscle tension and autonomic nervous system activity (the body's fight-or-flight response). It teaches self-regulation of bodily functions that react to stress, which are usually involuntary, such as heart rate, blood pressure, and digestion. Importantly, biofeedback can provide the ability to control that part of the nervous system activated by both pain and stress.

There are many different meditation strategies that can help manage stress and affect pain positively. Serene sounds (rain on a tin roof, soothing music or waves crashing on a beach, for example) may help to calm listeners suffering from excessive stress. Similar to biofeedback, meditation has been shown to lower heart rate, and blood pressure, alleviate anxiety and anger, and ease pain. Mindfulness-based stress reduction programs help to separate the sensory experience of pain from the emotional response to it. Just an eight-week meditation course has shown the capacity of the brain to "rewire" itself by decreasing gray matter (brain's nerve cells) in the amygdala, a part of the brain responsible for stress and fear.

Although most of us can benefit from reducing the stress in our daily routines, we must also accept the fact that a certain amount of stress is part of life. Getting enough sleep and eating a healthy diet greatly improve how we handle stress. Regular exercise is particularly vital in managing stress effectively, as it raises endorphin levels and lowers our levels of stress hormones such as cortisol and epinephrine (adrenaline). Research has shown that some runners release substances called endocannabinoids, marijuana-like chemicals produced in the body to dampen pain, and also release endorphins. Both may combine to fuel that "runner's high" that many athletes talk about.

Leading a balanced life with multiple supportive relationships and healthy hobbies and interests outside work also helps us process stress effectively. A person is more vulnerable to devastation from the loss of a job, for instance, if that job was the individual's sole source of identity and fulfillment. The same is true of the loss of a loved one if that person was an individual's only source of love and support. Individuals without close families or circles of friends should consider getting a cat or a dog to hold and love to help meet their need for comfort. Animal therapy is discussed in Chapter 22, Harnessing the Human Biofield.

## Understanding Emotional Health and Pain Prevention

Pain caused by emotional distress can actually be felt more deeply and for a longer period of time than pain caused by physical injuries, as documented in the journal *Psychological Science* in 2008. Advances in neuroimaging have uncovered the dynamic interplay between our mental state (mind) and our brain. For instance, as noted earlier in the chapter, anticipating pain, imagining pain, or empathizing with someone else's pain activates the same regions in the brain that are involved with processing a physically painful event like burning your finger.

## Emotional Health and Pain

Emotional pain can be experienced as social isolation, grief, or guilt. It can be triggered by a single event like a breakup or the death of a loved one or by a combination of circumstances involving disappointment or rejection. It may also result from a biochemical imbalance involving low serotonin levels, with no apparent cause.

Emotional pain that has not yet progressed to depression can manifest as physical pain in many different ways, depending on an individual's specific vulnerabilities. Physical disorders with emotional causes can include anything from migraines and back pain to nausea and spastic colon. Experiencing physical pain can trigger the memory of an emotionally painful event, and reliving emotionally painful events can trigger the physical pain all over again, making many treatments for pain less effective.

If left untreated, emotional pain may lead to depression. Some depression becomes so severe that patients begin to see suicide as the only way to end the pain. In this situation, seeking the help of a mental health professional is critical. As with sleep deprivation, there is a reciprocal relationship between chronic pain and depression: Chronic pain can lead to depression and depression intensifies

pain. Although emotional pain alone can cause serious physical distress, most patients who experience chronic pain together with a psychiatric illness do have a physical rather than a purely emotional basis for their pain. However, treating the depression will speed recovery from physical pain and make it less likely to recur.

People who suffer from depression often feel fatigued, worn out, mentally foggy, and even unworthy of life. They often blame themselves for their condition, thinking that if they just prayed more or became stronger that they would feel better. Even if they have much to live for, their brains often cannot see past their current feelings.

## Managing Emotional Pain

It is possible to heal from emotional pain, however, especially given enough time. Patients should try to replace painful memories with good ones, while not struggling against the urge to cry or grieve actively. While many resist crying as too painful or as a sign of weakness, it can be a wonderful way to release pain, bitterness and fear, and ultimately to facilitate healing.

Numbing pain with drugs, alcohol, irresponsible sex, or other self-destructive behavior can be very tempting but ultimately inhibits and delays healing. Instead, patients should work to honestly confront their feelings and move past them. It is important that patients evaluate their relationships and distance themselves from people who are overly critical, judgmental, or otherwise negative, while surrounding themselves with positive and encouraging people. The key is to collect those people who boost your energy, make you feel safe, and lift you up. Avoid the narcissists, victims, and passive–aggressive people. They will drain your energy, so set clear limits and boundaries with them.

Carrie, a loving wife and mother, describes her depression as "living in a glass tube"; she could see the world but was unable to connect with it in any meaningful way. Nothing was particularly wrong in her life, but her condition became so severe that she attempted suicide three times.

For Carrie, the physical pain involved in her condition was just part of her problem. The most dangerous phase of her illness was when she felt nothing. The absolute numbness and isolation from the rest of the world was terrifying and almost proved fatal. Fortunately, after her third suicide attempt, Carrie underwent electroconvulsive therapy (ECT). A light pulse of electricity was passed through her brain while she was under anesthesia, and the results were life-transforming. Most patients see a positive response within four treatments, but Carrie began to feel noticeably better after her first session. She experienced some minor side effects—mild aches in her neck and shoulders and small deficits in her short-term memory—but these disappeared within a few weeks.

Carrie's husband supported her recovery by writing her encouraging notes and by reaching out a group of friends to help him ensure she was rarely alone or without a listening ear. Loved ones can help a person struggling with emotional pain or depression by listening and offering kind, supportive words as well as helping them to obtain professional treatment if necessary. Importantly, showing self-compassion promotes our own emotional healing. Our main relationship in life is with ourselves, so being kind, loving, and encouraging to ourselves is therapeutic and represents a self-management approach to healing emotional wounds.

# Hope for Emotional Pain Relief

Emotional pain, stress, and depression are extremely complicated issues that express themselves differently in every individual. Reaching out to mental health specialists, such as psychologists or psychiatrists, is an important step toward feeling better, particularly in cases of suicidal thoughts or significant depression.

The good news is that medical research is continuing to offer us greater understanding of how to effectively deal with and prevent these problems. Safeguarding our emotional health as vigilantly as we would safeguard our physical health will go a long way toward helping us live long, pain-free lives.

You can learn more about sleep, stress, and emotional health by listening to the related episodes of my weekly radio program, *Aches and Gains*. You can find the broadcasts on sleep, stress, and emotional health at the following URLs.

**Sleep and Pain**
http://paulchristomd.com/sleep-pain

**Stress**
http://paulchristomd.com/stress-pain
http://paulchristomd.com/stress-pain-2

**Emotional**
http://paulchristomd.com/emotional-pain

# Suggested Further Reading

Bianchi, Matt T. *Sleep Deprivation and Disease: Effects on the Body, Brain and Behavior.* (n.p.): Springer, 2016. This book covers sleep physiology, experimental approaches to sleep deprivation and measurement of its consequences as well as the health and operational consequences of sleep deprivation. https://tinyurl.com/y7ou7xyq

Burch, Vidyamala, Penman, Danny. *You Are Not Your Pain: Using Mindfulness to Relieve Pain, Reduce Stress, and Restore Well-Being—An Eight-Week Program.* (n.p.) Flatiron

Books, 2015. This book reveals a simple eight-week program of mindfulness-based practices to reduce pain. https://tinyurl.com/y8k3cegm

Carney, Colleen, Manber, Rachel. *Quiet Your Mind and Get to Sleep: Solutions to Insomnia for Those with Depression, Anxiety or Chronic Pain.* (n.p.): New Harbinger, 2009. This workbook discusses cognitive behavior therapy to optimize your sleep pattern by using methods to calm your mind and help you identify behaviors that contribute to insomnia. https://tinyurl.com/y9o376lp

## Other Resources to Explore

Everydayhealth.com medically reviewed article about eliminating stress to relieve pain.

The National Sleep Foundation website is dedicated to improving health and well-being through sleep education and advocacy, including articles on pain-related sleep loss.

PainScience.com article about the role of sleep deprivation in chronic pain, specifically muscle pain.

Psychology Today article discussing the connections between emotional stress, trauma and physical pain.

Spine-Health.com peer reviewed artocle about chronic pain and incomnia.

# 19

# Mind-Body Techniques for Pain Relief

Since ancient times, philosophers and religious leaders have suggested that how we think affects how we feel, while skeptics have dismissed the idea. Now, modern neuroimaging studies are beginning to verify and reveal the depth of the relationship between our thoughts and our physical sensations. As we discussed in Chapter 18, Sleep, Stress, and Emotional Health, the anticipation, memory, or fear of pain can activate the same areas of the brain that physically painful stimuli activate.

## Understanding the Mind-Body Connection

The profound effect that the mind can have on the body has tremendous implications for pain management and relief. The relationship between our mental state and our pain is complicated because chronic pain often leads to persistent negative thoughts. Pain can change our mood, our relationships, and even our self-perception. The brain is responsible for processing painful signals that travel from the body, though the spinal cord, and on to specific regions of the cerebral cortex. It's the brain that interprets the meaning of pain and triggers emotional responses, such as sadness, anger, and fear. Because the brain is so active in this process, it's receptive to mind-based techniques for addressing pain.

This chapter discusses three techniques for pain self-management: biofeedback, cognitive behavioral therapy (CBT), and hypnosis. The effectiveness of these techniques does not mean that the pain is "all in the head" of the patient, suggesting that their pain was imaginary. Instead, it demonstrates the degree to which our response to pain determines how it is processed, how long and intensely it is felt, and how disabling it becomes. These techniques have virtually no side effects, so anyone suffering from chronic pain should strongly consider giving them a try. It's my hope that these mind-body strategies will enable you to discover within yourself the resources for reshaping the experience of pain. I've seen it happen for patients of mine.

## Biofeedback

Biofeedback may sound futuristic or mysterious, but it has actually been in use since the 1960s. In short, biofeedback involves using standard medical equipment to measure a patient's basic physiological functions, such as heart rate, blood pressure, and muscle tension. Once these assessments are made, the therapist shows the measurements to the patient (usually on a computer screen) and explains what they mean. The therapist then teaches the patient various techniques to begin to exercise a degree of control over these functions, most of which were once thought to be completely beyond voluntary control.

As patients learn to influence their breathing, heart rate, and muscle tension, they begin to reduce the response of their brains to pain and stress. For instance, studies show that biofeedback can be quite effective for treating migraine headaches in adults and children, and other research has demonstrated its benefit in tension headache, jaw pain (TMJ, for example), and fibromyalgia. Patients with arthritis, irritable bowel syndrome, neck pain, and pelvic pain can benefit from biofeedback as well. Most recently, a study on chronic back pain found that biofeedback alone or in addition to physical therapy or pain psychology (such as cognitive behavioral therapy; see the next section of this chapter) improved pain intensity, muscle tension, depression, and coping ability. Biofeedback can be used alone or to enhance other kinds of treatment such as pain medication or physical therapy. It can be a terrific alternative when medicines are not recommended such as during pregnancy or childhood.

Clarissa was a retired anesthesiologist who suffered from temporal arteritis, which is inflammation of an artery in the head that causes headaches, scalp tenderness, and jaw pain. She was also diagnosed with polymyalgia rheumatica, which caused her substantial muscle pain in her upper back, shoulders, and hip as well as Crohn's disease that caused abdominal pain, psoriasis, and migraines.

Temporal arteritis usually resolves with treatment, but Clarissa suffered from continual tenderness over the eyebrow even after treatment. Her sheer number of pain conditions would cause most patients and doctors to feel exasperated and simply give up. Clarissa found her pain completely debilitating, and after chronic use of oral steroids and several other medications failed to bring her relief, she knew she needed a different approach. Clarissa did not limit her search for relief. She was open to Eastern medicine and had a feeling that stress was a component of her symptoms.

## Biofeedback and Pain Relief

Biofeedback sessions teach patients the skill of self-regulation through breathing and cognitive techniques. Patients learn to exercise control over their physiological functions with the ultimate goal of reducing autonomic arousal—often referred to as the fight-or-flight response—and muscle tension, both of which exacerbate pain. As we discussed in Chapter 18, Sleep, Stress, and Emotional Health, the brain initially treats pain as a threat, activating the body's defense system. Patients implement biofeedback techniques to bypass this response, calming their muscles instead of tensing them in the face of pain. Biofeedback is a concrete example of how we can channel our thoughts to positively affect our body; the mind gains control of the part of the nervous system that both pain and stress activate.

Clarissa began sessions with Jim Cahill, the founder of Mindfulness-Based Biofeedback Therapy (MBBT), which utilizes Western medical equipment to measure physiological processes and Eastern mindfulness techniques to teach patients how to regulate these functions. Mindfulness—a cultivated state of nonjudgmental awareness of one's emotions, thoughts, and bodily functions—originated with Buddhism and has recently gained a great deal of popularity in the West.

During Clarissa's first session, Cahill explained some of the theory behind biofeedback, and then Clarissa was connected to an EKG machine with sensors on her chest, wrists, and fingers. Many patients may also wear an elastic sensor around their abdomens. Other therapists use EMG (electromyography, which measures muscle activity), respiratory, or heart rate variability biofeedback for treating chronic pain. After a few minutes, Clarissa was shown her heart rate and rhythm on a computer screen.

Cahill instructed Clarissa how to focus on her breathing—slowing its pace, exhaling completely, and breathing from her abdomen rather than her chest. After she had practiced the controlled diaphragmatic breathing for a few minutes, she was shown another readout from the EKG, which revealed that her heart rate too had slowed and become more regular. The heart rate wave had now coordinated with the breathing wave on the monitor. Clarissa also learned about meditation and special exercises for progressive muscle relaxation. (Progressive muscle relaxation is a relaxation technique that involves deliberately tensing muscle groups and then releasing the tension and paying attention to the contrast between tension and relaxation.)

After each session, Clarissa was given homework to practice the skills she had learned each day. The goal was to teach her to detect and control these physical functions on her own, without the equipment.

The purpose of looking at the feedback from the machine is to recognize the connection between particular painful sensations and what is actually going on in the body. This kind of subtle mental control takes time to learn and refine, but with regular practice, it is possible. Patients are encouraged to practice at least 10 minutes a day, twice a day, ideally in the morning and evening.

Some people learn to make the physical adjustments to their bodies independent of the biofeedback machines in as few as five guided sessions, but most patients benefit from 10 or 20 in order to see a therapeutic response. Biofeedback sessions typically last about an hour and can cost between $75 and $150 per hour with a therapist. Insurance companies vary in their coverage, but many won't cover biofeedback. Because biofeedback is both subtle and complex, it's important to find a qualified biofeedback therapist. Ask about training and experience.

Board certification does exist. Patients seeking biofeedback can consult the Biofeedback Certification International Alliance (BCIA).

---

Clarissa began seeing improvement after the first one or two sessions and felt an escalating benefit after each session. Today, she feels much better and practices the techniques on her own for about 20 minutes a day. She doesn't tense up her muscles anymore and feels that the benefits build over time as her skills continually improve. Clarissa now has the ability to control her response to the pain, and it's been "a life changer" for her. She has more fun, less stress, and less pain. She recommends that patients begin biofeedback right after they are diagnosed, rather than waiting.

Cahill believes that patients can achieve about 50% pain reduction in general, but the therapy needs to be maintained. He also mentions that side effects are very minimal. Relaxation-induced anxiety can occur, but it's rare. He also notes that patients who "can't sit still" are less likely to do well with biofeedback.

---

Newer applications of biofeedback include heart rate variability coherence biofeedback (HRVCB). In a pilot study, this technique improved pain, stress, and activity limitations among veterans with chronic pain due to injuries. The principle behind HRVCB is that the heart can be "trained" to send more vagus nerve impulses to the spinal cord, which then suppresses the flow of pain signals travelling to the brain.

### Biofeedback and Other Pain Therapies

Biofeedback doesn't interfere with other treatments, including nerve blocks and medication, and may increase their effectiveness. Some patients use biofeedback to reduce their need for medications as well. Biofeedback may be used in conjunction with physical therapy or cognitive behavioral therapy, especially for back pain. It's encouraging to see that some research even suggests that these combinations may result in even greater improvement in wellbeing.

# Cognitive Behavioral Therapy

Pain is processed and interpreted in various regions of the brain: Thoughts and images are activated in the somatosensory cortex, and certain emotions are formed in the limbic system, particularly the anterior cingulate cortex. Functional MRIs of the brain suggest that persistent negative beliefs and mental images can both prolong and amplify the pain experience.

Cognitive behavioral therapy (CBT) focuses on the relationship between our thoughts and our pain. Some CBT therapists also incorporate biofeedback techniques into their treatment. CBT gives us the tools to reshape our thinking, develop realistic alternatives to negative thoughts, and change how we perceive pain.

Neema developed complex regional pain syndrome (CRPS) after a workplace accident. A crushing pain that begin in her injured arm spread across her back to her other arm and caused her fingers to go numb, the hair on her arms to fall out, and her fingernails to become thin and brittle. Shower or tub water hurt her skin so much that sponge bathes were the only way she could clean her body. As the pain became unbearable, she lost her job and friends, and her husband divorced her. "I couldn't work anymore or contribute to the family income, needed to see doctors, took medicines, and couldn't get out of the chair," she said. "My husband couldn't take it anymore." Friends though she was faking her symptoms and stopped seeing her.

Although Neema found some relief from various medications, she also experienced terrible side effects. The opioids and medications such as gabapentin (Neurontin) and topiramate (Topamax) helped at first, but the side effects clouded the relief. In her ongoing quest for something that worked, she tried physical therapy, several sympathetic nerve blocks in her neck, epidurals, and an implanted spinal cord stimulator. The stimulator worked for a few years, but then the CRPS spread to her entire body, including regions not covered by the device. Finally, an implanted pain pump delivering hydromorphone (Dilaudid) and baclofen (Lioresal, Gablofen) for pain and spasms helped her cut back on the oral medications and provided her 40%–50% pain relief. (See Chapter 15, Pain Relieving Devices, for more information about neurostimulation and pain pump therapies.)

Yet Neema still felt her life was slipping away. She experienced negative thoughts about herself and the future. She was constantly reminded of how the pain had ruined her life and felt that she had nothing to live for. She lost interest in doing things, and slept all day in front of the TV. Neema thought about suicide, but she also had a desire to return to the life she once had. That's why she made a decision to try CBT, even though it was five years after her diagnosis. Neema felt that CBT might enhance the other pain relief methods she was utilizing, and, in fact, she found that CBT greatly increased the effectiveness of her pain pump by changing the way her brain processed the pain of CRPS. This in turn gave her enough relief to begin moving again and doing more physical therapy.

Like biofeedback, cognitive behavioral theory works to alter the way our brains process pain by changing the thought patterns associated with pain. As we've mentioned in previous chapters, chronic pain can make patients feel hopeless, depressed, fearful, and even suicidal. These negative thoughts are referred to as "maladaptive" because they are so counterproductive and actually make the pain worse.

Neuroimaging confirms that different types of statements and thoughts about ourselves can enhance or reduce activity in areas of the brain associated with processing pain (the "pain neuromatrix"). In short, negative thoughts increase pain neuromatrix activity and positive thoughts decrease it. Patients who cultivate positive, optimistic thinking can learn to modulate the severity of their pain. CBT therapists are trained to help patients learn different thinking patterns that we refer to as adaptive thoughts.

What people believe about the cause of their pain directly affects how they deal with it. Many times, patients unknowingly develop a fixed view of their suffering. When they receive a diagnosis of a particular disease or injury, they may assume that there is nothing they can do about the symptoms. For example, nerves may be damaged from an injury causing burning pain. The nerve damage certainly contributes to the pain, but patient *reaction* to the nerve damage contributes to the perception of pain too. CBT offers a different perspective, challenging patients to think about what they *can* do and to stay away from limiting statements and thoughts, such as, "The pain will always feel like this. I'll never get better."

Many of our thought patterns are so habitual they become almost automatic or part of our subconscious. Negative thinking can occur without us even knowing it. Negative thoughts that become automatic can become self-fulfilling prophecies. The beliefs become manifest in daily life. We may end up losing friends, losing a job, feeling more pain, or skipping activities. Just as biofeedback helps patients become aware of bodily processes that are largely involuntary, CBT helps patients recognize their subconscious thoughts and beliefs and evaluate whether those thoughts and beliefs are helpful or detrimental to their pain.

CBT patients are often encouraged to keep a diary of their pain as well as their feelings and thoughts in response to that pain. These strategies help them monitor their thoughts and replace negative thoughts with adaptive thoughts more quickly. Involving a supportive spouse or family member can also be very helpful. Loved ones can help by learning how to recognize maladaptive thinking and steer the patient toward a healthier response.

## Resilience, Catastrophizing, and Cognitive Behavioral Therapy

For some patients, an illness or injury is their first real experience with hardship, so they have not had a previous opportunity to develop much resilience. They have trouble adapting to the changes the pain brings. The longer the pain persists, the more they develop an image of themselves as disabled; every pain signal triggers a cascade of negative thoughts. That is why it is best to begin CBT as soon as possible after a diagnosis of chronic pain, rather than waiting until every other therapy has failed. Having a psychologist work on preventing any reinforcing, maladaptive pain thoughts from emerging can minimize the impact of the pain experience at the outset.

Some patients in pain catastrophize—ruminate obsessively, consider all of the worst-case scenarios, and predict that the pain will wreck their lives. Research using functional MRI (fMRI) scans shows that this type of behavior increases brain activity in areas that deal with attention to pain, anticipation of pain, and the emotional response to pain. Other studies indicate that catastrophizing interferes with our capacity to cope by amplifying pain and interfering with treatment. Needless to say, it's critical to limit this type of thinking, and CBT can be quite helpful in doing so.

CBT is not an exercise in fantasy: It requires patients to be honest about their pain and then examine how they are reacting to it. The positive adaptive thoughts must be realistic or they do not help the patient cope with reality. Patients must take ownership of their situations and commit to doing all they can to feel better, which can be quite challenging for people who feel helpless and hopeless. Neema admits that she had to face some hard truths, namely that her life wasn't going to be the same as it was before the injury. "That's the tough love part of CBT," she said. But she's been able to craft a new life, and that has made all the difference.

CBT is also not a matter of suppressing negative thoughts. It is a matter of recognizing negative thoughts and replacing them with more positive yet realistic thoughts that will reframe the patient's worldview. A lot of emotional distress and self-defeating behavior is based on inaccurate thinking, but this can be challenging to communicate to people in pain without making them feel that others are blaming them or failing to sympathize with what they are experiencing.

Many patients find that shifting their energy away from finding a cure to engaging in activities despite the pain enables them to achieve new goals. For example, Neema feels hopeful, more motivated and goal-oriented now. "I can set and meet goals which give me a sense of accomplishment that I haven't had since I was hurt," Neema said. I let my patients know that they may not function at the same level, but CBT can help them have the hope and energy to rearrange their activities, pace themselves, and set realistic goals to make their lives meaningful.

Effective treatment can also include talking with a vocational counselor. A counselor can help patients who have been unemployed because of their pain find a new profession or a related job. Both working and retired patients often benefit from finding new recreational pursuits and learning new skills and hobbies.

It is very important that those in pain know that they have people who love them and that they have a value to the world. For example, Neema felt that the pain robbed her of her identity and added such an emotional burden to her life. CBT gave her back a sense of self, making her feel empowered to act. "CBT changed my mental attitude and that rules over everything. Pain is a 50/50 deal—50% actual pain and 50% how you *deal* with it," she said.

> Neema found that she needed to develop her CBT skills intentionally and consistently. Each morning, she worked to come up with a positive statement. These could be affirmations like "The pain is not as bad as it was yesterday and it will be better tomorrow" or "The sun is shining and I am feeling good." Sometimes this was very difficult due to the intensity of the pain, but she continued to work at it, not giving up. She also learned to visualize the pain melting away or leaking out of her body and onto the carpet. And she learned skills similar to those covered in the biofeedback section, including meditation, controlled breathing, and progressive muscle relaxation. Neema used these techniques to heal herself. "I used my mind to help my body heal," she said.

## Cognitive Behavioral Therapy and Cognitive Restructuring

Neema learned to identify and combat the negative thoughts that were pervading her subconscious thinking, including the idea that her pain would never end, her life was over, she would never be happy again, and that her pain would kill her. She began replacing them with positive and realistic thoughts, such as the idea that life was just beginning, the pain would be better tomorrow, and that she was going to die, but she was not going to die today.

This process is known as cognitive restructuring, and it takes time and deliberate effort. It took about six to twelve months for Neema to see noticeable results, but they have been well worth it. Neema is now much more engaged in life; she has a job, a lot of friends, experiences much less mental anguish, anxiety, and particularly less depression. She was once unable to move her hands very much, and she now crochets regularly and teaches others to crochet as well. "I found my passion again," she said. "I *thought* I'd never crochet again, and now I'm teaching it." In short, she feels like her humanity is restored.

On the practical side, CBT has allowed Neema to stop diazepam (Valium) and alprazolam (Xanax) and given her an additional 30%–40% pain relief. She continues to use her pain pump, though. Her quality of life has improved 100%. "I'd never be crocheting, working, or walking without

CBT." Often, after three to five months of completing CBT therapy, old habits begin to reappear, so periodic refresher sessions are recommended to prevent relapses, maybe every three to four months. Neema still sees a pain psychologist every two to three weeks, to help her keep her CBT skills sharp.

Cognitive behavioral therapy can cost $95–$135 per hour with a PhD-trained psychologist. Sessions run 45 to 60 minutes on average. Unfortunately, insurance coverage has dwindled, so co-pays and deductibles have risen. Nurses and other health professionals trained in CBT principles can offer first-line care, which may improve access.

## Cognitive Behavioral Therapy and Pain Relief

Fibromyalgia, headaches, and low back pain can respond well to CBT. Studies over the past 30 years support the benefit of CBT for headaches, arthritis, chronic back pain, and orofacial pain. Children and older adults report improvements too. CBT holds particular appeal in these groups because it's such a safe alternative to medication therapy or surgery. It has also provided relief and benefits to countless individuals whose specific pain conditions haven't been widely studied with CBT.

We may see more CBT delivered through telemedicine (diagnosing and treating patients remotely using computers and mobile devices, for example) and web-based chronic pain management programs in the future. One such program found that patients with various pain conditions showed benefits in pain for up to six months after treatment. Other promising work is revealing that text messaging supportive statements or engaging in virtual reality distraction on a smartphone can even reduce pain.

Given its potential for improvement, low risk, and opportunity for self-management, I would recommend that anyone with a chronic pain condition certainly seek out CBT. We're learning that we have the ability within ourselves to change how the brain perceives pain. That is, changing how we think changes pain-inducing brain activity.

# Hypnosis

Hypnosis has been around for centuries and, in modern times, it has been used successfully for medical purposes in surgery and dentistry. Often stigmatized as the territory of entertainers and charlatans, hypnosis is used less frequently than other mind-body techniques, even though there has been compelling evidence for its effectiveness in both acute and chronic pain for decades. As a matter of fact, people from different cultures over the centuries have used hypnosis to treat every pain condition imaginable.

Hypnosis takes mind-body healing to another level by bypassing the brain's conscious judgment and screening mechanisms. According to research findings, it changes neural activity in areas of the brain and spinal cord that process pain. That is, it reduces the spinal cord processing of pain in the dorsal root ganglia (the cluster of nerve cells that conveys sensory information to the spinal cord), reduces the awareness of pain in the primary somatosensory cortex of the brain (the area where the intensity, location, and duration of painful signals is analyzed), and decreases the emotional response to pain in a region of the brain called the anterior cingulate cortex.

Hypnotic analgesia (applying hypnosis for pain relief) has been applied effectively to manage acute pain during dental procedures, childbirth, surgeries, burn trauma, biopsies, and headaches and to manage chronic pain from conditions including cancer and irritable bowel syndrome. Furthermore, a 1996 National Institutes of Health (NIH) panel stated that there was strong evidence for hypnosis in alleviating chronic pain from cancer and other chronic pain conditions.

When looking more closely at chronic pain, studies show that hypnosis is effective for low back pain, osteoarthritis, sickle cell disease, temporomandibular pain (TMJ), pain from breast and bone cancer, and chemotherapy-induced nausea and vomiting. The pain reduction can last for several months as well.

Marco was working in commercial real estate in Seattle when cardiac problems prompted his doctors to implant a pacemaker in his chest. Unfortunately, the surgery left Marco with frequent painful attacks in his back, shoulders, and the upper left side of his chest. It was so severe that it would cause him to double over in pain. Diagnosed with frozen shoulder as well, Marco tried physical therapy but found it did not help at all.

Marco had heard that hypnosis had worked for others with similar pain conditions, and, at this point, he was willing to try anything. In the hypnotherapist's office, Marco sat in a comfortable chair while the therapist told him a calming story designed to induce a trance. Marco did not lose consciousness, but he did feel completely relaxed. Then the therapist told a different story, which included customized suggestions that Marco's pain was dissipating and that he'd regain full motion of his shoulder. The session lasted about 40 minutes. The therapist recorded the session for Marco and instructed him to listen to it every day for a month. Over that time, Marco found his pain gradually subsiding until it stopped altogether and never returned.

## Choosing Hypnotic Analgesia

A trance is often defined as a state between consciousness and unconsciousness, but it can also be understood as a special learning state where the brain is more receptive than normal. Many of us have daydreamed or concentrated on something to the point where we became unaware of our surroundings, which are both everyday examples of a trance. The normal judgment and screening functions performed by the frontal lobe are suspended during a trance, making the brain much more open to suggestion.

Hypnotic analgesia is best understood as a cooperative effort between the therapist and the patient. This relationship incorporates the trance state as a way to lessen the impact of painful messages sent from the body to the brain. In a typical 30-minute session, the therapist takes the patient through the following phases:

1. *Attention:* Traditionally we think of a hypnotist using a swinging watch during this phase, but in practice the therapists will often tell a story to focus patients' attention away from their surroundings.

2. *Relaxation:* As with other mind-body techniques, the therapist will often ask the patient to focus on his or her breathing.

3. *Deepening:* This often involves the therapist counting or asking the patient to visualize going down a set of steps or riding down an elevator; the idea is that each step or number takes the patient "deeper" into the trance.

4. *Suggestion:* This is where the therapist accesses areas of the brain involved with pain modulation and makes suggestions about reducing pain intensity or lifestyle changes.

For example, the therapist may suggest that a painful sensation be replaced by a warm or cool feeling or tell the patient to look into the future and see himself or herself in less pain.

5. *Alert:* This brings the patient out of the trance; it is important that this step be done properly or the patient may experience headaches or confusion after treatment.

Brain imaging performed during hypnosis reveals a series of changes that take place during this process. As you might expect, the part of the brain that processes attention lights up during the first phase. It also seems that the influence of the left hemisphere over the right hemisphere becomes weaker, a state associated with a greater capacity for fantasy and imagination. As the therapist makes suggestions, changes can often be observed in the somatosensory cortex (which interprets pain intensity, location, duration) and anterior cingulate cortex (which interprets emotions and suffering).

The suggestion phase requires the most skill and training for therapists to get the desired results—it's the art of hypnosis. Depending on the source of the pain the patient is experiencing, suggestions must be made with careful wording or they will be less effective. Some patients, particularly those with neuropathic pain (diabetic peripheral neuropathy, or amputation, for example), respond better to suggestions for the pain to be less intense. Others, particularly those with chronic musculoskeletal pain, respond better to suggestions to suffer less, strengthen themselves, and make positive lifestyle changes.

Although many people are concerned that hypnotists can exert mind control over their subjects once they are hypnotized, repeated studies have shown that this is not the case. In decades past, various organizations and governments attempted to hypnotize people to become assassins or do other things they would not normally do without any success. The silly things people do during stage hypnosis like quacking like a duck result from the person's overall willingness to be part of a fun act.

## Hypnosis and Pain Relief

Hypnosis can be a godsend for patients who cannot tolerate certain pain medications or injections or who have a higher risk of side effects, including children and older adults. However, about 10%–20% of people may not benefit from hypnosis. It's not completely clear why some people are more able to be hypnotized than others, but there is likely a genetic component. In addition, many environmental factors influence the ability to be hypnotized such as motivation, curiosity, and a rich imagination. Interestingly, children are good subjects for hypnosis probably because they have rich fantasy lives and display more curiosity and open-mindedness than adults.

Pain relief from hypnosis varies a great deal by individual and the type of pain condition. In general, patients can expect about a 30% reduction in pain. For some, the relief may only last a few hours, but that can extend to several months, a year, or even continually if practiced regularly at home.

Trained therapists can be found through the American Society of Clinical Hypnosis or the American Association of Professional Hypnotherapists. Hypnotherapy is the use of hypnosis as a therapy technique. One hypnotherapy session may be sufficient for acute pain, while chronic pain like Marco's

may require ongoing treatment, generally about four to 10 sessions. Sessions typically cost between $100 and $200 and may be partially covered by insurance depending on the plan.

Self-hypnosis is an important feature of hypnotherapy, allowing patients to reduce their discomfort after the sessions end. You may just need 20 minutes in a quiet space. If you're especially talented, five minutes may be sufficient. Some welcome positive "side effects" of hypnotherapy include better sleep, greater sense of control, increased sense of well-being, and improved satisfaction with life.

Hypnosis is not recommended when pain is communicating an important message, such as the presence of an infection (appendicitis, for example), and should be used judiciously in patients who have undergone childhood trauma.

Marco found tremendous pain relief and without side effects. He regretted waiting to start hypnosis. He thought it was practical, safe, and as effective as taking a pain pill. "I think it's underutilized because people have apprehensions about what it might do," he said. Given his results, Marco now highly recommends hypnosis for managing pain.

Hypnotic analgesia offers the amazing potential to transfer pain to the background of our perceptions while providing a strong motivation for self-care and

enhanced activity. In the future, we can expect to see hypnotherapists harnessing virtual reality technology to facilitate a trance and aid in the therapeutic process.

# Other Sources of Information about Mind-Body Techniques for Pain Relief

You can learn more about biofeedback, cognitive behavioral therapy, and hypnosis by listening to the related episodes of my weekly radio program, *Aches and Gains*. You can find the broadcasts on biofeedback, cognitive behavioral therapy, and hypnosis at the following URLs.

**Biofeedback**
http://paulchristomd.com/biofeedback

**Cognitive Behavioral Therapy**
http://paulchristomd.com/CBT
http://paulchristomd.com/CBT-2

**Hypnosis**
http://paulchristomd.com/hypnosis

# Suggested Further Reading

Dibra, Sebhia Marie, Micozzi, Marc S. *Overcoming Acute and Chronic Pain: Keys to Treatment Based on Your Emotional Type.* (n.p.): Healing Arts Press, 2017. A holistic approach that reveals how pain should be understood as a dynamic condition—an interaction between mind and body. https://tinyurl.com/ycqhop7g

Kabat-Zinn, Jon. *Mindfulness Meditation for Pain Relief.* (n.p.): Sounds True, 2010. An audiobook that explains how mindfulness practice can help with pain management. https://tinyurl.com/yddlpzt8

Swingle, Paul G. *Biofeedback for the Brain: How Neurotherapy Effectively Treats Depression, ADHD, Autism, and More.* (n.p.): Rutgers University Press, 2008. This book describes how neurofeedback procedures work through numerous case examples. https://tinyurl.com/y9smdm2v

Thorn, Beverly E. *Cognitive Therapy for Chronic Pain: A Step-by-Step Guide.* (n.p.): The Guilford Press, 2004. A hands-on book providing a complete cognitive-behavioral treatment program for readers suffering from chronic pain. https://tinyurl.com/ybuwldtn

# Other Resources to Explore

Familydoctor.org is operated by the American Academy of Family Physicians and includes articles about the mind and body connection and how your emotions affect your health.

Medical News Today's article describing what biofeedback therapy is and how can benefit from it.

National Institute of Health Medline Plus magazine's directory of past articles about emotions and health and the mind-body connection.

The University of Minnesota Center for Spirituality and Healing's website offers a list of body-mind therapies, patient support groups, cognitive-behavioral therapy, mediation, yoga, biofeedback, and more.

WebMD's overview of biofeedback and how biofeedback therapy works.

# 20

# Alternative Medicine and Pain Relief

For centuries, Western medicine has focused primarily on the physical aspects of illness and considered only treatments that have been proven to be effective using the Western scientific method. Western medicine typically relies on surgical intervention and pharmacological therapies developed in laboratories and tested in large, randomized clinical trials. With these methods, Western medicine has been remarkably successful in increasing life expectancy and preventing death from traumatic injuries and infection.

But Western medicine has its limitations. For millennia, Eastern medicine—a general term used to described care strategies developed since ancient times in places such as China and India—has focused on holistic wellness. Holistic medicine is characterized by the treatment of the whole person, taking into account mental and social factors, rather than just the physical symptoms of a disease. Traditionally, Eastern medicine has taken the view that humans are spiritual and emotional as well as physical beings, and has focused on preventative medicine as well as healing.

Healers in ancient times did not have the means to see into the body with x-rays, MRIs, or CT scans or to perform blood analysis or large clinical trials, but they did have a body of knowledge passed down orally or in writing from their predecessors. These "clinical notes" recorded what did and didn't work in certain cases and gave rise to many practices still in use today. Ancient healers may not have had scientific evidence to support their treatments, but many of those treatments had positive effects on patients.

This chapter explores how some alternative treatments and innovative approaches to wellness are becoming integrated into modern Western medicine. We'll examine how Western doctors are beginning to address the whole person (rather than just the physical aspects of illness), the use of herbal remedies, and the ancient Chinese practice of acupuncture.

## Holistic Medicine

Holistic medicine looks at treating the whole person in order to achieve balance and well-being. Holistic medicine incorporates nutrition, the environment, and emotions as well as social, spiritual, and lifestyle modifications in order to help heal people and help them attain a state of wellness. Holistic medicine does not require a rejection of Western medicine, but rather involves an incorporation of some Eastern techniques into the therapeutic plan.

Country music star Naomi Judd unknowingly contracted hepatitis C, a potentially fatal liver disease, from an infected needle during her early career as a nurse. When Judd was diagnosed in 1991 after two years of experiencing worsening symptoms, her Grammy Award–winning singing career came to a crashing halt. She describes her experience with the disease-like having a severe case of the flu all the time. Her bones seemed to ache, she had a constant headache and low-grade fever, and she struggled daily with fatigue and depression. At one point, she was confined to a wheelchair and given three years to live.

But Naomi fought back. Under her doctor's guidance, she gave herself interferon injections—a combination of proteins designed to boost her body's ability to fight the hepatitis C virus—three times a week. Like others receiving such treatment, she experienced terrible side effects, so she began researching other ways to stimulate her immune system. Her quest for knowledge and hope led her to many alternative medicine techniques, and she tried an array of them—acupuncture, aromatherapy, biofeedback, chiropractic adjustments, music, meditation, massage, affirmations, visualizations, and guided imagery. She also found that the emotional release and deep breathing involved with singing supported her healing process.

Naomi continued to give herself the interferon injections, relying on alternative medicine to help her through the almost unbearable side effects. Finally, an improved form of interferon helped her body defend itself from the virus and put her hepatitis C into remission. She used a holistic approach to counterbalance the traditional means of treating disease and educated the public on the mind, body, spirit link. Naomi also added that instead of looking for Mr. Right, women should look for Dr. Right when dealing with pain. In other words, make sure the doctor is open to integrative strategies and doesn't dismiss your pain experience. Judd is the author of several self-help books and has been a spokesperson for Partners Against Pain.

Naomi Judd's story is a good example of how holistic medicine can complement conventional therapy. Patients give up on treatments such as chemotherapy (as Naomi almost gave up on interferon) because the side effects can be terrible. But Naomi integrated prayer, meditation, and visualization of her body fighting the virus, and these strategies enabled her to continue a full course of treatment.

## Holistic Medicine and Pain Relief

Modern brain imaging and other measurements of physical functions reveal that holistic medicine strategies (like the mind-body techniques discussed in Chapter 19, Mind-Body Techniques for Pain Relief), can have measurable physical benefits. For many years, doctors and nurses have noted anecdotally how cheerful patients with strong support systems seem to have much better chances of surviving an illness compared to lonely and depressed individuals with the same diagnosis.

More and more adults, even older adults, are finding holistic medicine useful for common musculoskeletal conditions, such as low back pain and arthritis. Complementary and integrative therapies are increasingly popular among adults; surveys indicate that about 33% of adults report using them. The most commonly used are herbals and dietary supplements.

I have had patients facing intense pain and frightening diagnoses, for example, who have found comfort and even pain relief in the Serenity Prayer, written by Reinhold Niebuhr and used by many 12-step programs, including Alcoholics Anonymous:

*God, grant me the serenity to accept*
*the things I cannot change,*

*The courage to change the things I can,*

*And the wisdom to know the*
*difference.*

For people of many different religious backgrounds, this prayer becomes a form of adaptive meditation, helping them let go of the desire to control the illness itself, and empowering them to take charge of their healing. I've had patients tell me that they use this prayer as a means of comfort just to get through each day.

A "take charge" self-help attitude can lead to less pain and disability, and less need for analgesics among patients with back and neck pain according to one study. The holistic care model can empower patients to reframe negative images of their health in favor of positive thinking about their own ability to manage their health and wellness. Numerous patients of mine, as well as Naomi Judd, have harnessed this positive, relaxed, and distracted mind-set to reduce pain sensitivity.

## *Choosing Holistic Medicine*

For various reasons, some patients are reluctant to consider a holistic approach, even if the methods have the potential for benefits and very few side effects. This can result from a low tolerance for ambiguity—preferring certainty and guarantees—or because they don't have the patience for the length of time that alternative therapies can take to work. In these cases, patients may need extensive education, including information about the growing body of scientific evidence for the non-physical components of pain covered in Chapter 18, Sleep, Stress, and Emotional Health—before they will agree to try mind-body techniques or similar integrative therapies.

Naomi Judd ultimately credits her triumph over hepatitis C to several factors including her spirituality, her supportive relationships, and her sense of humor. She also stayed close to nature, got the right amount of rest and exercise, ate healthy foods, and promoted a belief system that was open to new ideas.

# Herbal Remedies

Many plants have medicinal properties and these plants have been used for millennia for treating disease and easing pain. The World Health Organization (WHO) estimates that 4 billion people, or 80% of the world population, use herbal medicine for some aspect of their primary health care.

Recent clinical studies have supported the effectiveness, dismissed by conventional medicine for years, of some herbs to treat certain conditions. Improved analysis of ingredients has also allowed for the production and packaging of pharmaceutical grade herbals, in which the listed ingredients are accurate to at least 2%. These developments have caused herbals to become more accepted as treatment options, often as complements to more conventional therapies or sometimes as replacements for more traditional medicines.

Herbals can be taken orally, topically, or even injected. Some patients receiving prolotherapy injections, such as those described in Chapter 16, Regenerative Biomedicine, receive a combination of herbals such as vitamin B-12, calcium, and magnesium.

The beneficial compounds in plants can be extracted in a number of ways. Essential oils (also discussed in Chapter 21, Aromas, Music, and Pain Relief) are formed by various methods of pressing. Other herbal medications are derived by drying and grinding various parts of the plant, such as the flowers, stem, leaves, or roots. Common herbal remedies include chlorophyll derived from green plants; many vitamins and minerals from various sources; herbs associated with cooking such as garlic, turmeric, and ginger; and compounds such as bee pollen.

## Herbal Remedies and Pain Relief

Some herbals have such profound anti-inflammatory properties that they are known as "natural NSAIDs" and are therefore taken to alleviate pain. These include boswellia, chaparral, skullcap, devil's claw, and arnica.

Studies of devil's claw demonstrated it is just as effective taken orally as rofecoxib (Vioxx) for relieving low back pain but without the harmful side effects that eventually took rofecoxib off the market. Patients with low back pain have also benefited from willow bark, the plant from which aspirin is derived. Studies have shown that oral willow bark, like devils' claw, provided as much pain relief as rofecoxib (Vioxx) in those with low back pain.

If you have osteoarthritis (OA), willow bark may benefit you as well, according to another study. Although willow bark may not have substantial benefit over aspirin, patients report that the effect of willow bark lasts longer. However, it also takes a bit longer for them to begin noticing the effect of willow bark. Preliminary studies of green tea tablets taken with a traditional nonsteroidal anti-inflammatory drug (NSAID) suggest better pain control and joint function in patients with knee osteoarthritis—encouraging information for patients living with mobility restrictions from knee pain. Another herb called boswellia shows promise as an anti-inflammatory supplement for osteoarthritis. This supplement substantially improved both knee function and pain in a couple of studies.

Headaches, muscle aches, and arthritis often respond positively to herbal supplements. Feverfew, a member of the daisy family with NSAID-like activity, has been shown to bind to receptors in the brain similarly to aspirin. It has been used to treat headaches, arthritis, and even menstrual cramps. Sarapin—a solution derived from the plant Sarraceniaceae (pitcher plant)—can be injected as an alternative to cortisone in painful joints. Some herbalists report that pancreatitis and malabsorption problems also respond positively to herbal supplements. Most people benefit from various combinations of herbals (rather than just one herbal), designed by herbalists to remedy a specific problem such as joint pain or inflammation.

## Choosing Herbal Remedies

Herbal remedies are usually much less expensive than traditional prescription medicines, but unfortunately they are rarely covered by insurance. The average cost of a month's supply of herbal medicines hovers around $30–$60. Although they can have fewer side effects than pharmacological medicines, some herbs may cause nausea, vomiting, and dyspepsia. For example, devil's claw can decrease blood glucose, lower blood pressure, and increase stomach acid. Further, there are several reports of lead poisoning related to boswellia, so be careful when taking these remedies. Certain supplements also don't have an appealing smell or taste, dissuading some patients from trying them. Like pharmaceutical NSAIDs, if taken at high enough doses for long periods of time, certain herbals may lead to liver or kidney abnormalities. The most serious side effect of herbals is an allergic reaction, which is rare. Because of the potential risks of interactions between herbals and traditional drugs, be sure to let your doctor know which herbals you're taking.

Not all herbal supplements are created equal. More expensive herbals are not necessarily more effective, and sometimes herbals may be sold in forms that are not likely to be absorbed well. For example, vitamin C is often taken orally when it is absorbed much more effectively when given intravenously. There isn't much interest in or need for intravenous vitamin C treatments, though. Interestingly, high intake of oral vitamin C is associated with pain relief, less cartilage loss, and slower disease progression in patients with osteoarthritis of the knee. More research is needed, however, to figure out exactly how dietary changes might modify the progression of knee osteoarthritis.

Because there is little regulation or oversight of the thousands of herbal supplements available, it is easy to get a product that's old, has an inaccurate description of ingredients or potency, or even one that contains heavy metals. Some lower quality supplements may be made from the right plant but the wrong part of the plant. Fortunately, the U.S. Pharmacopeial Convention (USP) does provide a list of verified dietary supplements, which are products that have been voluntarily submitted to the USP dietary supplement Verification Program and have successfully met the their standards.

On the horizon, we can expect new tests that more accurately reveal an individual's vitamin and mineral deficiencies. This will allow for more beneficial supplements and treatments, customized according to individual need.

## Acupuncture

Acupuncture is a Chinese treatment that has been used for over 2500 years to maintain wellness and treat pain. During acupuncture treatment, fine needles are inserted into specific points in the skin called meridians to restore the vital force known as qi (pronounced chee). Traditional Chinese medicine asserts that these meridians traverse the body and carry qi (life energy) from organs to the surface of the body. Blockages of flow through these meridians lead to inflammation and pain. Needling releases these blocks and restores flow.

Traditional Chinese medicine holds that the uninterrupted flow of qi is central to good health, and illnesses are caused by blockages in this flow. They believe that in a healthy individual, qi flows from the organs to the skin through 12 meridians. Furthermore, these meridians represent body systems that help regulate function. The 360 traditional acupoints (locations where needles are inserted into the skin) are the "off ramps" from the meridians to the skin; needle placement maintains the healthy flow of qi or removes blockages to restore it. Think of the meridians as highways of energy flow, and picture the acupoints distributed over the front and back of the limbs, face, head, neck, and trunk.

Since President Richard Nixon's visit to China in 1972 normalized relations between the United States and China, millions of Americans have used acupuncture to treat pain. One of those Americans is Lila, who battled plantar fasciitis—pain and inflammation of a thick band of tissue found in the arch of the foot—for two years. She saw multiple podiatrists and other specialists to no avail. Although afraid of needles, Lila tried acupuncture. After just seven treatments a week apart, her foot pain completely stopped and has remained so two years later. Patients in some of the plantar fasciitis research studies have not necessarily experienced such remarkable relief, but they have reported less heel pain when traditional therapies such as NSAIDs and stretching are combined with acupuncture.

Unfortunately, years later, Lila was also diagnosed with fibromyalgia. Her pain covered the entire back half of her body, from her neck to her feet. It woke her from sleep, preventing her from working or exercising, and soon caused her to gain weight. She would feel a shooting sensation down her back that travelled to the back of her leg too. Lila's doctor started her on a low dose of duloxetine (Cymbalta), and he also referred her to a doctor who practiced alternative medicine. The duloxetine reduced her pain and improved her depression and anxiety. Lila then tried trigger point injections (which didn't really help) as well as chiropractic treatments and massage. She also returned to acupuncture because she wanted to be more functional and feel less discomfort.

## Forms of Acupuncture

Lila's treatment was fairly typical of acupuncture sessions. During each medical acupuncture session, the doctor would listen carefully to Lila's description of the pain she was feeling, which would inform his placement of the needles. He placed between 30 and 50 needles into the skin of her head, neck, back, arms, wrists, or any areas where she was experiencing pain.

Stimulating acupressure points with needles only, and often twirling them to achieve an effect at the site of insertion, is called conventional acupuncture. Acupuncture needles are sterile, disposable, and incredibly fine—significantly thinner than those used in IVs. They are usually made of stainless steel. Japanese practitioners typically place the needle just a few millimeters into the skin, whereas Chinese practitioners place them half an inch deep or more, but placement depth also depends on the location in the body and the type of pain being treated.

Some practitioners add electrostimulation to acupuncture therapy by running a small electrical charge through the needles, which varies in strength between 2 Hz and 100 Hz. It's believed that patients get faster relief with electrical acupuncture. Electro-acupuncture also seems to be an effective complement to antidepressants when treating certain kinds of depression.

Other practitioners forgo the needles altogether, using transcutaneous electrical acupoint stimulation, whereby electrical impulses are transmitted through adhesive pads. Children, and those with needle phobia, may be more receptive to acupuncture when offered this way.

Even lasers can be used to activate acupuncture points. Patients of mine have also found that the process of moxibustion, burning a Chinese herb near an acupuncture point, adds to the stimulatory effect.

In auricular acupuncture, practitioners target parts of the ear to reduce pain by stimulating the auricular nerve, a branch of the vagus nerve. (See the discussion of the vagus nerve in Chapter 15, Pain-Relieving Devices). The meridians mentioned earlier travel through the ear as well. Acupuncturists can place five or so needles in the ear for about 20 minutes to modify pain. Not only that, auricular acupuncture can help support the treatment of drug addiction in hospital settings and substance abuse treatment programs. A few of my patients with difficult to treat conditions such as CRPS and phantom limb pain have done well with auricular acupuncture. They have felt much more comfortable with needles around their ears compared to anywhere else in the body.

### Acupuncture and Pain Relief

Let's examine how acupuncture relieves pain. It is thought that there are three primary levels of action as follows:

1.  Needle placement has a local anti-inflammatory effect, increasing circulation to painful areas and improving energy flow.

2.  Electro-acupuncture appears to stimulate the release of endorphins, the body's own natural painkillers. Interestingly, lower frequencies seem to trigger the release of endorphins, while higher frequencies trigger other natural painkillers referred to as dynorphins. Some practitioners believe that they can treat acute pain with one frequency and chronic pain with another one. And research in animals shows that acupuncture

not only releases endorphins but another pain fighting chemical called adenosine.

3. Functional MRI (fMRI) imaging of the brain shows significant changes in brain activity when needles are placed in certain areas. Acupuncture appears to quiet the limbic system, the seat of our emotional response to pain discussed in the last chapter, and to lower autonomic arousal (the body's "fight or flight" response). Even more fascinating is that it may be able to reverse the abnormal changes in the brain's processing of pain, according to fMRI research in patients with carpal tunnel syndrome.

Studies are currently underway to determine if acupuncture may also produce an endocrine effect, stimulating or suppressing the release of particular hormones.

Interestingly, Western medicine affirms the usefulness of many of the 360 traditional acupoints. Many acupoints closely correspond to common myofascial trigger points—tense, tight, hypersensitive bands of muscle. Needle placement may help to deactivate trigger points and reduce pain that way. Some myofascial pain is also associated with spontaneous electrical activity in the connective tissues, and putting a needle in the area can normalize that activity.

We also know that acupoints have higher concentrations of nitric oxide than other areas in the body. Nitric oxide dilates blood vessels and is important in signaling between cells. The meridians do not correspond to blood vessels or lymph nodes, but the meridians do seem to correspond anatomically to connective tissue planes. The acupoints are the spots on the body where these connective tissue planes come together. Needling releases nitric oxide, and it is possible that instead of following nerves or blood vessels, nitric oxide flows to other acupoints along the connective tissue planes or the meridians, thereby sending messages to the spinal cord and brain in a unique fashion.

As we just noted, placing needles in some acupoints demonstrates definite changes in the brain, which are detectable on fMRI scans. There are specific points for modifying pain too. Needle placement in both Large Intestine 1 (an acupoint found between the first and second finger) and Stomach 36 (found on the shin) shows a very specific ability to reduce certain areas of brain hyperactivity associated with pain. For example, Stomach 36 might be accessed for knee arthritis or neuropathic pain in the legs.

Practitioners who treat patients with acupuncture listen to the patients' descriptions of their symptoms and look for patterns of tenderness along specific meridians. Large intestine points are generally needled for pain in the upper body, and stomach points are needled for pain in the lower body. Some practitioners place needles directly into the region of pain (into the scalp or neck if pain is located in those areas, for example).

Acupuncture is quite safe. A group in Germany studied almost 230,000 patients receiving physician-administered acupuncture and found that 8.6% had at least one side effect; bleeding and pain were the most frequent.

## Choosing Acupuncture

There is evidence that acupuncture improves bioelectrical signals travelling between tissue planes and triggers pain-relieving processes in the skin, spinal cord, and brain. If you read the literature, you'll find some doubt over the value of acupuncture for pain. Yet, several large, high-quality scientific reviews do describe benefit for low back and neck pain, migraine, knee osteoarthritis, shoulder pain, and fibromyalgia. Recent clinical guidelines from the American College of Physicians recommend acupuncture for acute and chronic low back pain. Patients of mine have found acupuncture helpful for low back pain, migraine headaches, and fibromyalgia. Patients with upper back pain can respond well to acupuncture therapy as well as those with tennis elbow, menstrual cramps, and pain after dental surgery too. I even have patients with chronic facial pain who have found traditional and auricular acupuncture helpful in reducing the intensity of their pain.

If you suffer from any of these conditions, consider acupuncture alone or in addition to other treatments because it could make a meaningful difference in your life. The benefits of acupuncture tend to be cumulative—each treatment builds on the previous one—so patients should give it about 10 sessions to evaluate effectiveness. It's not easy to wait that long, so patients often concurrently use medications or nerve blocks if appropriate. I've found that integrating acupuncture into a comprehensive treatment program produces good results.

To treat her fibromyalgia, Lila started with a 20-minute session—both traditional and electro-acupuncture—twice a week for the first month. Then she started tapering down. By her fourth session, she was feeling significant improvement, especially in her neck and shoulders. After her sessions, she would feel a little sore but relaxed and even a little lethargic. Other unexpected benefits were stress relief and anxiety reduction. Actually, the treatments were so relaxing that she would fall asleep during each one. She even found that acupuncture regulated her menstrual cycle. Now Lila goes for acupuncture once a month and enjoys about 70% relief from her fibromyalgia pain. At this point, she has been able to wean off duloxetine (Cymbalta). She continues the treatment to maintain the positive effects on stress and anxiety and reiterates that acupuncture requires time; the results aren't instantaneous.

Acupuncture does not interfere with other medications or treatments. The cost per session (which can last anywhere from 20 minutes to an hour) can range from $20 to $35 for community acupuncture (sessions are tailored to individual needs but occur with other clients in the same space) to an average of $93 per session for a private visit. This can be costly, but some insurance companies will cover at least part of the cost. Both physicians and other healthcare providers perform acupuncture. To find a qualified and licensed acupuncturist, visit medicalacupuncture.org (the web site for the American Academy of Medical Acupuncture) or nccaom.org (the web site for the National Certification Commission for Acupuncture and Oriental Medicine).

## Other Sources of Information about Alternative Medicine and Pain Relief

You can learn more about holistic medicine, herbal remedies, and acupuncture by listening to the related episodes of my weekly radio program, *Aches and Gains*. You can find the broadcasts on holistic medicine, herbal remedies, and acupuncture at the following URLs.

**Holistic**

http://paulchristomd.com/holistic-approaches

**Herbals**

http://paulchristomd.com/herbal

**Acupuncture**

http://paulchristomd.com/acupuncture

http://paulchristomd.com/acupuncture-2

# Suggested Further Reading

Chevallier, Andrew. *Encyclopedia of Herbal Medicine.* (n.p.): DK, 2016. A home reference on the healing benefits of plants. https://tinyurl.com/ybpmj4nn

De la Foret, Rosalee. *Alchemy of Herbs: Transform Everyday Ingredients into Foods and Remedies That Heal.* (n.p.): Hay House Inc., 2017. This book teaches readers the healing properties of various herbs. https://tinyurl.com/ycg48yf7

Kennedy, Anne. *Herbal Medicine Natural Remedies: 150 Herbal Remedies to Heal Common Ailments.* (n.p.): Althea Press, 2017. This book offers effective natural remedies that can be used to treat common ailments, without the risk of potentially harmful pharmaceuticals. https://tinyurl.com/y8c2b9ab

Ma, Yun-tao. *Biomedical Acupuncture for Sports and Trauma Rehabilitation: Dry Needling Techniques.* (n.p.): Churchill Livingstone, 2010. Through evidence-based research acupuncture expert Yun-tao Ma shows how biomedical acupuncture will enhance athletic performance, accelerate recovery after intensive workouts, and speed trauma rehabilitation after injuries or surgeries. https://tinyurl.com/y9gyh5a5

Pursell, J. J. *The Herbal Apothecary: 100 Medicinal Herbs and How to Use Them.* (n.p.): Timber Press, 2015. This book profiles 100 medicinal plants with instructions for making herbal teas, tinctures, compresses, and salves to treat everything from muscle strain to the common cold. https://tinyurl.com/y9w3frav

# CHAPTER

# 21

# Aromas, Music, and Pain Relief

We associate pain most often with our sense of touch, but pain, and chronic pain in particular, is a highly emotional experience too. Pain extends to other dimensions of our lives and can take us down the path of depression, cognitive impairment, or insomnia. Our memory can be affected, which can in turn lower our self-confidence and lead to despair. Along with touch, other senses may be deeply involved in modifying pain. The relationships between our senses and pain have yet to be fully explored. This chapter discusses aromatherapy, which involves our sense of smell, and music therapy, which involves our sense of hearing. (Aromatherapy can also be understood as a component of herbal therapy, discussed in Chapter 20, Alternative Medicine and Pain Relief.) These holistic techniques can be wonderful supplements to conventional therapies and can offer surprising relief and comfort for even the most severe pain.

## Aromatherapy

Odors are all around us and most of us are quite sensitive to smell. Odors can be foul, steering us away from spoiled food or toxic chemicals. Pleasant odors, however, such as spices or flowers, can trigger pleasant emotions and memories, give us a burst of energy, and lift our spirits. But could aromatherapy actually treat a serious disorder? That idea might sound farfetched, but Amanda and Lana found relief through aromatherapy after decades of suffering from debilitating migraines and chronic sinusitis, respectively.

More and more people in the United States and around the world are turning to aromatherapy—the medicinal therapeutic use of highly concentrated essential oils from plants or the peel of citrus fruits—as an option for alleviating pain, managing stress, and enhancing relaxation. It is important to note when discussing aromatherapy, that synthetic fragrances from soaps and candles are not essential oils and are not recognized as aromatherapy. Real essential oils are produced by a process of steam distillation, which separates the essential oil from the plant, producing the extract called an essential oil. Oils such as lavender, peppermint, and chamomile are inhaled or rubbed into the skin. Under the guidance of a certified medical aromatherapist, they can also be taken orally as tinctures or as rectal or vaginal suppositories. Most commonly, though, patients inhale the oils or apply them topically.

Since her mid-twenties, Amanda had suffered from chronic sinus infections, bronchitis and asthma, which led to pounding pressure and pain in her right ear and eye. She had to "mouth breathe," developed ear infections, and couldn't concentrate. A nasal steroid resolved many of her symptoms, but Amanda was afraid of its detrimental effect on her glaucoma. After years of taking over-the-counter medications such as Allegra-D (for allergy and congestion) and Mucinex (an expectorant), she began taking even stronger prescription antihistamines and decongestants. Unfortunately, these left her tense and interfered with her sleep, and, eventually, her glaucoma forced her to discontinue her prescription medications because of their side effects.

Lana, a retired administrator, suffered for 50 years from migraine headaches. A typical headache would leave her bedridden for two to three days. She'd feel the pain in the back of her neck and forehead, experience blurred vision, nausea, and eventually "couldn't function as a normal human being." Lana took countless prescription medications including beta blockers, nortriptyline (Pamelor), and verapamil (Calan), but still experienced migraines almost weekly, despite injections as well.

Both Lana and Amanda were introduced to aromatherapy later in their lives but found its positive effects to be more potent than they could have imagined. Initially, Amanda was skeptical of aromatherapy because she had already discovered that certain perfumes and fragrances aggravated her medical conditions. But under the guidance of a doctor trained in aromatherapy, she tried a tincture—an oral dose of essential oils—made up of black pepper, peppermint, lavender, clove bud, frankincense, and lemongrass oil. In addition to taking the tincture twice a day, she also rubbed essential oils on the skin of her forehead and inserted a cotton swab with the oils into each nostril.

Amanda didn't like the process at first, and for the first several days, applying the oils seemed like a strange ritual, but after about two weeks, her congestion dissipated almost completely. Within two months, she had completely weaned herself off all her prescription and over-the-counter medications. Lab tests confirmed that her histamine levels dropped from 900 to about 190. For the first time in over 25 years, Amanda felt relaxed, calm, and able to breathe freely. The tincture reduced the number of right ear infections too. Both her ear and eye pain went away along with the pressure pain she felt in her sinuses.

And the effects have lasted. As long as Amanda sticks to her essential-oil regimen, she finds that her sinusitis resurfaces only when she is exposed to heavy levels of smoke, dust, or pollen. "If I forget to use the aromatherapy, the stuffiness can return, but I can even exercise for an hour now without getting winded," she said.

Amanda notices no side effects; however, in some cases, essential oils can cause slight skin irritation but seem to be regarded as safe by the FDA. Rarely, essential oils can cause photosensitivity (bad sunburn) if taken orally in large amounts. Similar to reports of patients in research studies, Amanda experiences a lot less anxiety as well. Aromatherapy studies have found that patients feel less depressed and better satisfied with their treatment too.

Lana has a similar success story. She began to rub a combination of peppermint, black pepper, lavender, lemongrass, clove bud, and frankincense oils behind her ears, on the back of her neck, and on her temples and forehead whenever she felt a migraine was imminent. This amounted to applying aromatherapy oils a couple of times per week. Incredibly, Lana finds that this allows her to elude the onset of the migraine more than 95% of the time. She's discovered that applying the oils soon after sensing the migraine prevents it from becoming a debilitating headache. The oils need just five to 10 minutes to take effect before the headache goes away.

Her ability to fend off the headaches that used to keep her in bed for days has freed Lana up to live her life much more fully than before. For example, she can perform daily tasks at home and have a normal day. "It's wonderful," she said. "I'd be bedbound during the migraines if I didn't have the aromatherapy." Like Amanda, Lana has experienced no side effects even after three years of regular treatment.

## Aromatherapy and Pain Relief

Several studies have found beneficial effects of either topical or inhalational aromatherapy for reducing a variety of painful conditions. When used on the skin, an essential oil is often combined with a carrier oil—olive or almond oil—and then delivered by massage. Oils can be applied to the skin without massage too, as Amanda and Lana experienced.

The evidence indicates that aromatherapy may be effective for a host of painful conditions. These conditions include the following (the method of delivery is listed in parentheses):

◆ Chronic back and neck pain (massage)

◆ Knee pain (massage)

◆ Menstrual pain (abdominal massage)

◆ Episiotomy pain (topical)

◆ Hemodialysis needle stick pain (inhaled)

◆ Multiple sclerosis (massage at pain site)

◆ Kidney pain (inhaled)

◆ Pediatric pain from blood draw and after tonsillectomy (inhaled)

That's not to say aromatherapy is ineffective for other conditions such as migraine or sinusitis. As Lana's and Amada's stories indicate, people who suffer from these conditions have also found relief with aromatherapy. Some patients with cancer pain, post-stroke shoulder pain, and women in labor or after Cesarean section assert that aromatherapy helps manage their discomfort as well.

Aromatherapy is one of the oldest healing arts, dating back to ancient Egypt and is found in virtually every healing culture around the world. French doctor Jean Valnet popularized it during the 1950s. His book, *The Practice of Aromatherapy: A Classic Compendium of Plant*

*Medicines and Their Healing Properties*, was published in 1980. In the United States, several states include clinical aromatherapy as a holistic option for nursing care and practice.

## Understanding Aromatherapy

Medical aromatherapy probably alleviates pain in at least a couple of different ways. First, as a patient inhales the odor, the molecules travel through the nose and to parts of the brain known as the hippocampus and amygdala (parts of the limbic system) by way of the olfactory nerve. These brain regions help to process pain and may reduce unpleasant sensations. They also regulate emotions of pleasure and reward. For instance, studies have shown that in less than one second, inhaled clove can begin to change hormones and neurotransmitters that amplify pain. It may be that the odor suppresses pain by reaching the pleasure center of the brain. Furthermore, scents activate specific memories when they reach the hippocampus. Aromatherapy may trigger pleasurable memories and the release of endorphins, both of which make us feel better and alter pain sensations.

Second, when an essential oil, such as thyme, is inhaled, the molecules of the odor travel into the lungs, often opening airways and making breathing easier.

Pleasant odors often cause our breathing to slow and deepen, and research suggests that this change in breathing pattern induced by aromatherapy reduces pain perception. In addition, slow, deep breathing can suppress the sympathetic nervous system (part of the autonomic nervous system that is responsible for our fight-or-flight response), which in turn influences pain processing.

Unlike artificial fragrances, essential oils are small and chemically simple compounds, made mostly from carbon and hydrogen. They are extracted from plants through distillation, or in the case of citrus peels, through pressing. Oils that are rubbed into the skin can absorb into the bloodstream transdermally (through the skin), but are also vaporized by body heat and thus inhaled. Once in the lungs, the odor molecules are absorbed into the capillaries and enter the blood stream that way.

Essential oils produce pain-relieving effects in unique ways. For instance, clove has been shown to stimulate the production and release of GABA, a neurotransmitter that interferes with nerve firing and controls pain transmission. Clove has been used as a local anesthetic before needle insertion, and applying one drop of clove oil on a cotton swab tip can help with toothaches.

Eucalyptol—the active agent found in eucalyptus, rosemary, and other plants—has a direct pain relieving effect, but studies show it also suppresses the release of inflammatory compounds such as interleukins and leukotrienes. Furthermore, eucalyptol can be a digestive aid as well. By improving digestive function, it reduces over-stimulation of the pancreas and the excessive release of insulin.

Other essential oils that offer pain relief include the following:

- German chamomile has actually been shown to alter the adrenal glands' production of cortisol and DHEA, which in turn alters mood. It seems that it can act like an opioid pain reliever as well as block the effects of opioids.

- Oil made from grapefruit increases the release of epinephrine (adrenaline) and acts as a natural antidepressant.

- Lemon oil produces a cheering effect.

- Frankincense is anti-inflammatory along with stress-relieving.

- Peppermint oil stimulates cold receptors in the skin that takes away the heat from inflammation. Consider applying it after a sunburn.

- Birch and oil of wintergreen both contain large amounts of salicylic acid, very similar to aspirin, which can soothe arthritic pain.

- In cases of muscle spasm in the low back, marjoram has been shown to have effective anti-spasmodic qualities and also increases GABA.

- Pelvic pain associated with premenstrual syndrome (PMS) or dysmenorrhea can be decreased with yarrow, chaste tree berry, sage, and German or Moroccan chamomile massaged into the skin. These seem to reduce inflammation and histamine release as well as balance estrogen and progesterone.

- Several oils massaged on the skin or taken orally can be useful for fibromyalgia too. These include eucalyptus, lavender, geranium, fennel, and clary sage.

Overall, peppermint, clove, lemongrass, eucalyptus, and German chamomile have the best track record for relieving pain. Eucalyptus may be more effective for inflammatory pain, while clove may better modify nerve pain. Rose, balsam fir, German chamomile, lavender, and fennel can have positive effects on bone pain, and rose might be particularly helpful in metastatic cancer pain.

## Choosing Aromatherapy

Inhaling essential oils offers relief within seconds, but the effects of inhalation also last for the briefest duration. Oils can be inhaled safely every one to two hours when placed on a cotton ball or cotton swab. Alternatively, oils can be placed in a diffuser, allowing patients to vaporize the scent continuously. Effects from rubbing essential oils into the skin are felt within minutes and should last for several hours, after which oils can be reapplied. When essential oils are taken orally—which is typically done two to three times a day under the guidance of a physician or certified medical aroma-therapist —it may take an hour or two for the onset of relief of symptoms, but relief should last for most of the day. There are also aromatherapy patches that can be worn on the skin. Parents can treat young children in pain by waving a cotton ball with essential oil near the nose, positioning it two feet away and bringing it gradually closer so it is not frightening. Even people without pain may find inhaling essential oils helpful for lessening anxiety and facilitating a meditative state of peace and calmness.

Perhaps the easiest way to inhale essential oils is with an ultrasonic diffuser (similar to a vaporizer) placed at home or in the office. An ultrasonic diffuser may also be helpful in postoperative recovery rooms. Two postoperative pain studies have demonstrated positive results with inhalation aromatherapy in patients after total knee replacement, and breast biopsy surgery. Heat damages the compounds in oils, thereby weakening their healing properties so avoid heating the oils when putting them in a diffuser.

Aromatherapy probably works best when combined with standard pain management therapies. It offers exciting possibilities for managing pain and stress as an inexpensive treatment with few side effects. Remember that essential oils are real chemical compounds and should be recommended for medicinal use by qualified aromatherapists. Certain forms of thyme and Holy Basil, for instance, can be toxic to the mouth and throat. Always ask practitioners for their certification.

# Music Therapy

Music has been used since ancient times to influence health and help people deal with pain and distress. Across all cultures, music sways human emotion and changes mood. We know that emotions and mood are both capable of lessening pain as well. Music's therapeutic use in the modern era began in psychiatric hospitals in 1930s and early work continued with World War II veterans a decade later.

Music has been shown to reduce pain during surgery and to have a positive effect on those with chronic pain or terminal illness. When compared to standard care or other non-drug therapies, studies have also shown that music reduces postoperative pain, anxiety, and analgesia consumption. Music has proven to be effective when patients are under general anesthesia too. Music interventions can involve patients listening to any kind of live or recorded music they enjoy, watching videos along with the music, or even playing or singing music themselves.

Musician and composer Tim Janis spent a month living in his car as he struggled to make it in the music industry. His first CD featured him singing original compositions, but he also decided to include one track that was entirely instrumental. Little did he know how that decision would change the course of his career.

Janis began to receive letters praising his first album. To his surprise, the instrumental track generated by far the most positive response, with many people telling him how calm and peaceful it made them feel. Janis took the feedback to heart and began focusing on composing instrumental music with simple, soothing melodies. Today, not only has he worked with many world-class musicians such as Billy Joel and Ray Charles, but his music is also played in operating rooms, delivery rooms, nursing homes, and palliative care settings across the country.

## Music Therapy and Pain Relief

Like aromatherapy, music therapy seems to relieve pain in diverse ways. Some research reports that music lowers levels of the fight-or-flight neurotransmitters epinephrine and norepinephrine, leading to a dampening effect on the sympathetic nervous system and reducing heart rate, blood pressure, and respiratory rate. Other studies have associated pleasurable music with activation of the nucleus accumbens (part of the brain's reward system and pain processing network) as well as other brain regions that regulate emotional, autonomic, and cognitive function.

Music also stimulates the release of another neurotransmitter in the nucleus accumbens and other parts of the brain called dopamine. Dopamine has a role in analgesia and we have data showing that an overall increase in dopamine levels can inhibit long lasting pain. Pleasant music has the ability to decrease pain perception by influencing neurotransmitters in the spinal cord as well.

Music can serve as a positive distraction from pain by capturing our attention and triggering pleasant memories and images. This prevents existing pain from being magnified by anxiety or distress and often shortens its duration. Soothing music like Janis's—with tempos between 60 and 80 beats per minute—also causes us to relax, relieving muscle tension. It's this slow, flowing tempo that seems to promote pain relief too.

Patients who sing or play wind instruments breathe deeply, which is associated with stimulating the parasympathetic nervous system in a way that slows the heart rate and decreases muscle tension. Music can even trigger the release of endorphins, the body's natural pain killers. Sometimes, musicians or those listening to an instrumental performance such as a symphony will experience euphoria, the feeling of intense joy associated with even higher endorphin levels.

Maria has battled decades of chronic spinal pain and finds a great deal of relief when she sings either by herself or with a group. She has learned that the more emotionally invested she is in the music, the greater the relief she feels. "The harmonies and lyrics take me to another place," she says. If the piece is particularly challenging, it will require greater concentration and distract her for longer periods. When she sings or performs with a group, the collective energy and companionship cheer her up, while the deep breathing needed to sing also relaxes her. The relief she experiences lasts anywhere from 20 to 30 minutes after performing or listening to music. If she could bottle the feelings of euphoria after singing and "take that out later, it would be great," she says.

Kate, a music therapist who often plays the keyboard or autoharp for her patients, will play a song at the tempo at which a patient is breathing and then gradually slow down. This can actually help slow the patient's breathing and have a calming effect. In her experience, the type of music doesn't matter as much as the patient's relationship to it. For example, some of her patients love gospel music, while others respond better to country.

Kate's experience as a music therapist includes countless success stories. She has seen multiple sclerosis patients not only improve their pain, but also improve the gait and cadence of their walk. She had a patient with cancer who was using such high doses of opioid in his intravenous patient controlled analgesia (IV PCA) pump that it reached toxic levels in his blood. After introducing music therapy to complement his pain medication, he needed far less opioid and never became toxic on the medication again. In my practice, I have met others who share Kate's positive experience with music and have found music therapy helpful in alleviating pain for patients in palliative care settings.

Evidence is mounting for the value of music therapy. Preliminary work in patients with neuropathic pain has shown lowered pain scores, and many patients who have access to music therapy reduce their need for medication and experience improved sleep. Listening to music helps reduce pain intensity for chronic conditions such as low back pain, arthritis, fibromyalgia, and cancer.

## Choosing Music Therapy

Music therapy sessions can range from 20 to 60 minutes in length with sustained benefit for up to two weeks after discontinuing the therapy according to one study. Surgical patients can use headphones to listen to music before, during, and after the procedure, which has been shown to reduce acute pain as described earlier. Some hospitals use audio pillows that have speakers inside of them instead of headphones.

If you have children who must have surgery, ask if music therapy is available. One recent study found that children listening to music or audio books while wearing headphones after surgery minimized their pain compared to those who had no intervention.

Music therapy doesn't interfere with medications or treatments. It's easy to administer, safe, and costs little to implement. The benefits are evident and I hope we see music therapy provided more often as a complementary treatment for acute and chronic pain management.

Eliana's mother led a very active life until she was hospitalized with pneumonia and chronic obstructive pulmonary disease (COPD). "She was dancing just a few weeks before her hospitalization," Eliana remarked. During her stay, Eliana's mother was intubated (had a breathing tube placed in her trachea) three times, which prevented her from talking. Being intubated, stuck with needles, and confined to bed led to tremendous emotional and physical pain, but this was made much more bearable by listening to Tim Janis's music and watching his accompanying videos daily.

The music helped Eliana's mother forget about the seriousness of her medical condition and occupied her mind while she was confined to bed. When listening to the music, she smiled, was interactive, had a calm facial demeanor, and didn't need much pain medication. "The music took my mom out of the hospital mentally and emotionally," she said. "The effects were immediate too." As her mother's caregiver and loved one, Eliana found the music comforting as well. She told me that she felt as if angels were caring for the two of them through Janis's healing music.

Unfortunately, due to a dispute with the insurance company, the music therapy was cut off after several weeks. Eliana immediately noticed a dramatic change in her mother for the worse. Her mother began groaning, asking for more pain medication, and became more demanding. "The pain started immediately after the music stopped, and my mom began to focus on her breathing and feeding tubes," she said. To Eliana, this was proof positive of the value of music therapy. Importantly, once the music was restored it transformed her mom's last weeks of life into a peaceful, calm, and hopeful experience.

Tim Janis has drawn much of his inspiration from film composers and Romantic composers such as Debussy and Rachmaninoff as well as from the natural beauty of his native state of Maine. His pieces are relatively short—usually between three and four minutes—and the melody is usually introduced within the first few seconds. He blends orchestral music and folk instruments to reach listeners deeply.

Janis believes it is the melody that supplies the energy and power to uplift and heal, and so he keeps his melodies simple and easy to learn. "Music motivates you to move (exercise) and keeps you going when your body gets tired," he said. My own patients have recognized that music inspires them to better engage in life by accomplishing even little things like going to physical therapy or taking a walk with friends. This correlates well with some of the research highlighting greater functional mobility in patients with fibromyalgia who engage in music therapy, for instance.

Janis has composed special music for wounded soldiers who often suffer from physical and emotional pain, depression, and anxiety as well as for military men and women serving overseas. They often write him to share the impact of his calming and comforting music, reminding them of home. Janis sees music as a sort of "nutrition for the soul," offering us a sense of well-being and peace in a world that is often full of turmoil. Most importantly, Janis believes, "it can open doors inside us that pain has closed."

# Other Sources of Information
## about Aromas, Music, and Pain Relief

You can learn more about aromatherapy and music therapy by listening to the related episodes of my weekly radio program, *Aches and Gains*. You can find the broadcasts on aromatherapy and music therapy at the following URLs.

**Aromatherapy**
http://paulchristomd.com/aromatherapy
http://paulchristomd.com/aromatherapy-2

**Music Therapy**
http://paulchristomd.com/audioanalgesia

Tim Janis

http://paulchristomd.com/melodic-medicine

http://paulchristomd.com/melodic-medicine-2

# Suggested Further Reading

*Essential Oils Natural Remedies: The Complete A–Z Reference of Essential Oils for Health and Healing.* (n.p.): Althea Press, 2015. Amazon's number one bestselling aromatherapy book outlining the healing properties of essential oils. https://tinyurl.com/y7tnjht3

Kennedy, Anne. *Aromatherapy for Natural Living: The A–Z Reference of Essential Oils Remedies for Health, Beauty, and the Home.* (n.p.): Althea Press, 2016. This comprehensive guide demystifies the chemistry and uses of essential oil remedies. https://tinyurl.com/yacaarrv

Korb, Christine. *The Music Therapy Profession: Inspiring Health, Wellness, and Joy.* (n.p.): Xlibris Corp, 2014. This book seeks to inform the general public and also musicians and students about music therapy written by former students. https://tinyurl.com/ycswumkf

Silverman, Michael J. *Music Therapy in Mental Health for Illness Management and Recovery.* (n.p.): Oxford University Press, 2015. This book informs readers of the psychotherapeutic research base and show how music therapy can effectively and efficiently function within a clinical scenario. https://tinyurl.com/ybzm6j4f

Worwood, Valerie Ann. *The Complete Book of Essential Oils and Aromatherapy, Revised and Expanded: Over 800 Natural, Nontoxic, and Fragrant Recipes to Create Health, Beauty, and Safe Home and Work Environments.* (n.p.): New World Library, 2016. This book offers readers tools to address a huge variety of health issues, including specific advice for children, women, men, and seniors, as well as self defense against microbes and contaminants, dealing with emotions, and specialist advice for athletes, dancers, travelers, cooks, gardeners, and animal lovers. https://tinyurl.com/yclvcr8g

## Other Resources to Explore

The Alternative Daily's list of essential oils for chronic pain relief.

American Music Therapy Association's official website offers information about the progressive development of the therapeutic use of music in rehabilitation, special education, and community settings.

Arthritis.org blog entry about aromatherapy for pain relief.

Base Formula, one of the UK's leading aromatherapy suppliers, lists the best aromatherapy oils for natural pain relief.

Everydayhealth medically reviewed article about music therapy in pain managements, how music can soothe, relax and provide a calming distraction to pain.

Practical Pain Management article highlighting the stories of five different patients who used music therapy to manage various types of pain.

# CHAPTER

# 22

# Harnessing the Human Biofield

Although the medications, nerve blocks, injection therapies, and neurostimulation devices discussed in Chapter 14, Pharmacological Therapies, and Chapter 15, Pain-Relieving Devices, can all be quite effective, they are limited; not everybody responds to them. Similarly, not everyone can benefit from the emerging state-of-the-art regenerative therapies discussed in Chapter 16, Regenerative Biomedicine. Accordingly, patients are seeking complementary approaches to aid in managing their pain. Although energy healing and biofield therapies are considered by most Western doctors to be a passing New Age fad with no scientific evidence to support their use or effectiveness, practitioners of healing arts, such as Jin Shin Jyutsu and Healing Touch have built up impressive track records of success. Now, a growing number of hospitals

are integrating such practices into the care they offer patients. In fact, energy healers practice in conjunction with conventional doctors and nurses in reputable hospitals and cancer centers around the country

In this chapter, we explore therapies that involve healing with touch and energy. Maybe the better term for biofield therapies such as energy healing (Healing Touch and chakra healing, for example) is "frontier medicine" given that the National Advisory Council for Complementary and Alternative Medicine (NACCAM) classifies them under this heading. In many ways, both energy therapies and regenerative therapies are truly "frontier medicine." It's not clear how these therapies work, so their use is controversial, but their potential is extraordinary.

# Healing with Touch and Energy

Energy healing traces its roots to the ancient healing arts in the East. In the ancient world, many religious, philosophical, and medical ideas were spread and exchanged between the great civilizations in India, China, and Japan. Thus, it is not surprising that we see so many similar concepts among the energy healing modalities that arose in these different areas, although each has its own special characteristics and practices.

So what is biofield therapy and how do energy and touch relate to pain? A common belief among the energy healing traditions is that all living things express *bio-energy* fields reflecting *bio-electrical* and *bio-electromagnetic* currents. These currents influence physiological processes. According to the biofield therapies, these energy fields (also called biofields) project beyond the skin's surface and interact with the environment, and practitioners can adjust the biofields to affect our body's internal system.

At first glance, this may seem unbelievable. Some feel that promoting mystical healing is nonsense and endangers the public's belief in solid biological treatments, especially if patients chose them over established treatments for disease. Yet, mainstream medicine is already

measuring bioelectric fields of the brain and heart with innovative, superconducting machines. For example, the heartbeat and chemical interactions inside cells, which are thought to create this biofield, have been measured in laboratory tests related to certain energy therapies. We unquestionably need more research to establish a scientific foundation for these therapies, but there is little harm to them and the benefits may astonish us. In fact, a large number of Americans have already been astonished based on a U.S. Gallup Poll indicating that 27% of respondents have experienced "a remarkable healing" with respect to their medical condition.

Scientifically, we are just beginning to understand energy healing. We know that electricity flows throughout the human body, and we're gradually gaining more insight into how to tap into biological energy fields to support health and soothe pain. We are not yet clear on the connection between these biofields and the subtler form of energy or "life force" described in ancient Eastern medicine as qi (China), prana (India), or ki (Japan). Nor do we have the capacity to actually measure the "aura," a field of luminous bioenergy, which is felt to surround an individual like a halo. Still there is clinical evidence to suggest that accessing the biofield can reduce pain.

Practitioners of the energy therapies influence the human energy field using non-contact or direct contact to restore flow and balance to the body. Similar to the theory behind acupuncture (discussed in Chapter 20, Alternative Medicine and Pain Relief), energy healing seeks to open blocks or disturbances in flow in order to heal pain, disease, or emotional and spiritual disruptions.

Within the context of pain, the concept is twofold: Pain interferes with a person's holistic balance and results from disruptions in the balance. Most energy healers begin a session by getting details about a patient's history and current symptoms. Practitioners, often trained through apprenticeship programs, typically use no touch, light touch, or gentle holds to release blockages to the circulation of energy—promoting health and possibly even supporting resistance to disease.

In my experience, I have seen patients incorporate energy therapies into conventional treatment, adding to the pain-relieving effect. Many energy therapies appear to help reduce the autonomic fight-or-flight response and enhance relaxation, a combination that is known to relieve pain. Some argue that energy therapy should simply be renamed relaxation

therapy. However, the benefits of relaxation alone don't explain why some individuals who have tried massage and other relaxation techniques without success are able to find relief from energy healing.

Scientific research on energy therapy can be difficult in general due to the placebo effect. (The placebo effect refers to positive results that are not due to the intervention being studied, which sometimes arise because patients believe in the effectiveness of a treatment.) However, some investigators have studied how energy healing affects cancer cells in the laboratory. Quite amazingly, researchers have noted that various forms of energy healing have inhibited cancer cell growth in test tubes, and similar results were seen in animal studies. We can't yet make reliable conclusions on the effects of energy healing for cancer, but the available information supports more extensive investigation. There may be a time when energy therapy has a place along with more conventional treatments for human cancers and cancer-related symptoms.

In this chapter, we explore several distinct but related energy healing therapies as well as the use of therapy animals to bring relief to those in chronic pain. As a side note, patients have reported that energy work offers them a significant emotional release, which can be so freeing when you have continual pain. Even patients who express skepticism about the mechanisms involved in energy therapies have benefited. Personally, I wonder whether some of the self-healing processes activated by the bioenergy therapies actually reflect, at least in part, the proposed cellular mechanisms involved in the regenerative therapies discussed in Chapter 16, Regenerative Biomedicine. It's an intriguing theory and one which well-developed experiments will help clarify.

## Chakra Healing

As a teenager, Ruby was in a serious car accident that left her with terrible whiplash and several pulled muscles. She spent three months in a neck brace and did a lot ofphysical therapy but still suffered from flare ups of severe neck and back pain.

As an adult, Ruby was in a horseback riding accident. She flew off the horse and landed sitting up. The riding accident left her with a vertebral body fracture in the upper part of her lower back, obviously making her pain even worse. "It felt like a knife piercing my back," she said.

After this accident, Ruby tried orthopedic inversion therapy, chiropractic adjustments, and massage therapy but still found her back and neck pain unrelenting. It became especially unbearable when she became cold or overly stressed. Emotionally she became more on-edge and impatient, and noticed that she was quick to interrupt others, for example. The pain spread into her arms and hands, and her neck would sometimes become so stiff that she could barely move.

Then Ruby's sister suggested she visit Kim Meisinger, an experienced chakra and energy healer. Ruby was about ready to give up, but she liked the concept of treating the whole person, so she contacted Kim.

Chakra balancing is an energy therapy rooted in the tantric and yoga traditions of Hinduism and Buddhism. The word *chakra* is derived from the Sanskrit word for wheel, which some healers visualize as a vortex of energy. The tradition teaches that there are seven main chakras, each connected to a physical place in the body that governs a certain set of organs or glands. The chakras represent energy sources that together form the human energy field.

Chakra healing practitioners believe that good health is associated with a balanced, steady flow of energy through the seven major chakras, which they evaluate in a number of ways. Kim Meisinger, the healer Ruby visited, is an empath, so she feels energy sensations travel to the surface of her hands as she places them over the body parts associated with the chakras, checking for blockage or congestion. For instance, Kim may feel a warmth over regions of a client's body that are painful or inflamed.

Tradition holds that the flow of energy between the chakras may be disrupted due to trauma or illness, and practitioners can help restore the normal flow of energy and support the body's ability to heal itself. To Meisinger, it feels like pain drains the energy fields. When she works with someone who is injured or in pain, she senses an underfunctioning of the chakras and a decrease in vitality.

Practitioners believe they are channels or conduits for healing energy to flow into a patient. In chakra healing, there is a focus on tapping our innate ability to heal ourselves. Healers such as Meisinger facilitate a patient's ability to engage this inner wisdom. "We are more than we imagine ourselves to be. The world today is so busy and out of tune with the internal part of ourselves that we miss the full journey that could be ours," Meisinger asserts. She has seen her clients feel less discomfort and redefine themselves in ways that are separate from the "pain identity."

Meisinger has seen a good response with chakra healing for patients suffering from irritable bowel syndrome, fibromyalgia, and those recovering from traumatic injuries. She has not seen favorable results in patients with metastatic cancer pain to the bone. There are few side effects, although on occasion, getting to sleep can be tough because patients feel so energized.

Ruby began each session lying comfortably on a massage table. Kim Meisinger would run her hand over Ruby's body to get a "read" on her chakras and energy flow. Her hands would then hover over various places on Ruby's body, based on what she sensed. Sometimes, Meisinger grasped her feet. Ruby told me she felt the sensation of lava flowing through her body and her feet, or she'd feel as though she were on a roller coaster or riding a wave—nothing scary, just a calming feeling. After the session, which lasted between 45 and 90 minutes, Ruby felt much better, more at ease, and centered.

Ruby experienced significant physical and emotional relief after her first session, and about 90% enduring relief after six of them. She still experiences occasional flare-ups of pain, particularly when life becomes stressful, but she no longer needs sessions on a regular basis. She goes occasionally for a maintenance session to preempt health problems, but otherwise, Ruby is living her life almost pain free.

Chakra healing sessions typically run between $60 and $150 an hour, depending on the experience level of the practitioner. The degree of pain relief depends on a patient's internal resources, lifestyle changes, and specific medical conditions, but Kim Meisinger says it's rare for somebody to not experience any relief.

Like many energy healers, Meisinger works in cooperation with physicians and other healthcare providers. She actually prefers that patients see a physician before consulting her for help. Meisinger often sees patients who, after medical assessments and interventions, hope that changes in energy flow will furnish additional quality of life benefits. She enjoys working in concert with healthcare providers.

Critics will point out that there seem to be no anatomical or physiological regions that correspond to the location of the chakras and that no "life force" energy or aura has ever been detected using modern instruments. There have been relatively few studies on the practice, but Dr. Valerie Hunt spent seven years studying energy healer Rosalyn L. Bruyere at the University of California, Los Angeles, in an attempt to document the existence of human energy fields. The study, while not able to measure the energy itself, did demonstrate a correlation between the energy sensed by Bruyere and physiological processes in the patients themselves.

## Healing Touch

Healing Touch is a form of energy therapy developed by Janet Mentgen, RN, BSN, in 1989. Mentgen, a nurse and experienced energy healer, standardized the scope of care and training program for Healing Touch practitioners. There is a formal Healing Touch curriculum, including a one-year mentorship that culminates in certification. The foundations of Healing Touch derive from therapeutic touch (the ancient practice of laying-on of the hands), other healing practices, and techniques developed by Mentgen herself.

Healing Touch shares many characteristics of chakra healing. Practitioners assess a patient initially by moving their hands either on or above the body and determining which energy centers may be imbalanced. They then direct energy to improve health or to treat a specific dysfunction by altering the biofield. Healing Touch acknowledges the seven chakras, the meridians of acupuncture, and the human aura. As with chakra healing, touch is not necessary to restore normal energy flow, but many practitioners use it to communicate empathy and positive change.

Darla was diagnosed with scoliosis at the age of 12. She wore a back brace for three years and had corrective surgery at age 18. Although her pain worsened after the surgery, she was able to do martial arts and enjoyed running. Over time, however, Darla experienced low back pain, sciatica, and back spasms that would render her motionless, sometimes for days. She couldn't lift or twist without pain, and for years she relied on ibuprofen (Advil) or acetaminophen (Tylenol), massage, and heat to manage the pain. Despite these measures, she often had to lie down flat on the floor when a back spasm hit her.

Darla had her doubts about Healing Touch but wanted to explore non-drug treatments that weren't too invasive. It appealed to her as natural and wholesome healing. Before her session, Darla was told to dress comfortably and that she would need to remove her shoes, lie face up on a massage table, and take deep breaths during the session. After scanning Darla's body, Nancy Lester, a certified Healing Touch practitioner and instructor, would begin the session by holding her ankles and feet. Nancy would then gradually work her way up the body to the top of Darla's head, gently touching Darla over various energy centers while continuously moving her hands. The practice is believed to recreate energy flow and achieve balance to the body.

As Nancy worked, Darla experienced a sensation like a warm blanket being placed over her body. She also felt a light tingling at times, and she said it took a while before she could sense the energy centers opening. According to Darla, when the centers do open, "it's like warm water spreading through a joint or area of your body. The pain flows down the legs and is released from the energy centers." Following her first session, Darla felt much more relaxed but didn't recognize any pain relief until several hours or even days later. Today, she experiences immediate relief after a session.

After several sessions, Darla's sciatica was gone, and her muscle spasms had greatly decreased in frequency and intensity. Darla hasn't had symptoms of sciatica for about five years now. She experienced an overall 90% reduction in pain and can exercise, garden, and participate in many other family activities she loves. "You wouldn't even know that I had scoliosis. I feel whole, centered, and confident in handling stress," Darla remarked. Nancy taught Darla to channel her own energy at home as a self-help intervention for pain flare-ups. When pain resurfaces, Darla places her hands on a painful part of her body, senses the energy field, and then sends positive, caring messages, which help to dampen the pain.

Healing Touch practitioners believe they are transferring energy from their own biofields to the patient's biofield. This supports and optimizes the body's ability to heal and elicits a deep relaxation by engaging the parasympathetic nervous system. Nancy has seen impressive results in patients with acute pain, and other practitioners have noted the same in children with cancer.

Healing Touch has been studied in cancer pain, postsurgical pain, and chronic pain conditions such as fibromyalgia and headaches. It often results in decreased pain, less pain medication usage, and lower frequency of opioid dosing. Encouraging work in patients with knee osteoarthritis has shown not only pain reduction, but improvement in joint function. As with chakra healing, the benefits are believed to be cumulative. Sessions are typically an hour and cost around $80. To find a practitioner, visit healingtouchprogram.com.

# The Japanese Healing Art of Jin Shin Jyutsu

Contrary to what you might be thinking, Jin Shin Jyutsu (JSJ)—which means the Way of the Compassionate Spirit—is a Japanese form of energy healing, not a martial art. Jin Shin Jyutsu was developed by a Japanese philosopher and healer named, Jiro Murai in the twentieth century. Principles of this technique are said to predate the Buddha (circa 500 BCE), and it is closely related to Tibetan, Hindi, and Native American healing traditions. Jin Shin Jyutsu also shares common roots with acupuncture and acupressure (discussed in Chapter 20, Alternative Medicine and Pain Relief).

According to Jin Shin Jyutsu, pain represents blocks of energy that can be opened to facilitate flow. Jin Shin Jyutsu practitioners use gentle hand touch on vital energy points in the human body, usually two at a time, to release areas of accumulated pain, stress, and disease. JSJ practitioners also teach their clients to perform certain holds at home for self-healing and maintenance.

Elisabetta had a terrible horseback riding accident, which left her with five shattered ribs, a dislocated shoulder, and a collapsed lung. The horse flipped over backwards and pinned Elisabetta against the stall. In the hospital, Elisabetta became nauseated from the intravenous morphine, but felt tremendous relief once a thoracic epidural catheter was placed. Unfortunately, after several days, the epidural was removed. She was then left with a feeling that her chest was filled with shards of glass that stabbed her every time she tried to breathe. The pain was intense and made her sob.

Elisabetta had absolutely no faith in energy healing, but she was in such terrible discomfort that she knew she needed help. A certified Jin Shin Jyutsu practitioner named Jennifer Bradley, who worked at the hospital, treated Elisabetta for 30 minutes, after which Elisabetta's pain completely resolved. She remembers Bradley performing a variety of gentle holds on her feet, hands, around her neck and near her hips, and then feeling a sudden release and the pain draining away. "It was like a muscle cramp relaxing," she remembers. Elisabetta was so startled by the relief that she remembers asking Bradley if she was a witch doctor.

The pain did return after a few days, and Elisabetta was sent home from the hospital with oral opioids and muscle relaxants. However, after seeing Bradley three more times over the course of three weeks, she was able to wean off the opioid pain medication. Each session lasted 30 minutes and Elisabetta felt progressively more relief after each session. She was able to drive, return to work, and ultimately return to riding the horses she loves. She will occasionally feel pain when she rolls over in bed onto the side where her ribs were shattered, but it does not last.

Elisabetta has returned to Bradley for numbness in her hand due to a pinched nerve in her neck as well as arthritic pain in her ankles and knees. Her hand numbness went away and the arthritis improved after the Jin Shin Jyutsu sessions. The self-help hand holds taught to her by Bradley reduce episodic pain by about 75% for several hours, but they are not as effective as a session with Bradley. According to Elisabetta, there is a component to the sessions that gives her an emotional boost too.

Jin Shin Jyutsu acknowledges both the chakras and the meridian system of acupuncture. It specifically teaches that there are 26 energy locks on each side of the body that act like circuit breakers, turning "off" a segment of the body's bioenergy in response to trauma or disease. JSJ practitioners often hold two of these energy lock sites at once, until they feel that the tension or congestion is released.

The Jin Shin Jyutsu energy locks are often located on joints, and they can be thought of as spheres of energy, approximately the size of the palm of your hand.

The energy locks are like trigger points in conventional medicine or acupoints in acupuncture. They are located on the body's energy circulation flows and are similar to meridians that move through the body and somewhat like the nervous or circulatory systems in conventional medicine.

According to Jin Shin Jyutsu, when stress accumulates and pain escalates, the disease process accelerates without any intervention to restore harmony. In the Jin Shin Jyutsu intervention, the practitioner applies harmonizing sequences to unblock certain pathways and restore energy flow. Unlike acupuncture or acupressure, Jin Shin Jyutsu uses only light touch, not pressure, massage, or needles.

When we look at the literature, it seems that Jin Shin Jyutsu may benefit patients with conditions such as breast cancer, heart transplants, and multiple myeloma. One study noted that Jin Shin Jyutsu decreased heart rate and blood pressure in stroke patients. One explanation is that this energy therapy triggered the relaxation response in the autonomic nervous system (responsible for our fight-or-flight response). Jin Shin Jyutsu might, therefore, reduce the future risk of cardiovascular disease among stroke patients.

Jin Shin Jyutsu practitioners often assess patients' bodies by having them lie clothed on a massage ,table and lifting their legs one at time. They "listen to" the pulse at the wrists to determine the initial cause of disharmony before holding particular areas of the body.

Jin Shin Jyutsu practitioner Jennifer Bradley has used Jin Shin Jyutsu to reduce pain from radiation therapy in patients with head and neck cancer, breast cancer, and postsurgical pain as well as neuropathic pain conditions such as chemotherapy-induced peripheral neuropathy. In her own private practice, she's

seen Jin Shin Jyutsu benefit patients with autoimmune diseases, diabetic peripheral neuropathy, fibromyalgia, sciatica, and overuse sports injuries. There is also some thought that Jin Shin Jyutsu can be helpful for musculoskeletal conditions in sports medicine. Bradley has even successfully treated babies in the neonatal intensive care unit going through withdrawal after exposure to various drugs before they were born.

To heal low back pain, a Jin Shin Jyutsu practitioner might use simple holds on the fingers and toes, spending two to three minutes on each finger and toe combination. For arthritis, the base of the neck and the inside of the elbow are held. According to Jin Shin Jyutsu theory, this reopens those safety locks and allows the energy to flow freely again. Some people feel their body relax first, and then their mind. Others feel a shift in their body and some don't feel anything.

Jin Shin Jyutsu practitioners may keep a certain hold for five minutes and even up to 20 minutes, until they feel the pathway open. Bradley experiences this process as gentle pulsations in the pads of her hands, which synchronize when the opening is complete. Many of the cancer and postsurgical patients she treats report better range of motion as well as less fluid retention or lymphedema and less fatigue. They are also able to wean off their opioid medications more quickly than those who don't receive treatment. JSJ sessions are typically between 50 and 60 minutes, and cost around $60. To find a practitioner, visit jsjinc.net.

## Distance Healing

Of all the forms of energy healing, distance (or distant) healing may seem the most farfetched and the furthest outside the realm of traditional Western medicine. To understand it, we must suppose that some healing arts are not bound by physical limitations (such as distance and time), and we must allow for the possibility that some universal force such as God provides human beings with avenues to connect with each other for healing purposes. In this worldview, thought, as a form of energy, can connect with this universal force and can manifest as physical changes in health and well-being. Despite the tremendous advances in medical science over the years, some phenomena remain inexplicable, yet compelling and successful in their outcome.

Scientifically, distance healing, along with the other energy healing traditions, is viewed as non-medical healing; however, there is growing acceptance of these interventions as a part of holistic and humanistic movements in health care. For example, about 7% of people in the United States have reported trying some form of spiritual healing based on a study of complementary and alternative medicine. And the National Institute for Healthcare Research concluded that spiritual and religious involvement has been consistently linked to positive health outcomes.

Distance healing refers to the conscious mental effort made by one person for the benefit of another person's physical and emotional well-being undertaken at a distance. It's interesting to note that the world's major religions including Christianity, Islam, Buddhism, and Hinduism practice distance healing, most commonly in the form of prayers for the sick.

There have been some studies and reports of distance healing showing health benefits. Some have shown positive effects for patients with heart disease and AIDS. There have also been a few studies of distance healing on the chronic pain of fibromyalgia, rheumatoid arthritis, and injury. Those with pain had good improvement over the course of one to two months of distance healing.

After being diagnosed with breast cancer, Edina underwent a difficult series of chemotherapy and radiation treatments. Later that year, she was also in a serious car accident that caused a disc herniation with severe low back pain and a hot, burning, tingling sensation down her left leg. Despite all these health problems, speaking with an energy healer over the telephone made a world of difference for her.

Edina was struggling with nausea, insomnia, constipation, extreme joint pain, and headaches from chemotherapy, and none of the medications her doctors prescribed were helping. Physical therapy and medications had not been effective either, and she was left unable to work and hobbling on one leg. A friend recommended Kim Meisinger, the energy healer mentioned in the chakra healing section of this chapter, but Edina lived in Salt Lake City, Utah, and Meisinger was in Kansas. Edina had never tried energy healing and was a little skeptical, but she felt desperate so she contacted Meisinger.

About 15 minutes before each session, Edina would begin deep breathing and meditation to clear her mind of distractions. Then she would lie on the floor comfortably and put the phone on speaker. She and Meisinger started each session with a conversation, and Edina would answer simple questions about how she was feeling and where it hurt most. Meisinger would then mentally "scan" her body and ask Edina more questions about tension or pain that she sensed. As Meisinger began to work, Edina felt a sensation like warm oil being poured all over her back. She felt her anxiety release, and when she got up she felt deeply refreshed, as if she had had a good night's sleep. "I felt peace and relaxation as if I had taken a deep breath," she said. Edina continued to call Meisinger for about five more sessions, and gradually her painful symptoms from cancer treatment began to fade away.

Edina's skin was very fair and sensitive, but despite 26 rounds of radiation over six weeks, her skin did not become pink or blister (a common side effect of radiation). She had no pain from radiation when many patients experience skin sensitivity, sunburn-like pain, or blistering. She had no more nausea or constipation from chemotherapy, and she was able to sleep well at night. Edina's headaches and joint aches were also greatly reduced. After further sessions with Meisinger, Edina's back and leg symptoms substantially improved as well. She felt significantly better after the first session, and subsequent sessions further alleviated these particular symptoms. "It felt like the pain went from my low back and drained out of my feet," she said.

Edina's doctors reacted in different ways. Her oncologist was thrilled she had found effective support and urged her to continue as long as she needed to. Her radiation oncologist was astounded that she didn't have any radiation side effects and was delighted with her results. Her pain doctors were doubtful and were certain that the credit lay with the pain medications they were prescribing her.

Still, there is no question in Edina's mind that the distance healing sessions with Meisinger have not only prolonged her life, but also helped get her back to full health after cancer. "Chemotherapy in conjunction with Kim's intervention helped me get the 'all clear' sign. I wouldn't replace the traditional treatments with distance healing, but energy healing helps with the emotional upheaval that builds up in the body. Traditional medicine is not helpful here. Kim works with the physical and emotional, which go hand in hand. Keep an open mind to another pathway of healing," she added. Edina continues to talk to Meisinger monthly for stress management.

In addition to seeing clients in person, Meisinger has used phone sessions to treat patients from all over the country and around the world. What happens during a distance healing session from Meisinger's perspective? She explains that she begins by learning as much as she can about the client, looking at a picture if possible and doing a detailed intake of symptoms and experiences. She can even tune in energetically to a person by the sound of his or her voice. She then begins to feel connected to what they feel physically and emotionally. Meisinger has even worked with people she's never spoken to personally when she has been asked to intervene on a patient's behalf by a family member.

The process that Meisinger and other distance healers describe involves making contact with the patient's inner mind to sense the nature of the injury or disease. The healers form a mental image of the patient's body completely healed and whole. They then send or request the transfer of healing energy to the patient and instruct the patient's inner mind how to access the energy for healing to occur.

Meisinger does believe that the healing process through which she guides her clients involves joining with a divine and benevolent higher power. And although people do not need to believe in energy healing to benefit from it, she does believe they need to desire healing and be open to whatever form it may take. As an empath, Meisinger feels what the client feels (pain, longing, agitation, for example). Meisinger says she's been able to see a client's pain leaving her own hand followed by the patient telling her that the pain is less intense. If patients have an emotional component to their pain, that particular component usually resolves faster than the physical element during distance healing.

In Meisinger's experience, each healing session offers benefits, and those benefits are cumulative. Meisinger asks her clients to carefully monitor their symptoms during and after the distance sessions, and record in detail any changes.

This is how she tracks improvement. People are now reaching out to her earlier in their illnesses. She used to see more patients once they reached the limits of medical care, but that's changing. The ability or the experience of the healer matters as well—the broader the experience, the better according to Meisinger. She's seen success with fibromyalgia, headaches, and nerve pain from trauma. If there's an imbalance of the autonomic nervous system (fight-or-flight system), she can also help rebalance it through distance healing.

If a client does not show any improvement in three to four sessions, Meisinger will try to help them find another modality of healing. Her initial session is $200 for two hours and subsequent sessions range from $100 to $160 per hour. She can be reached at www.kchealer.com. You can also contact the National Federation of Spiritual Healers to locate other practitioners of distance healing.

## Animal Therapy

Animal therapy, more accurately called animal-assisted therapy, involves the use of animals, usually dogs specifically trained to be obedient, calm, and comforting. Animal therapy could be considered a form of energy healing. Similar to a biofield therapy, animal therapy involves not only the sense of touch, but perhaps the so-called sixth sense as well. This is highlighted by a patient who said, "the dog seemed to know right where my worst pain was and went right to it.

After having him by the pain, it seemed to get much better."

Animal-assisted therapy also addresses the non-physical components of pain that can be so influential—stress, fatigue, irritability. Most of us have felt the soothing sensations of stroking the fur of our pets, especially dogs and cats. Published studies show that animal-assisted therapy optimizes healing, and therapy dogs provide benefits across a broad range of medical conditions, including pain.

A terrible car accident left Ted with a fractured skull, neck vertebra, collarbone, elbow, and pelvis as well as with a torn carotid artery, a punctured lung, and lacerations all over his body. He was in a coma for weeks, then rehabilitated on the brain injury unit. Needless to say, his road to recovery was fraught with frustration and tremendous pain, but his dog Maisy—a German shepherd, Chow, and Labrador retriever mix—helped him fight back and begin living again.

Taking care of Maisy as a puppy got Ted moving, even when he didn't feel like it. Maisy helped Ted's hip pain feel better by forcing him to walk rather than remain immobile, which would have just resulted in more stiffness and discomfort. Other patients have noticed the benefits that petting a dog's fur provides on mobilizing stiff joints and exercising the muscles and joints of both the fingers and wrist.

Maisy improved Ted's mood and helped him get out of his house to socialize with others. Stroking her and cuddling with the dog helped regulate Ted's emotions, something traumatic brain injury makes it so difficult for patients to do. Maisy seemed to know when Ted was sick or in pain and would come over and rub against him to comfort him at those times. "Maisy was in tune with my emotions and would stay beside me when I needed to stay in bed," he said. Maisy seems to feel protective of Ted, and always likes to stay close to him.

Ted has also used craniosacral therapy, prolotherapy, and acupuncture to help him with the ongoing pain from his injuries, but he feels that Maisy increases his pain relief by at least an additional 30%. The greatest effect comes from snuggling with his dog and holding her. To a certain degree, he prefers contact with Maisy to contact with humans because he doesn't have to talk about anything related to his accident. It's easier and more beneficial in many ways, according to Ted. He also credits Maisy with helping him ward off the depression and despair that so often accompany chronic pain. The idea of getting out of the cycle of just focusing on himself, and redirecting his energy to care for a pet resonates with Ted too. "I don't worry about what I can't do because I'm responsible for taking care of this animal," he said.

Being able to love and stroke a pet has been shown to decrease blood pressure, heart rate, and stress hormones, such as cortisol, and increase endorphin levels, leading to natural pain relief. Interestingly, a study examining patients following total joint replacement showed that hospitalized patients were able to lower their need for oral opioids after just five to 15 minutes of dog-assisted therapy. Many people also believe that the unconditional love and acceptance that domestic animals offer contributes to their calming effect on human beings. Patients without pets of their own can still benefit from time spent with therapy animals— usually dogs—which have been trained to interact positively with strangers.

Specifically, patients with low back pain, fibromyalgia, headaches, abdominal pain, and myofascial pain have shown to benefit from time with a therapy dog. These patients not only report lower levels of pain and distress, but also are more likely to keep up with an exercise program and get better sleep. Even just five to 15 minutes with a therapy dog is enough for many people to demonstrate a significant drop in stress, aggravation, and sadness. Patients don't necessarily have to touch the animal either. The health benefits can arise from the mere interaction between person and animal. Often the benefits outlast the time with the animal as well, perhaps due to the physical and chemical changes that occur in the brain.

Many different dog breeds have been shown to make good therapy animals because they want to bond with humans. Most people are not allergic to dogs, but if allergies are a problem, there are some dog breeds that are hypoallergenic. Although dogs are by far the most common choice for therapy animals, cats and rabbits have been used therapeutically too. Similarly, dolphins and horses have been used successfully to engage people with autism.

Animal therapy is just another holistic approach to pain relief that takes into account our need for touch, love, and emotional comfort. They can offer a pleasant distraction from painful symptoms in the hospital or outpatient setting, and at home. Particularly for patients who live alone, animals can be a wonderful complement to other pain treatments.

## Other Sources of Information about Harnessing the Human Biofield

You can learn more about biofield therapies by listening to the related episodes of my weekly radio program, *Aches and Gains*. You can find the broadcasts on biofield therapies at the following URLs.

**Chakra Healing**
http://paulchristomd.com/chakra-healing

**Distance Healing**
http://paulchristomd.com/energy-healing
http://paulchristomd.com/energy-healing-2

**Healing Touch**
http://paulchristomd.com/healing-touch

**Jin Shin Jyutsu**
http://paulchristomd.com/jin-shin-jyutsu
http://paulchristomd.com/jin-shin-jyutsu-2
jsjinc.net

**Animal Therapy**
http://paulchristomd.com/animals

## Suggested Further Reading

Alcantra, Margarita. *Chakra Healing: A Beginner's Guide to Self-Healing Techniques that Balance the Chakras.* (n.p.): Althea Press, 2017. This book offers chakra healing techniques in addition to a variety of other therapeutic methods including Meditations & Visualizations, Crystals, Essential Oils, Yoga, Food & Diet, and more to address ailments and concerns such as Asthma and Allergies, Back Pain, Fatigue, Digestive Issues, Neuropathy, Skin Issues, Headache, and more. https://tinyurl.com/y9agaqm2

Angelo, Jack. *Distant Healing: A Complete Guide.* (n.p.): Sounds True, 2008. A step-by-step guide to the art of distant healing. https://tinyurl.com/y8jwxc9f

Dale, Cyndi. *The Complete Book of Chakra Healing: Activate the Transformative Power of Your Energy Centers.* (n.p.): Llewellyn Publications, 2009. A guide to chakra healing with true stories from the author's healing practice and illustrations of the energetic nature of diseases. https://tinyurl.com/ydbz6k9z

McKenzie, Eleanor. *The Reiki Bible: The Definitive Guide to Healing with Energy.* (n.p.): Sterling, 2009. This book provides a comprehensive guide to the ancient spiritual system of Reiki from origins and development to the energy and body systems, and the three levels of Reiki. https://tinyurl.com/yb6vc48n

Quest, Penelope. *Reiki for Life: The Complete Guide to Reiki Practice for Level 1, 2 & 3.* (n.p.): Tarcher Perigee, 2016. A handbook containing everything readers need to know about the healing art of Reiki, including basic routines, details about the power and potential of each level and special techniques for enhancing Reiki practice. https://tinyurl.com/y7cqk9ky

## Other Resources to Explore

Everydayhealth medically reviewed article on how pets can ease chronic pain.

Mayo Clinic's consumer health article about pet therapy healing depression and fatigue.

The Institute of Noetic Sciences' frequently asked questions about distance healing.

The National Fibromyalgia and Chronic Pain Association's page on animal assisted therapy.

Orthology.com article on pain reduction through pet therapy.

# CHAPTER

# 23

# Pain Relief through Movement

Musculoskeletal pain is perhaps the most common kind of pain, affecting at least 30% of adults. Myofascial pain alone, which is pain felt in the muscles and does not include the bones and joints, affects up to 85% of the general population. Both traumatic and overuse injuries affect our bones, muscles, joints, and connective tissue. The more we move, stand, and sit, and the older we get, the more aches and pains we expect. But is musculoskeletal pain really a necessary part of life?

A growing body of research suggests that we can treat musculoskeletal pain and greatly reduce our risk of future injuries by improving our flexibility, balance, posture, and proprioception (our awareness of the placement of our body in space). Many people suffering from all sorts of painful conditions have found relief in practices that address strength, posture, and alignment.

Greater flexibility helps to ensure a greater range of motion in our limbs and allows us to stay mobile as we age. Improved balance helps to prevents falls. Better posture helps to prevent pain associated with sitting or standing for long periods of time. Engaging the body helps to reframe chronic pain into an experience that reinforces our sense of resiliency, confidence, and ability to progress. This chapter covers a variety of activities and exercises that offer both pain relief and pain prevention by improving flexibility, balance, posture, and proprioception. The therapies addressed include yoga as well as lesser-known posture-correction therapies that have brought relief to more people than you might imagine.

# Yoga

Yoga is an ancient practice that is one of the most popular non-conventional therapies pursued for health benefits. Historically, yoga centered on inner development—promoting tranquility of the mind and body and leading participants on a path toward enlightenment. Yoga participation has exploded in America during recent years. Along with massage and Pilates, U.S. consumers rate yoga as high as prescription medications in its effectiveness for easing pain.

Patients with chronic low back and neck pain, fibromyalgia, osteoarthritis, and rheumatoid arthritis have all found relief by practicing yoga. It has shown an effect in teenagers with irritable bowel syndrome and seems promising for children with chronic pain and stress-related conditions. The 2017 clinical practice guideline from the American College of Physicians listed yoga as one of several noninvasive treatment recommendations for chronic low back pain.

Antonio, an investment banker, was injured in a serious motorcycle accident that shattered his tailbone, tore muscles in his buttocks, and left him with worse low back pain than he had experienced after disc herniation surgery three years earlier. Sitting became very painful; this was especially problematic since his job required 12 to 15 hours in front of a computer each day. His back muscles would tighten up too. After a few epidural steroid injections for the shooting leg pain, Antonio relied on regular doses of ibuprofen (Motrin) to control the sciatica and back stiffness that resulted from the extended time he had to spend at his desk. But the muscle relaxants, chiropractic therapy, and the ibuprofen were all unable to provide him with meaningful relief.

In addition to distracting him at work, the persistent back pain eventually caused Antonio to step away from almost all his athletic pursuits. After being active his entire life, these new limitations robbed him not only of the activities that kept him moving, but also a lot of his regular social interactions. He became more introverted and detached from life.

Antonio knew he needed to do something, so he tried simple exercises on his own. However, like many busy people, he struggled to stretch and move consistently. Finally, at his wife's urging, he attended a yoga class with her. Right away, he was shocked at what a challenging workout the class offered. He was accustomed to aggressive gym work outs with weights. This was definitely different, but Antonio noticed that the fluid motion of the exercises felt "safe" for his sensitive back. It was good for developing his physique as well. Even without weights, he felt like every muscle in his body was being activated and challenged. At times, he was drenched in sweat and working hard to keep up.

## Understanding Yoga

Yoga consists of three main elements: postures and poses; breath control; and meditation and relaxation. It's a form of moving meditation and exercise. The multifaceted nature of yoga offers patients pain relief, stress management, social connection, and physical activity. Certain patients who see me for chronic pain report that the deep stretching along with deep rhythmic breathing makes them feel better. I've recommended yoga as a supplement to injection therapies and medications when appropriate as well as an alternative form of exercise.

There are several styles of yoga instruction available in the United States. The most common, and perhaps the most ancient, is Hatha: a series of classical Indian poses most often associated with the term "yoga" in the United States. Iyengar Yoga, named for its founder, utilizes the Hatha poses but emphasizes the precise alignment and posture of the body as well as breath control. Bikram Yoga is typically practiced in a room heated to about 104 degrees. Bikram yoga participants generally feel that the sweating helps release toxins.

Vinyasa Yoga emphasizes a smooth flow between movements in a particular sequence and rhythm. It's quite physical and popular in the United States because it's identified with a good work out. Power Yoga challenges participants to hold poses for longer periods of time, focusing on strength and the attainment of muscular awareness. Gentle Yoga is a good option for patients with injuries and pain because it focuses on simple, easy stretches and utilizes props to help patients attain the right positions. Restorative Yoga emphasizes mental calm; it also uses straps, props, guided meditation, and a limited number of poses to help release tension in the body. It's the equivalent of "spa therapy" yoga.

In addition to different schools of yoga, different studios and instructors all bring unique styles and approaches to their classes. Most studios have several options geared toward every interest and athletic ability. Classes range in length from about 45 to 105 minutes, although an hour is the most common. Various organizations and community centers offer free or donation-based yoga classes but more private instruction starts around $15–$20 a class. Costs increase depending on instructor experience and location.

Most yoga classes begin with breathing and meditation exercises. Students may be asked to chant as well as close their eyes to reduce distraction. They will be instructed to breathe deeply from their bellies, as opposed to their chests. As mentioned in earlier chapters, this diaphragmatic breathing slows the heart rate and calms the mind. The positive effect on the heart rate comes from an activation of the parasympathetic nervous system—the "rest and relax" part of the autonomic nervous system. (In contrast, the fight-or-flight component of the autonomic nervous system is the sympathetic nervous system.)

Instructors then lead students through different position changes depending on the type of yoga. Students are coached to keep their breathing steady and regular as they change poses. Participants may sit with blocks or rolled up blankets to support their posture and elongate their spines. Most classes involve several positional changes—the length of time each pose is held varies—and incorporate flexion, extension, and rotation, while building strength and flexibility. Standing poses improve proprioception and balance by strengthening stabilizing muscles. There are specialized poses for the spine, reducing tight muscles, strengthening abdominal and thoracic cavities, and correcting vertebral curvatures.

## Yoga and Pain Relief

Several studies of low back pain have demonstrated symptom reduction with improvements in fatigue and functional disability for those participating in yoga. In the research on low back and neck pain, there seems to good evidence for short-term effectiveness. Other data support an increase in flexibility, coordination, and strength among yoga participants, as well as elevated mood and a reduction in anxiety and stress. Women who practice yoga find that they are able to draw upon its techniques during childbirth to ease pain, stay calm, and control their breathing. There are even yoga poses that can help when a baby is past its due date. If you have discomfort from muscle soreness or computer usage, the studies support strong positive effects from yoga.

Like Antonio, many new students are surprised by how much exercise yoga can involve. Intermediate and advanced classes test range of motion in the body's joints and muscles to a greater degree, but they shouldn't be attempted until students have mastered correct body placement in basic poses. As with any exercise program, new yoga students should calibrate their expectations and remember not to push themselves too hard when they are beginning. In a class setting, it can be tempting to watch students who are more experienced and try to imitate them. The best way to avoid injury and excessive post exercise soreness is to take it slowly, especially at first.

Like other exercise regimes that require equal levels of exertion, yoga can occasionally cause injury. I caution patients with neck pain or cervical disc disease to avoid poses such as headstands, handstands, and shoulder stands, since these are more often associated with injuries. Backward and forward bends need to be performed cautiously if you have lumbar spine disease or have had spine surgery. If your pain worsens or you experience new neurological symptoms such as pins and needles sensations, seek medical attention. Remember that poses can be uncomfortable, but shouldn't be painful.

When Antonio began yoga, the closest he could come to touching his toes was placing his fingertips on his shins. Now, he can bend forward with straight legs and lay his palms flat on the floor. He does three sets of forward bends at home that relieve tension in his back and give him the feeling of being active physically. The more consistently he attends yoga, the less he needs ibuprofen (Motrin) to keep his back pain in check. He also notices that if he doesn't make it to class, his back and neck become much stiffer and tighter. "I feel like yoga is a better workout than the gym. I do push-ups and abdominal work, and I strengthen my arms and legs," he says. There's a toning and endurance component that he enjoys, equating it to swimming. According to Antonio, once you see results, you'll want to see more of them, but have realistic expectations. You'll be disappointed if you think that all of your pain will go away. The benefits are incremental, not instant.

Overall, Antonio feels he gets 50% or more relief from his back and neck pain by practicing yoga twice a week. He warns that you many feel worse when first attending yoga class because the practice strains muscle. He advises people to know their limits and take breaks. For Antonio, yoga is also a great way to spend time with his wife, and they have met many friends in class with whom they enjoy socializing. He also believes that the concentration required in yoga helps him clear his mind of the stress associated with his job, giving him greater peace and improving his overall quality of life. In general, yoga provides positive effects as a supportive and relatively inexpensive treatment.

## Pain Relief through Posture and Movement

We spend our days standing, sitting, and moving. Sometimes the way we do these basic activities actually exacerbates pain and puts us at greater risk for injury. Poor posture can lead to muscle imbalance, joint instability, and even lower metabolism and cause bone density loss.

Continual pain frequently changes patterns of movement, and this leads to new locations of pain or prolongs chronic pain. Many people have found relief from pain in relearning how to stand, sit, and move in ways that promote proper alignment of the skeleton and efficient, graceful movement. The Feldenkrais Method, the Egoscue Method, Revolution In Motion, and the Gokhale Method all reflect approaches to pain relief and prevention that address the need for proper skeletal alignment and posture. These methods seek to teach us to move in ways that are compatible with our bodies' design. Although I am less personally familiar with these techniques, I still encourage patients to be open to exploring and researching these methods and others similar to them that offer a legitimate basis for managing pain. The rest of this chapter describes these methods in greater detail.

The Feldenkrais Method, the Egoscue Method, Revolution in Motion, and the Gokhale method all view the body as a single unit. Even when practitioners are assisting patients with acute injuries or complaints in particular parts of the body, the focus is on the body as a whole. These methods may offer benefit to patients with fibromyalgia and other chronic pain conditions, although it may take some time for people with such conditions to see results. The aim of these practices is to make people more aware of how they stand, sit, and move so that they can move in ways that will keep them as healthy as possible. If patients can recognize that they can be physically active despite persistent pain, they can accomplish more in life—that's the ultimate benefit.

## The Feldenkrais Method

The Feldenkrais Method is a gentle movement-education therapy named for its founder, Moshe Feldenkrais. The method's goal is to increase patients' overall functioning by increasing their ease and range of motion, improving their flexibility and coordination, and making all their movements more efficient and painless.

People can participate in the Feldenkrais Method in two primary forms. Functional Integration is one-on-one therapy in which the instructor takes over the work of the muscles through gentle touch and instruction. Patients relearn healthy patterns of movement that help them improve their overall function. The second form, Awareness Through Movement, is offered in a class setting where a group of individuals is guided through a series of movements designed to deepen awareness of body placement in ways that decrease effort and increase efficiency. For instance, imagine turning your head to the left. If you simultaneously rotate your shoulder forward, then you're limiting the movement of your upper skeleton and increasing the chances of neck pain. The Feldenkrais Method addresses the entire pattern of motion. Both forms of the Feldenkrais Method are designed to improve how we function in life, at work, and in recreation.

While the Feldenkrais Method is not an exercise program, participants assert that the method enhances and improves whatever exercise they choose to participate in. Runners, for example, may be able to improve their speed without expending extra energy. The Feldenkrais Method can also help people recover from acute injury, often fairly quickly. Even though it takes time to notice benefit, those with chronic pain can enhance their quality of life by participating in the Feldenkrais Method.

Tabitha suffered from terrible neck and shoulder pain after a kayaking mishap left her with bulging discs in her neck and a torn rotator cuff in her shoulder. The most intense symptoms focused around her shoulder blade and the region between the shoulder blade and spine. The pain prevented her from sleeping more than three hours a night, and she was unable to wash her own hair or dress herself. Limited ability to lift her arm or reach forward made driving tough as well. "I felt like everything locked up. My posture worsened, I guarded my left arm, and felt unsteady," she said. Traditional treatments such as muscle relaxants and tramadol (Ultram) along with acupuncture and massage eased the pain, but she needed more relief. She hoped to avoid surgery so she tried the Feldenkrais Method at her acupuncturist's suggestion.

In her one-on-one session, the Feldenkrais Method instructor evaluated Tabitha as she stood up and then lied down on a massage table. The instructor pushed gently on various parts of her body, watched her response, and asked her detailed questions about the pain she was experiencing. The instructor then began to speak to her about how she was holding her body and moving, including simple motions like turning her head to one side or the other.

The instructor explained to Tabitha that her shoulder injury had caused her to keep certain parts of her body immobile, leading her to move differently than she normally would. This kind of change in normal movement often prolongs the pain or even leads to secondary injuries. Much of Tabitha's early Feldenkrais sessions were devoted to teaching her how to stop guarding her injured shoulder and to move without pain. Her instructor would show her which roadblocks to remove for efficient motion. She then learned how to relax portions of her body during movement so that motion wouldn't elicit pain.

Group Feldenkrais Method classes focus on movement awareness through guided exercises performed lying on mats or standing. Tabitha participated in group classes too and now practices the techniques she learned in class at home. The process allows students to tune into every aspect of each motion while cultivating muscle memory of pain-free movement. Overall, Feldenkrais Method students believe that the skills improve kinesthetic (activity-based) and proprioceptive self-awareness, which allows them to transform unhealthy movements into ones that promote comfort during day-to-day activities.

Tabitha's pain improved within the first two weeks, and after five months, she felt 98% pain free, with the range of motion in her shoulder immensely improved as well. Research supports Tabitha's experience. Positive changes have been demonstrated in a study for patients with neck and scapular pain.

Tabitha is now able to reach forward, perform her job without difficulty, and do those things she did before the kayaking accident. It took work on her part, though. She participated in sessions three times a week for a while, then two times a week, and finally once a week over several months. Feldenkrais requires consistency and commitment, but it is a low-risk technique and participation is rarely painful.

One study has shown that the Feldenkrais Method results in faster reductions in pain intensity and pain perception (compared to a intervention protocol called back school that involves teaching skills about back care, body mechanics, posture and prevention) among patients with low back pain. There are also reports of diminished neck and shoulder pain, headache, and post-injury pain. There's evidence that older adults with osteoarthritis who practice the Feldenkrais Method have better balance and mobility. Preliminary research on the Feldenkrais Method also shows reduced pain, less fatigue, and better sleep in patients with fibromyalgia.

Patients trying the Feldenkrais Method should allow four to five sessions before expecting noticeable relief. It's important to build on small improvements and not give up. Private one-on-one sessions (Functional Integration) run between $40 and $200 each, depending on the experience of the teacher. Group classes (Awareness Through Movement) cost between $5 and $15 per session. Feldenkrais Method is covered by insurance in some states. You can find qualified instructors through The Feldenkrais Guild of North America Member Directory at www.feldenkrais.com.

## The Egoscue Method

The Egoscue Method is a unique exercise therapy program that focuses on posture realignment. It was developed by anatomical physiologist, Pete Egoscue, and it focuses on improving chronic musculoskeletal pain due to workplace and sports injuries, accidents, and aging. Egoscue's clients include elite athletes such as golfer Jack Nicklaus. The cornerstone of the technique involves encouraging patients to move the part of the body that's painful. The Egoscue Method believes that just as a broken bone or cut will heal on its own, joint problems and other musculoskeletal problems can do the same if posture is corrected. The Egoscue Method views the body as a complete, functional unit. Treatment is given only in a one-on-one therapy setting.

Injured as a marine in Vietnam, Egoscue used his own journey to healing to develop his method for correcting posture for both acute and chronic pain. He interprets pain as the body's method of communicating important information. During Egoscue Method sessions, patients are asked to move the part of the body that is causing pain, listen to what the body is telling them, and relearn how to move the body part healthily. Interestingly, this process not only conditions muscles but is thought to redevelop neural connections in the brain, which ultimately eases pain.

Rod Susman, a retired professional tennis player, suffered from osteoarthritic hip pain that made it hard for him to walk or play any tennis. He didn't see himself taking medicines or having surgery. Physical therapy made some difference, but according to Rod, it was the Egoscue Method that diminished his pain and helped him regain his function. Initially, Rod noticed subtle changes in pain and his ability to move, and after seven months of sessions, he noticed substantial benefits from postural realignment. Rod believed that the Egoscue Method treated the "Big Picture"—the entire musculoskeletal system. "It's an ongoing project. You need to continue the technique to maintain the benefits," he said. Today, he feels less vulnerable to musculoskeletal pain, more energetic, and more in control.

Patients who want to try the Egoscue Method are offered an initial session, during which an instructor does a detailed intake of history and symptoms and then performs a very comprehensive postural evaluation. The instructor then prepares and leads the student through a series of exercises that are customized to the patient's needs and specific injury compensations. If patients think the method will work for them, they have the option to sign up for more sessions. When I spoke to Egoscue on my radio show, he explained that most patients choose eight one-hour sessions for $1495, but his organization typically doesn't turn people away for financial reasons. Egoscue feels that corrections to posture usually require eight sessions. He reports that he's seen good results for those with back pain, temporomandibular joint disorder (TMJ), migraine headaches, and plantar fasciitis, among other disorders.

The Egoscue Method is a gradual process that requires commitment to and consistent application of its principles. Participants report not only decreased pain, but also improved activity levels, energy, and mood, according to Egoscue. He has seen some patients wean off pain medications and avoid joint replacement or other orthopedic surgeries. If postural corrections are not relieving painful symptoms, however, patients are encouraged to seek a different modality of treatment. Clinics can be found at egoscue.com.

### Revolution In Motion

Revolution In Motion (RevInMo) is an exercise system developed by Dr. Edythe Heus, a chiropractor and kinesiologist. It integrates Eastern and Western thought to enhance the physical, emotional, and spiritual core. Heus asserts that the technique conditions our proprioception, the sense we have of our body parts in space and next to each other. Students can learn the Revolution In Motion exercises in a private or class setting. Exercises are performed barefoot on slanted boards, pipes, balance discs, and other unstable surfaces. Students also use light weights and other props to perform motions that seem simple but actually require a great deal of balance and coordination.

The Revolution In Motion technique begins with the feet, moves to the lower abdomen to lengthen the spinal muscles, and then reaches the shoulder muscles. The program is designed to activate muscles we are typically less aware of, such as the lower abdominal and pubic muscles, as well as other stabilizing muscles that support larger muscle groups. By strengthening these muscles and deepening an awareness of them, students improve their posture, balance, and coordination. They also fine tune their proprioception, making them less vulnerable to falls and other injuries.

Selena, a filmmaker, had foot and hip pain. Her friend recommended Revolution In Motion after it helped him improve an injury. In sessions, Selena found herself using gymnastic balls and props filled with water, which was sort of dazzling.

Over just a two-week period, Selena realized that she no longer needed her foot orthotics and noticed that her footprint appeared different on the bathtub rug. When she walked, her gait had changed too; it was more fluid and stable. "I felt like Edythe's system re-booted the sensory parts of my body. I began accessing muscles I used a child," she said. Selena has a refined sense of awareness, lowered stress, and a greater sense of well-being today. The aches and pains she once experienced in her leg are gone.

Edythe Heus explains that the RevInMo program is painless and designed to achieve very fast results. It fine-tunes the proprioceptors located in the inner ear and muscles. She believes that her technique helps to heal fascia (the thin sheaths of fibrous tissue enclosing muscles) that are damaged from overuse injuries or other painful conditions. Patients can generally expect to achieve noticeable improvement in chronic or acute pain after one to three private sessions, or six to 10 class sessions. Clients typically pay $25–$50 per class and private sessions run $120.

Some people who have tried Revolution In Motion are very pleased with the results. A stuntman from the Broadway show *Spider-Man: Turn Off the Dark* incorporated RevInMo into his recovery after a 30-foot fall that left him in a body cast with multiple broken bones. He was able to heal several weeks faster than doctors had predicted, returning to the production far ahead of schedule.

Ultimately, Heus believes that Revolution In Motion can free us from pain by organizing the body for optimal posture and movement. "Pain is an indicator that we need to change something. Revolution In Motion permits that change," she said. It provides a playful environment for exercise too. Those interested in finding a class can visit revinmo.com.

## The Gokhale Method

Yeji, director of search quality at a well-known international company, spends more than 60 hours a week sitting in front of a computer or on an airplane. So many of us do the same, shifting from computer screen, to smartphone screen, and then to television screen. This lifestyle combined with injuries sustained as an acrobat earlier in his life, led to growing tension and tightness in Yeji's neck, shoulders, and lower back. The pain became serious enough that he had to limit his time surfing—his favorite pastime—and he began choosing only recreational activities that wouldn't aggravate his pain. Like many others in chronic pain, he slowly stopped doing what he loved to do.

Yeji tried physical therapy and yoga, and he bought several books on posture, sensing intuitively that his problem had to do with posture and flexibility. His solution came from taking a class from the so-called posture guru of Silicon Valley, Esther Gokhale. There he learned the theory behind Gokhale's approach to posture realignment and benefited from practical instruction and hands-on adjustment from Gokhale herself.

Esther Gokhale, who has a background in both biochemistry and acupuncture, developed her method after suffering from terrible back pain associated with a herniated disc during her first pregnancy. She later had surgery, but the symptoms recurred. "None of the alternative methods worked, and it felt like I had an ice pick in my back for an entire year," she said. Gokhale's approach is based on the idea that bad posture is culturally learned and that we need to return to our "primal posture," a way of sitting and standing seen worldwide in young children and in people of all ages in nonindustrial societies. "Other cultures keep this posture into adulthood which correlates to a pain-free structure," she says.

What is this ideal posture? Imagine yourself standing with your chest open, shoulders back, neck tall, and back "J-shaped." The J shape depicts a spine that's upright, relaxed, and without much curve. It engages muscles around the torso. Take a look at how children stand and walk and you'll understand the concept of primal posture. The more typical "S-shaped" spine we see in Western adults is associated with an 85% incidence of back pain, according to Gokhale.

Gokhale's research took her all over the world, and her books and seminars are full of images of children and adults in other countries sitting and standing in a way that counters the slouch that occurs so naturally to many in the West. Take a look at people around you. You'll see this hunched over position is very common. In Gokhale's seminars, students compare photos taken of their own posture to these pictures of properly aligned posture to guide their repositioning. Gokhale also uses detailed pictures of human anatomy and guided movements and stances to help students regain their primal posture.

Gokhale's instruction is designed to be incorporated immediately into everyday life, and does not involve any extra exercises one must perform outside of class.

Yeji did not find the Gokhale realignments painful, although some clients do report feeling uncomfortable or awkward at first. With his busy schedule, Yeji appreciated that he could apply the principles to his daily activities, rather than having to set aside extra time to stretch and exercise. In a condensed course with 20 students, Yeji spent four to five hours a day learning the theory and practice of the Gokhale method.

In class, Yeji learned a different way to lie down on his surfboard, which immediately eliminated the pain he experienced while surfing. Within two to three months of sitting the new way he was taught, he experienced about a 70% reduction in back pain. He's developed safer ways to lift and move objects too. It required remembering how to change his body position more than exerting a lot of effort to do so. And rather than relying on ergonomically correct equipment, Yeji can sit comfortably in regular chairs now.

Although our modern sedentary lifestyle is blamed for a multitude of health problems, Gokhale points out that in traditional societies, workers (potters and weavers, for example) sit for long periods of time as well, but do not develop the same pain complaints as those in postindustrial societies. She believes it is the misaligned posture, not the length of time sitting or standing that causes the greatest amount of harm.

Gokhale asserts that her approach can benefit anyone who has bad posture and the chronic pain that comes from, or is made worse by it. These include people with many kinds of hip, foot, back, neck, and knee problems. Gokhale believes that her method can even assist women with endometriosis although she notes that her technique is not as beneficial for those who have had multiple surgeries or who are extremely obese.

The Gokhale method is a six-lesson workshop. Individual sessions are 45 minutes each and the cost is $900 for the course. Group classes—restricted to eight people in a group so each person can get individualized attention—are 90 minutes long and the cost is $450 for the course.

For information on the workshops, visit gokhalemethod.com.

## Other Sources of Information about Engaging the Body

You can learn more about yoga and the other movement practices and pain-relief methods discussed in this chapter by listening to the related episodes of my weekly radio program, *Aches and Gains*. You can find the broadcasts on yoga and the other movement practices and pain-relief methods discussed in this chapter at the following URLs.

**Yoga**
http://paulchristomd.com/yoga
http://paulchristomd.com/yoga-2

**The Feldenkrais Method**
http://paulchristomd.com/feldenkrais

**The Egoscue Method**
http://paulchristomd.com/musculoskeletal-pain

**Revolution in Motion**
http://paulchristomd.com/revolution-in-motion

**Esther Gokhale: The Posture Guru**
http://paulchristomd.com/posture-guru
http://paulchristomd.com/posture-guru-2

## Suggested Further Reading

Boorstein Grossman, Gail. *Yoga Journal Presents Restorative Yoga for Life: A Relaxing Way to De-stress, Re-energize, and Find Balance.* (n.p.): Adams Media, 2014. This book teaches readers to practice a form of yoga that focuses on physical and mental relaxation, including treatment for ailments such as headaches, digestive issues, and anxiety, through specific yoga poses and sequences. https://tinyurl.com/ybrbxexx

Burns, Keith, Smith, William, Volgraf, Christopher. *Exercises for Perfect Posture: Stand Tall Program for Better Health Through Good Posture.* (n.p.): Hatherleigh Press, 2017. This book provides the physical and preventative education necessary to improve posture and health through a comprehensive fitness program for all ages. https://tinyurl.com/yas478jj. For more details visit GetFitNow.com.

Egoscue, Pete, Gittines, Roger. *Pain Free: A Revolutionary Method for Stopping Chronic Pain.* (n.p.): Bantam, 2000. An introduction to the system for eliminating chronic pain without drugs, surgery, or expensive physical therapy through a series of gentle exercises and stretches. https://tinyurl.com/y7hps4gu

Feldenkrais, Moshe. *Awareness Through Movement: Easy-to-Do Health Exercises to Improve Your Posture, Vision, Imagination, and Personal Awareness.* (n.p.): HarperOne, 2009. This book integrates physical and mental development through exercises for posture, eyes, and more. https://tinyurl.com/yd9qgocr.
See also https://tinyurl.com/yd7h7v8c.

Fishman, Loren. *Healing Yoga: Proven Postures to Treat Twenty Common Ailments—from Backache to Bone Loss, Shoulder Pain to Bunions, and More.* (n.p.): W. W. Norton & Company, Inc., 2015. This book unites medical knowledge with the practice of yoga to help treat twenty common conditions, including headache, weight gain, the common cold, scoliosis, PMS, stress, depression, and eight different types of back pain. https://tinyurl.com/y9rebnbw

Fishman, Loren, and Saltonstall, Ellen. *Yoga for Arthritis: The Complete Guide.* (n.p.): W. W. Norton & Company, Inc., 2008. A comprehensive, user-friendly medical yoga program designed for management and prevention of arthritis. https://tinyurl.com/y87cluhw

Porter, Kathleen. *Natural Posture for Pain-Free Living: The Practice of Mindful Alignment.* (n.p.): Healing Arts Press, 2013. This book provides easy-to-follow instructions for mindful alignment during daily activities that can offer relief from chronic pain and tension. https://tinyurl.com/yaeozp5v

Stiles, Tara. *Yoga Cures: Simple Routines to Conquer More Than 50 Common Ailments and Live Pain-Free.* (n.p.): Harmony, 2012. An A-to-Z guide of the poses you can do to target specific problems in the body, ranging from arthritis and fibromyalgia to jiggly thighs and hangovers. https://tinyurl.com/y9vazhuc

## Other Resources to Explore

The Egoscue Method uses  postural therapy to alleviate pain and return you back to an active, pain free lifestyle.  The website offers a list of resources an d a blog.

The Gokhale Method uses healthy posture and movement to help you restore your structural integrity and regain a pain-free life. This website offers free resources, videos, includes an online store and a blog.

YogaU is an online yoga education website offering a wellness blog including methods for pain relief, videos for at-home practice and online courses.

# CHAPTER

# 24

# Conclusion

Pain affects all of us at various points in our lives, regardless of age, race, gender, or nationality. When pain doesn't go away, it can touch every aspect of who we are and what we do, from our careers to our hobbies and our relationships. Pain can devastate us, not only physically, but emotionally, mentally, and even spiritually. I've seen too many patients who feel isolated, tormented, and on the verge of giving up because they view their lives as over. You don't have to let that happen because there is hope and there are treatments that can help ease pain and suffering.

If you have made it this far in the book, you have seen that whatever painful condition is affecting you or your loved ones, you are not alone. Millions have suffered, but many have found ways to feel better, typically through pursuing therapies and sometimes by restructuring their lives. These people are successfully living past their limitations and closer to their dreams. This book provides initial insight into our deepening understanding of pain and how to treat it more effectively. In light of this growing body of knowledge and information, I want to leave you with the following parting thoughts: Don't wait; reach out for the help you need; be open; and don't give up.

## Don't Wait

If you are in pain, seek treatment. The longer pain persists, the more difficult it can be to treat effectively. Research has shown us that repeated exposure to pain reduces the threshold for pain and amplifies our response to pain when events trigger it later. If you are experiencing acute pain that seems abnormal or chronic pain that clearly isn't going away, speak up! Talk to your doctor or healthcare professional, and if necessary, seek out a pain specialist.

Many patients let pain go on for far too long. Life gets busy, and they let precious months and years slip away, hoping their condition will get better on its own. Some have been told that the pain is all in their heads, and they feel embarrassed to seek help. During that time, the underlying condition transforms into the *disease* called chronic pain. Nerves in the tissue, spinal cord, and brain change the way they process and transmit painful signals until the body becomes more accustomed to pain as "normal."

As the previous chapters illustrate, pain is a highly individual experience. Two people may have identical illnesses, injuries, or surgical procedures and yet each person has a very different pain intensity, location, or sensation afterwards. One person may no longer experience pain one month later; the other may not understand why the pain hasn't gone away 10 months later. Some are able to manage just fine with over-the-counter medications, others may find that yoga is the silver bullet when it comes to addressing their pain, and still others will need specialized interventions.

Seeking treatment for your pain does not mean you are weak or that you have a low pain tolerance. It means that you value your quality of life and well-being enough to ensure you get your pain addressed properly. The same goes for advocating for a loved one. Keep searching until you find a physician, pain specialist, other healthcare professional, or alternative therapist who will believe you and put you on the path of progress.

## Reach Out for the Help You Need

In your pursuit of treatment, always reach out for the help that you need. Don't try to solve your problems alone. The emotional distress and helplessness that often accompany pain can be just as destructive as the physical aspects of the pain. Many times, loved ones may not know how to help. Don't expect them to read your mind: Pick up the phone, or send a text or an email and ask for help. Do what some of my patients have done and bring your relatives or friends to doctor's appointments so they can understand what you are going through. Talk to others who have passed through the same experience.

Surround yourself with positive, supportive people who will encourage you and extend a caring hand. Don't waste time or energy on people who are negative, critical, or draining. If you are caring for a loved one in pain, be sure to take care of yourself as well. Ask others for assistance so that you can have a break to avoid exhausting yourself.

There are local and national support groups for people in pain and for their loved ones, some of which are listed in this book. Be sure to check out any that may be relevant to you. The companionship of others is comforting, and often inspiring. There is no need to take the journey by yourself.

## Be Open

All of us have preconceived ideas about pain itself and how it should be treated. Some people are deeply suspicious of holistic therapies, while others are terrified of needles, staunchly against medications, or doubtful of electrical stimulation. Be open to the possibilities. Of course, you should always discuss with your doctor or healthcare provider the potential risks and benefits of any course of treatment. You want to begin with a full understanding of the possible side effects and with realistic expectations for success.

Patients of mine are distinctive in the manner they measure success. It might be based on the magnitude or length of relief, their capacity to regain function, or their renewed satisfaction with life. Sometimes, just small, incremental steps are possible, but taken together they lead to greater well-being.

When patients ask me for guidance, I first recommend treatments for which we have the greatest information from scientific research. Then I discuss other treatments that I believe might help based on available evidence, experience, and safety.

You should never agree to something that makes you feel very uncomfortable. However, if the treatments you have tried haven't brought you sufficient relief, consider other approaches that you may have initially ruled out. Some patients of mine are open to specific interventions only later during the course of care, and that's okay. For example, they may want to pursue injection therapies only after medications or physical therapy haven't helped.

We still don't fully understand the mechanisms of a variety of pain-relieving therapies, but that should not prevent you from trying them. I have had patients experience relief from a therapy that they never would have imagined trying before their suffering became unbearable. Their desperation led them to an approach that they had never considered, but they were so glad to have tried, retrospectively.

It is also critical to give treatments enough time to work. That's especially tough when you are in unrelenting pain. Several specific pain medications require days or weeks to produce the intended effects. Injection therapies can be quick, but not always. Yoga, acupuncture, a new diet, or a new exercise program may take months. And a single treatment may not be enough. You may need a combination of treatments, each of which address a separate pain generator. Give your chosen treatment the opportunity to have a positive effect, but if a treatment is not offering meaningful relief after allowing the appropriate amount of time, try something else!

As you've read in the previous chapters, some patients take years to find a treatment that worked for them. Others find a solution earlier, but that solution isn't always easy to find; they find it by educating themselves, researching their options, and aggressively pursuing their needs. Network and learn all you can about your condition and other patients who are in the same boat. Talk to others with a similar experience and find out what helped them. Be open-minded and self-directed.

## Don't Give Up

Pain can feel all encompassing, and sometimes after months, years, or even decades of unceasing suffering, it can be very tempting to give up. Fighting just seems too difficult, and some patients either resign themselves to a lifetime of perpetual suffering, or even contemplate and ultimately commit suicide. This is tragic and never the right course of action.

The scientific community is constantly working to advance both our understanding and treatment of pain. Many therapies available today would have been unimaginable not too long ago. Sometimes, just a new variation on an existing medicine is enough to dampen the pain for a new group of patients. Other times, a centuries old technique is revived and proves to be effective.

Hope is a vital part of overcoming pain. You must believe that things can get better, see yourself getting better, and remember that your life and health are worth the fight. Whether it comes from a cutting-edge new therapy or an age-old folk treatment, your answer may be just around the corner.

# Bibliography

Listed here are selected resources the author has consulted in the process of researching *Aches and Gains*. For the complete list of Dr. Christo's sources, please visit www.bullpub.com/downloads.

## Chapter 1

Afridi, S. K., Shields, K. G., Bhola, R., & Goadsby, P. J. (2006). Greater occipital nerve injection in primary headache syndromes—Prolonged effects from a single injection. *Pain, 122*(1–2), 126–129. doi:10.1016/j.pain.2006.01.016

Ashina, M. (2004). Neurobiology of chronic tension-type headache. *Cephalalgia, 24*(3), 161–172. doi:10.1111/j.1468-2982.2003.00644.x

Bajwa, J. H.; Smith, J. H. (2017). UpToDate: Preventive treatment of migraine in adults.

Barloese, M. C., Jurgens, T. P., May, A., Lainez, J. M., Schoenen, J., Gaul, C., . . . Jensen, R. H. (2016). Cluster headache attack remission with sphenopalatine ganglion stimulation: Experiences in chronic cluster headache patients through 24 months. *J Headache Pain, 17*(1), 67. doi:10.1186/s10194-016-0658-1

Becker, W. J. (2015). Acute migraine treatment in adults. *Headache, 55*(6), 778–793. doi:10.1111/head.12550

Bendtsen, L., Evers, S., Linde, M., Mitsikostas, D. D., Sandrini, G., Schoenen, J., & EFNS. (2010). EFNS guideline on the treatment of tension-type headache—Report of an EFNS task force. *Eur J Neurol, 17*(11), 1318–1325. doi:10.1111/j.1468-1331.2010.03070.x

Bendtsen, L., & Jensen, R. (2000). Amitriptyline reduces myofascial tenderness in patients with chronic tension-type headache. *Cephalalgia, 20*(6), 603–610. doi:10.1046/j.1468-2982.2000.00087.x

Bigal, M. E., Dodick, D. W., Rapoport, A. M., Silberstein, S. D., Ma, Y., Yang, R., . . . Lipton, R. B. (2015). Safety, tolerability, and efficacy of TEV-48125 for preventive treatment of high-frequency episodic migraine: A multicentre, randomised, double-blind, placebo-controlled, phase 2b study. *Lancet Neurol, 14*(11), 1081–1090. doi:10.1016/S1474-4422(15)00249-5

Cohen, S. P., Peterlin, B. L., Fulton, L., Neely, E. T., Kurihara, C., Gupta, A., . . . Zhao, Z. (2015). Randomized, double-blind, comparative-effectiveness study comparing pulsed radiofrequency to steroid injections for occipital neuralgia or migraine with occipital nerve tenderness. *Pain, 156*(12), 2585–2594. doi:10.1097/j.pain.0000000000000373

Colman, I., Brown, M. D., Innes, G. D., Grafstein, E., Roberts, T. E., & Rowe, B. H. (2005). Parenteral dihydroergotamine for acute migraine headache: A systematic review of the literature. *Ann Emerg Med, 45*(4), 393–401. doi:10.1016/j.annemergmed.2004.07.430

Diener, H. C., Kronfeld, K., Boewing, G., Lungenhausen, M., Maier, C., Molsberger, A., . . . Group, Gerac Migraine Study. (2006). Efficacy of acupuncture for the prophylaxis of migraine: A multicentre randomised controlled clinical trial. *Lancet Neurol, 5*(4), 310–316. doi:10.1016/S1474-4422(06)70382-9

Dodick, D., & Freitag, F. (2006). Evidence-based understanding of medication-overuse headache: Clinical implications. *Headache, 46 Suppl 4*, S202-211. doi:10.1111/j.1526-4610.2006.00604.x

Dodick, D. W., & Capobianco, D. J. (2001). Treatment and management of cluster headache. *Curr Pain Headache Rep, 5*(1), 83–91.

Dodick, D. W., Schembri, C. T., Helmuth, M., & Aurora, S. K. (2010). Transcranial magnetic stimulation for migraine: A safety review. *Headache, 50*(7), 1153–1163. doi:10.1111/j.1526-4610.2010.01697.x

Fontaine, D., Lazorthes, Y., Mertens, P., Blond, S., Geraud, G., Fabre, N., . . . Lanteri-Minet, M. (2010). Safety and efficacy of deep brain stimulation in refractory cluster headache: A randomized placebo-controlled double-blind trial followed by a 1-year open extension. *J Headache Pain, 11*(1), 23–31. doi:10.1007/s10194-009-0169-4

Gabai, I. J., & Spierings, E. L. (1989). Prophylactic treatment of cluster headache with verapamil. *Headache, 29*(3), 167–168.

Gantenbein, A. R., Lutz, N. J., Riederer, F., & Sandor, P. S. (2012). Efficacy and safety of 121 injections of the greater occipital nerve in episodic and chronic cluster headache. *Cephalalgia, 32*(8), 630–634. doi:10.1177/0333102412443335

Holle-Lee, D., & Gaul, C. (2016). Noninvasive vagus nerve stimulation in the management of cluster headache: clinical evidence and practical experience. *Ther Adv Neurol Disord, 9*(3), 230–234. doi:10.1177/1756285616636024

Jackson, J. L., Shimeall, W., Sessums, L., Dezee, K. J., Becher, D., Diemer, M., . . . O'Malley, P. G. (2010). Tricyclic antidepressants and headaches: Systematic review and meta-analysis. *BMJ, 341*, c5222. doi:10.1136/bmj.c5222

Johnson, J. L., Hutchinson, M. R., Williams, D. B., & Rolan, P. (2013). Medication-overuse headache and opioid-induced hyperalgesia: A review of mechanisms, a neuroimmune hypothesis and a novel approach to treatment. *Cephalalgia, 33*(1), 52–64. doi:10.1177/0333102412467512

Johnstone, C. S., & Sundaraj, R. (2006). Occipital nerve stimulation for the treatment of occipital neuralgia-eight case studies. *Neuromodulation, 9*(1), 41–47. doi:10.1111/j.1525-1403.2006.00041.x

Karadas, O., Gul, H. L., & Inan, L. E. (2013). Lidocaine injection of pericranial myofascial trigger points in the treatment of frequent episodic tension-type headache. *J Headache Pain, 14*, 44. doi:10.1186/1129-2377-14-44

Law, S., Derry, S., & Moore, R. A. (2016). Sumatriptan plus naproxen for the treatment of acute migraine attacks in adults. *Cochrane Database Syst Rev, 4*, CD008541. doi:10.1002/14651858.CD008541.pub3

Linde, K., Streng, A., Jurgens, S., Hoppe, A., Brinkhaus, B., Witt, C., . . . Melchart, D. (2005). Acupuncture for patients with migraine: A randomized controlled trial. *JAMA, 293*(17), 2118–2125. doi:10.1001/jama.293.17.2118

Lipton, R. B., Dodick, D. W., Silberstein, S. D., Saper, J. R., Aurora, S. K., Pearlman, S. H., . . . Goadsby, P. J. (2010). Single-pulse transcranial magnetic stimulation for acute treatment of migraine with aura: A randomised, double-blind, parallel-group, sham-controlled trial. *Lancet Neurol, 9*(4), 373–380. doi:10.1016/S1474-4422(10)70054-5

Nesbitt, A. D., Marin, J. C., Tompkins, E., Ruttledge, M. H., & Goadsby, P. J. (2015). Initial use of a novel noninvasive vagus nerve stimulator for cluster headache treatment. *Neurology, 84*(12), 1249–1253. doi:10.1212/WNL.0000000000001394

Nestoriuc, Y., Rief, W., & Martin, A. (2008). Meta-analysis of biofeedback for tension-type headache: efficacy, specificity, and treatment moderators. *J Consult Clin Psychol, 76*(3), 379–396. doi:10.1037/0022-006X.76.3.379

Schmidt-Wilcke, T., Leinisch, E., Straube, A., Kampfe, N., Draganski, B., Diener, H. C., . . . May, A. (2005). Gray matter decrease in patients with chronic tension type headache. *Neurology, 65*(9), 1483–1486. doi:10.1212/01.wnl.0000183067.94400.80

Schoenen, J., Jacquy, J., & Lenaerts, M. (1998). Effectiveness of high-dose riboflavin in migraine prophylaxis. A randomized controlled trial. *Neurology, 50*(2), 466–470.

Schreiber, C. P., Hutchinson, S., Webster, C. J., Ames, M., Richardson, M. S., & Powers, C. (2004). Prevalence of migraine in patients with a history of self-reported or physician-diagnosed "sinus" headache. *Arch Intern Med, 164*(16), 1769–1772. doi:10.1001/archinte.164.16.1769

Silberstein, S. D., Mannix, L. K., Goldstein, J., Couch, J. R., Byrd, S. C., Ames, M. H., . . . Toso, C. (2008). Multimechanistic (sumatriptan-naproxen) early intervention for the acute treatment of migraine. *Neurology, 71*(2), 114–121. doi:10.1212/01.wnl.0000316800.22949.20

Silberstein, S. D., & Rosenberg, J. (2000). Multispecialty consensus on diagnosis and treatment of headache. *Neurology, 54*(8), 1553.

Simpson, D. M., Hallett, M., Ashman, E. J., Comella, C. L., Green, M. W., Gronseth, G. S., . . . Yablon, S. A. (2016). Practice guideline update summary: Botulinum neurotoxin for the treatment of blepharospasm, cervical dystonia, adult spasticity, and headache: Report of the Guideline Development Subcommittee of the American Academy of Neurology. *Neurology, 86*(19), 1818–1826. doi:10.1212/WNL.0000000000002560

Sun, H., Dodick, D. W., Silberstein, S., Goadsby, P. J., Reuter, U., Ashina, M., . . . Lenz, R. (2016). Safety and efficacy of AMG 334 for prevention of episodic migraine: A randomised, double-blind, placebo-controlled, phase 2 trial. *Lancet Neurol, 15*(4), 382–390. doi:10.1016/S1474-4422(16)00019-3

## Chapter 2

Aker, P. D., Gross, A. R., Goldsmith, C. H., & Peloso, P. (1996). Conservative management of mechanical neck pain: systematic overview and meta-analysis. *BMJ, 313*(7068), 1291–1296.

Apkarian, A. V., Sosa, Y., Sonty, S., Levy, R. M., Harden, R. N., Parrish, T. B., & Gitelman, D. R. (2004). Chronic back pain is associated with decreased prefrontal and thalamic gray matter density. *J Neurosci, 24*(46), 10410–10415. doi:10.1523/JNEUROSCI.2541-04.2004

Arroll, B., & Goodyear-Smith, F. (2005). Corticosteroid injections for painful shoulder: A meta-analysis. *Br J Gen Pract, 55*(512), 224–228.

Bannuru, R. R., Schmid, C. H., Kent, D. M., Vaysbrot, E. E., Wong, J. B., & McAlindon, T. E. (2015). Comparative effectiveness of pharmacologic interventions for knee osteoarthritis: A systematic review and network meta-analysis. *Ann Intern Med, 162*(1), 46–54. doi:10.7326/M14-1231

Bellamy, N., Campbell, J., Robinson, V., Gee, T., Bourne, R., & Wells, G. (2006). Intraarticular corticosteroid for treatment of osteoarthritis of the knee. *Cochrane Database Syst Rev* (2), CD005328. doi:10.1002/14651858.CD005328.pub2

Bicket, M. C., Horowitz, J. M., Benzon, H. T., & Cohen, S. P. (2015). Epidural injections in prevention of surgery for spinal pain: Systematic review and meta-analysis of randomized controlled trials. *Spine J, 15*(2), 348–362. doi:10.1016/j.spinee.2014.10.011

Biondi, D., Xiang, J., Benson, C., Etropolski, M., Moskovitz, B., & Rauschkolb, C. (2013). Tapentadol immediate release versus oxycodone immediate release for treatment of acute low back pain. *Pain Physician, 16*(3), E237–246.

Blaine, T., Moskowitz, R., Udell, J., Skyhar, M., Levin, R., Friedlander, J., . . . Altman, R. (2008). Treatment of persistent shoulder pain with sodium hyaluronate: a randomized, controlled trial. A multicenter study. *J Bone Joint Surg Am, 90*(5), 970-979. doi:10.2106/JBJS.F.01116

Carette, S., Moffet, H., Tardif, J., Bessette, L., Morin, F., Frémont, P., . . . Blanchette, C. (2003). Intraarticular corticosteroids, supervised physiotherapy, or a combination of the two in the treatment of adhesive capsulitis of the shoulder: A placebo-controlled trial. *Arthritis Rheum, 48*(3), 829–838. doi:10.1002/art.10954

Chou, R., Deyo, R., Friedly, J., Skelly, A., Hashimoto, R., Weimer, M., . . . & Grusing, S. (2016). Noninvasive treatments for low back pain.

Cohen, S. P., Bicket, M. C., Jamison, D., Wilkinson, I., & Rathmell, J. P. (2013). Epidural steroids: a comprehensive, evidence-based review. *Reg Anesth Pain Med, 38*(3), 175–200. doi:10.1097/AAP.0b013e31828ea086

Cohen, S. P., Chen, Y., & Neufeld, N. J. (2013). Sacroiliac joint pain: a comprehensive review of epidemiology, diagnosis and treatment. *Expert Rev Neurother, 13*(1), 99–116. doi:10.1586/ern.12.148

Cohen, S. P., Huang, J. H., & Brummett, C. (2013). Facet joint pain—Advances in patient selection and treatment. *Nature Reviews Rheumatology, 9*(2), 101–116.

Cohen, S. P., Williams, K. A., Kurihara, C., Nguyen, C., Shields, C., Kim, P., . . . Strassels, S. A. (2010). Multicenter, randomized, comparative cost-effectiveness study comparing 0, 1, and 2 diagnostic medial branch (facet joint nerve) block treatment paradigms before lumbar facet radiofrequency denervation. *Anesthesiology, 113*(2), 395–405. doi:10.1097/ALN.0b013e3181e33ae5

Cooper, B. C., & Kleinberg, I. (2007). Examination of a large patient population for the presence of symptoms and signs of temporomandibular disorders. *Cranio, 25*(2), 114–126. doi:10.1179/crn.2007.018

Deer, T. R., Skaribas, I. M., Haider, N., Salmon, J., Kim, C., Nelson, C., . . . Washburn, S. N. (2014). Effectiveness of cervical spinal cord stimulation for the management of chronic pain. *Neuromodulation, 17*(3), 265–271; discussion 271. doi:10.1111/ner.12119

Desai, M. J., Kapural, L., Petersohn, J. D., Vallejo, R., Menzies, R., Creamer, M., & Gofeld, M. (2016b). Twelve-month follow-up of a randomized clinical trial comparing intradiscal biacuplasty to conventional medical management for discogenic lumbar back pain. *Pain Med.* doi:10.1093/pm/pnw184

Engquist, M., Löfgren, H., Öberg, B., Holtz, A., Peolsson, A., Söderlund, A., . . . Lind, B. (2013). Surgery versus nonsurgical treatment of cervical radiculopathy: A prospective, randomized study comparing surgery plus physiotherapy with physiotherapy alone with a 2-year follow-up. *Spine (Phila Pa 1976), 38*(20), 1715–1722. doi:10.1097/BRS.0b013e31829ff095

Fritzell, P., Hägg, O., Wessberg, P., Nordwall, A., & Group, Swedish Lumbar Spine Study. (2001). 2001 Volvo Award Winner in Clinical Studies: Lumbar fusion versus nonsurgical treatment for chronic low back pain: A multicenter randomized controlled trial from the Swedish Lumbar Spine Study Group. *Spine (Phila Pa 1976), 26*(23), 2521–2532; discussion 2532–2524.

Hellum, C., Johnsen, L. G., Storheim, K., Nygaard, O. P., Brox, J. I., Rossvoll, I., . . . Group, Norwegian Spine Study. (2011). Surgery with disc prosthesis versus rehabilitation in patients with low back pain and degenerative disc: two year follow-up of randomised study. *BMJ, 342*, d2786.

Hochberg, M. C., Altman, R. D., April, K. T., Benkhalti, M., Guyatt, G., McGowan, J., . . . Rheumatology, American College of. (2012). American College of Rheumatology 2012 recommendations for the use of nonpharmacologic and pharmacologic therapies in osteoarthritis of the hand, hip, and knee. *Arthritis Care Res (Hoboken), 64*(4), 465–474.

Kwon, Y. W., Eisenberg, G., & Zuckerman, J. D. (2013). Sodium hyaluronate for the treatment of chronic shoulder pain associated with glenohumeral osteoarthritis: A multicenter, randomized, double-blind, placebo-controlled trial. *J Shoulder Elbow Surg, 22*(5), 584–594. doi:10.1016/j.jse.2012.10.040

Liddle, S. D., Baxter, G. D., & Gracey, J. H. (2004). Exercise and chronic low back pain: What works? Pain, 107(1–2), 176–190.

List, T., Axelsson, S., & Leijon, G. (2003). Pharmacologic interventions in the treatment of temporomandibular disorders, atypical facial pain, and burning mouth syndrome. A qualitative systematic review. *J Orofac Pain, 17*(4), 301–310.

Machado, G. C., Ferreira, P. H., Harris, I. A., Pinheiro, M. B., Koes, B. W., van Tulder, M., . . . Ferreira, M. L. (2015). Effectiveness of surgery for lumbar spinal stenosis: a systematic review and meta-analysis. *PLoS One, 10*(3), e0122800. doi:10.1371/journal.pone.0122800

Mekhail, N., Vallejo, R., Coleman, M. H., & Benyamin, R. M. (2012). Long-term results of percutaneous lumbar decompression mild(®) for spinal stenosis. *Pain Pract, 12*(3), 184–193. doi:10.1111/j.1533-2500.2011.00481.x

Menzies, R. D., & Hawkins, J. K. (2015). Analgesia and improved performance in a patient treated by cooled radiofrequency for pain and dysfunction postbilateral total knee replacement. *Pain Pract, 15*(6), E54–58. doi:10.1111/papr.12292

Michalsen, A., Klotz, S., Lüdtke, R., Moebus, S., Spahn, G., & Dobos, G. J. (2003). Effectiveness of leech therapy in osteoarthritis of the knee: a randomized, controlled trial. *Ann Intern Med, 139*(9), 724–730.

Monticone, M., Cedraschi, C., Ambrosini, E., Rocca, B., Fiorentini, R., Restelli, M., . . . Moja, L. (2015). Cognitive-behavioural treatment for subacute and chronic neck pain. *Cochrane Database Syst Rev* (5), CD010664. doi:10.1002/14651858.CD010664.pub2

Moreland, L. W. (2003). Intra-articular hyaluronan (hyaluronic acid) and hylans for the treatment of osteoarthritis: mechanisms of action. *Arthritis Res Ther, 5*(2), 54–67.

Prager, J., Deer, T., Levy, R., Bruel, B., Buchser, E., Caraway, D., . . . Stearns, L. (2014). Best practices for intrathecal drug delivery for pain. *Neuromodulation, 17*(4), 354–372; discussion 372. doi:10.1111/ner.12146

Raynauld, J. P., Buckland-Wright, C., Ward, R., Choquette, D., Haraoui, B., Martel-Pelletier, J., . . . Pelletier, J. P. (2003). Safety and efficacy of long-term intraarticular steroid injections in osteoarthritis of the knee: A randomized, double-blind, placebo-controlled trial. *Arthritis Rheum, 48*(2), 370–377. doi:10.1002/art.10777

Schnitzer, T. J., Posner, M., & Lawrence, I. D. (1995). High strength capsaicin cream for osteoarthritis pain: Rapid onset of action and improved efficacy with twice daily dosing. *J Clin Rheumatol, 1*(5), 268–273.

Seminowicz, D. A., Wideman, T. H., Naso, L., Hatami-Khoroushahi, Z., Fallatah, S., Ware, M. A., . . . Stone, L. S. (2011). Effective treatment of chronic low back pain in humans reverses abnormal brain anatomy and function. *J Neurosci, 31*(20), 7540–7550. doi:10.1523/JNEUROSCI.5280-10.2011

Tempelhof, S., Rupp, S., & Seil, R. (1999). Age-related prevalence of rotator cuff tears in asymptomatic shoulders. *J Shoulder Elbow Surg, 8*(4), 296–299.

Wiggins, M. E., Fadale, P. D., Barrach, H., Ehrlich, M. G., & Walsh, W. R. (1994). Healing characteristics of a type I collagenous structure treated with corticosteroids. *Am J Sports Med, 22*(2), 279–288. doi:10.1177/036354659402200221

## Chapter 3

Ajeganova, S., van Steenbergen, H. W., van Nies, J. A., Burgers, L. E., Huizinga, T. W., & van der Helm-van Mil, A. H. (2016). Disease-modifying antirheumatic drug-free sustained remission in rheumatoid arthritis: An increasingly achievable outcome with subsidence of disease symptoms. *Ann Rheum Dis, 75*(5), 867–873. doi:10.1136/annrheumdis-2014-207080

Anderson, J. J., Wells, G., Verhoeven, A. C., & Felson, D. T. (2000). Factors predicting response to treatment in rheumatoid arthritis: The importance of disease duration. *Arthritis Rheum, 43*(1), 22–29. doi:10.1002/1529-0131(200001)43:1[22::AID-ANR4]3.0.CO;2-9

Avouac, J., Gossec, L., & Dougados, M. (2007). Efficacy and safety of opioids for osteoarthritis: a meta-analysis of randomized controlled trials. *Osteoarthritis Cartilage, 15*(8), 957–965. doi:10.1016/j.joca.2007.02.006

Bonilla-Hernán, M. G., Miranda-Carús, M. E., & Martin-Mola, E. (2011). New drugs beyond biologics in rheumatoid arthritis: the kinase inhibitors. *Rheumatology (Oxford), 50*(9), 1542–1550. doi:10.1093/rheumatology/ker192

Busso, N., & So, A. (2010). Mechanisms of inflammation in gout. *Arthritis Res Ther, 12*(2), 206. doi:10.1186/ar2952

Choi, H. K., Atkinson, K., Karlson, E. W., Willett, W., & Curhan, G. (2004a). Alcohol intake and risk of incident gout in men: A prospective study. *Lancet, 363*(9417), 1277–1281.

doi:10.1016/S0140-6736(04)16000-5

Choi, H. K., Liu, S., & Curhan, G. (2005). Intake of purine-rich foods, protein, and dairy products and relationship to serum levels of uric acid: The Third National Health and Nutrition Examination Survey. *Arthritis Rheum, 52*(1), 283–289. doi:10.1002/art.20761

Chou, R., Turner, J. A., Devine, E. B., Hansen, R. N., Sullivan, S. D., Blazina, I., . . . Deyo, R. A. (2015). The effectiveness and risks of long-term opioid therapy for chronic pain: a systematic review for a National Institutes of Health Pathways to Prevention Workshop. *Ann Intern Med, 162*(4), 276–286. doi:10.7326/M14-2559

Donahue, K. E., Gartlehner, G., Jonas, D. E., Lux, L. J., Thieda, P., Jonas, B. L., . . . Lohr, K. N. (2008). Systematic review: Comparative effectiveness and harms of disease-modifying medications for rheumatoid arthritis. *Ann Intern Med, 148*(2), 124–134.

Fransen, M., McConnell, S., Hernandez-Molina, G., & Reichenbach, S. (2010). Does land-based exercise reduce pain and disability associated with hip osteoarthritis? A meta-analysis of randomized controlled trials. *Osteoarthritis Cartilage, 18*(5), 613–620. doi:10.1016/j.joca.2010.01.003

Friedewald, V. E., Bennett, J. S., Christo, J. P., Pool, J. L., Scheiman, J. M., Simon, L. S., . . . Roberts, W. C. (2010). AJC Editor's consensus: Selective and nonselective nonsteroidal anti-inflammatory drugs and cardiovascular risk. *Am J Cardiol, 106*(6), 873–884. doi:10.1016/j.amjcard.2010.04.006

Hochberg, M. C., Martel-Pelletier, J., Monfort, J., Möller, I., Castillo, J. R., Arden, N., . . . Group, MOVES Investigation. (2016a). Combined chondroitin sulfate and glucosamine for painful knee osteoarthritis: A multicentre, randomised, double-blind, non-inferiority trial versus celecoxib. *Ann Rheum Dis, 75*(1), 37–44. doi:10.1136/annrheumdis-2014-206792

Jutkowitz, E., Choi, H. K., Pizzi, L. T., & Kuntz, K. M. (2014). Cost-effectiveness of allopurinol and febuxostat for the management of gout. *Ann Intern Med, 161*(9), 617–626. doi:10.7326/M14-0227

Khanna, D., Fitzgerald, J. D., Khanna, P. P., Bae, S., Singh, M. K., Neogi, T., . . . Rheumatology, American College of. (2012). 2012 American College of Rheumatology guidelines for management of gout. Part 1: systematic nonpharmacologic and pharmacologic therapeutic approaches to hyperuricemia. *Arthritis Care Res (Hoboken), 64*(10), 1431–1446. doi:10.1002/acr.21772

Khanna, D., Khanna, P. P., Fitzgerald, J. D., Singh, M. K., Bae, S., Neogi, T., . . . Rheumatology, American College of. (2012). 2012 American College of Rheumatology guidelines for management of gout. Part 2: Therapy and antiinflammatory prophylaxis of acute gouty arthritis. *Arthritis Care Res (Hoboken), 64*(10), 1447–1461. doi:10.1002/acr.21773

Klareskog, L., Catrina, A. I., & Paget, S. (2009). Rheumatoid arthritis. *Lancet, 373*(9664), 659–672. doi:10.1016/S0140-6736(09)60008-8

Mason, L., Moore, R. A., Edwards, J. E., McQuay, H. J., Derry, S., & Wiffen, P. J. (2004). Systematic review of efficacy of topical rubefacients containing salicylates for the treatment of acute and chronic pain. *BMJ, 328*(7446), 995. doi:10.1136/bmj.38040.607141.EE

McInnes, I. B., & O'Dell, J. R. (2010). State-of-the-art: Rheumatoid arthritis. *Annals of the rheumatic diseases, 69*(11), 1898–1906.

Neogi, T., Chen, C., Niu, J., Chaisson, C., Hunter, D. J., & Zhang, Y. (2014). Alcohol quantity and type on risk of recurrent gout attacks: An internet-based case-crossover study. *Am J Med, 127*(4), 311–318. doi:10.1016/j.amjmed.2013.12.019

Osteoarthritis: National clinical guideline for care and management in adults. In Conditions. NCCfC (Ed), Royal College of Physicians, London 2008.

Richette, P., Doherty, M., Pascual, E., Barskova, V., Becce, F., Castañeda-Sanabria, J., . . . Bardin, T. (2017). 2016 updated EULAR evidence-based recommendations for the management of gout. *Ann Rheum Dis, 76*(1), 29–42. doi:10.1136/annrheumdis-2016-209707

Roddy, E., & Choi, H. K. (2014). Epidemiology of gout. *Rheum Dis Clin North Am, 40*(2), 155–175. doi:10.1016/j.rdc.2014.01.001

Schlesinger, N., Alten, R. E., Bardin, T., Schumacher, H. R., Bloch, M., Gimona, A., . . . So, A. K. (2012). Canakinumab for acute gouty arthritis in patients with limited treatment options: Results from two randomised, multicentre, active-controlled, double-blind trials and their initial extensions. *Ann Rheum Dis, 71*(11), 1839–1848. doi:10.1136/annrheumdis-2011-200908

Schlesinger, N., Norquist, J. M., & Watson, D. J. (2009). Serum urate during acute gout. *J Rheumatol, 36*(6), 1287–1289. doi:10.3899/jrheum.080938

Song, R., Lee, E. O., Lam, P., & Bae, S. C. (2003). Effects of tai chi exercise on pain, balance, muscle strength, and perceived difficulties in physical functioning in older women with osteoarthritis: a randomized clinical trial. *J Rheumatol, 30*(9), 2039–2044.

Sundy, J. S., Baraf, H. S., Yood, R. A., Edwards, N. L., Gutierrez-Urena, S. R., Treadwell, E. L., . . . Becker, M. A. (2011). Efficacy and tolerability of pegloticase for the treatment of chronic gout in patients refractory to conventional treatment: Two randomized controlled trials. *JAMA, 306*(7), 711–720. doi:10.1001/jama.2011.1169

Towheed, T. E., Maxwell, L., Judd, M. G., Catton, M., Hochberg, M. C., & Wells, G. (2006). Acetaminophen for osteoarthritis. *Cochrane Database Syst Rev* (1), CD004257. doi:10.1002/14651858.CD004257.pub2

Van der Heide, A., Jacobs, J. W., Bijlsma, J. W., Heurkens, A. H., van Booma-Frankfort, C., van der Veen, M. J., . . . Hofman, D. M. (1996). The effectiveness of early treatment with "second-line" antirheumatic drugs: A randomized, controlled trial. *Ann Intern Mede, 124*(8), 699–707.

Wallace, K. L., Riedel, A. A., Joseph-Ridge, N., & Wortmann, R. (2004). Increasing prevalence of gout and hyperuricemia over 10 years among older adults in a managed care population. *J Rheumatol, 31*(8), 1582–1587.

Whiting, P. F., Smidt, N., Sterne, J. A., Harbord, R., Burton, A., Burke, M., . . . Dieppe, P. (2010). Systematic review: accuracy of anti-citrullinated Peptide antibodies for diagnosing rheumatoid arthritis. *Ann Intern Med, 152*(7), 456–464; W155-466. doi:10.7326/0003-4819-152-7-201004060-00010

Yan, J. H., Gu, W. J., Sun, J., Zhang, W. X., Li, B. W., & Pan, L. (2013). Efficacy of Tai Chi on pain, stiffness and function in patients with osteoarthritis: a meta-analysis. *PLoS One, 8*(4), e61672. doi:10.1371/journal.pone.0061672

## Chapter 4

Apalla, Z., Sotiriou, E., Lallas, A., Lazaridou, E., & Ioannides, D. (2013). Botulinum toxin A in postherpetic neuralgia: A parallel, randomized, double-blind, single-dose, placebo-controlled trial. *Clin J Pain, 29*(10), 857–864. doi:10.1097/AJP.0b013e31827a72d2

Argoff, C. E., Cole, B. E., Fishbain, D. A., & Irving, G. A. (2006). Diabetic peripheral neuropathic pain: Clinical and quality-of-life issues. *Mayo Clin Proc, 81*(4 Suppl), S3–11.

Barad, M. J., Ueno, T., Younger, J., Chatterjee, N., & Mackey, S. (2014). Complex regional pain syndrome is associated with structural abnormalities in pain-related regions of the human brain. *J Pain, 15*(2), 197–203. doi:10.1016/j.jpain.2013.10.011

Bennetto, L., Patel, N. K., & Fuller, G. (2007). Trigeminal neuralgia and its management. *BMJ, 334*(7586), 201–205. doi:10.1136/bmj.39085.614792.BE

Bouhassira, D., Lantéri-Minet, M., Attal, N., Laurent, B., & Touboul, C. (2008). Prevalence of chronic pain with neuropathic characteristics in the general population. *Pain, 136*(3), 380–387. doi:10.1016/j.pain.2007.08.013

Boulton, A. J., Vinik, A. I., Arezzo, J. C., Bril, V., Feldman, E. L., Freeman, R., . . . Association, American Diabetes. (2005a). Diabetic neuropathies: a statement by the American Diabetes Association. *Diabetes Care, 28*(4), 956–962.

Breuer, J., Pacou, M., Gautier, A., & Brown, M. M. (2014). Herpes zoster as a risk factor for stroke and TIA: a retrospective cohort study in the UK. *Neurology, 83*(2), e27–33. doi:10.1212/WNL.0000000000000584

Bruehl, S. (2015). Complex regional pain syndrome. *BMJ, 351*, h2730.

Christo, P. J., & McGreevy, K. (2011). Updated perspectives on neurogenic thoracic outlet syndrome. *Curr Pain Headache Rep, 15*(1), 14–21. doi:10.1007/s11916-010-0163-1

Colhado, O. C., Boeing, M., & Ortega, L. B. (2009). Botulinum toxin in pain treatment. *Rev Bras Anestesiol, 59*(3), 366–381.

Collins, S. L., Moore, R. A., McQuayHJ, & Wiffen, P. (2000). Antidepressants and anticonvulsants for diabetic neuropathy and postherpetic neuralgia: a quantitative systematic review. *J Pain Symptom Manage, 20*(6), 449–458.

Cunningham, A. L., Lal, H., Kovac, M., Chlibek, R., Hwang, S. J., Díez-Domingo, J., . . . Group, ZOE-70 Study. (2016). Efficacy of the Herpes Zoster Subunit Vaccine in Adults 70 Years of Age or Older. *N Engl J Med, 375*(11), 1019–1032. doi:10.1056/NEJMoa1603800

de Vos, C. C., Meier, K., Zaalberg, P. B., Nijhuis, H. J., Duyvendak, W., Vesper, J., . . . Lenders, M. W. (2014). Spinal cord stimulation in patients with painful diabetic neuropathy: a multicentre randomized clinical trial. *Pain, 155*(11), 2426–2431. doi:10.1016/j.pain.2014.08.031

Drulovic, J., Basic-Kes, V., Grgic, S., Vojinovic, S., Dincic, E., Toncev, G., . . . Pekmezovic, T. (2015). The prevalence of pain in adults with multiple sclerosis: A multicenter cross-sectional survey. *Pain Med, 16*(8), 1597–1602. doi:10.1111/pme.12731

Finnerup, N. B., Attal, N., Haroutounian, S., McNicol, E., Baron, R., Dworkin, R. H., . . . Wallace, M. (2015). Pharmacotherapy for neuropathic pain in adults: A systematic review and meta-analysis. *Lancet Neurol, 14*(2), 162–173. doi:10.1016/S1474-4422(14)70251-0

Foley, P. L., Vesterinen, H. M., Laird, B. J., Sena, E. S., Colvin, L. A., Chandran, S., . . . Fallon, M. T. (2013). Prevalence and natural history of pain in adults with multiple sclerosis: systematic review and meta-analysis. *Pain, 154*(5), 632–642. doi:10.1016/j.pain.2012.12.002

Franklin, G. M., Fulton-Kehoe, D., Bradley, C., & Smith-Weller, T. (2000). Outcome of surgery for thoracic outlet syndrome in Washington state workers' compensation. *Neurology, 54*(6), 1252–1257.

Griebeler, M. L., Morey-Vargas, O. L., Brito, J. P., Tsapas, A., Wang, Z., Carranza Leon, B. G., . . . Murad, M. H. (2014). Pharmacologic interventions for painful diabetic neuropathy: An umbrella systematic review and comparative effectiveness network meta-analysis. *Ann Intern Med, 161*(9), 639–649. doi:10.7326/M14-0511

Harden, R. N., Kaye, A. D., Kintanar, T., & Argoff, C. E. (2013). Evidence-based guidance for the management of postherpetic neuralgia in primary care. *Postgrad Med, 125*(4), 191–202. doi:10.3810/pgm.2013.07.2690

Häuser, W., Klose, P., Langhorst, J., Moradi, B., Steinbach, M., Schiltenwolf, M., & Busch, A. (2010). Efficacy of different types of aerobic exercise in fibromyalgia syndrome: a systematic review and meta-analysis of randomised controlled trials. *Arthritis Res Ther, 12*(3), R79. doi:10.1186/ar3002

Häuser, W., Urrútia, G., Tort, S., Uçeyler, N., & Walitt, B. (2013). Serotonin and noradrenaline reuptake inhibitors (SNRIs) for fibromyalgia syndrome. *Cochrane Database Syst Rev* (1), CD010292. doi:10.1002/14651858.CD010292

Johnson, R. W., & Dworkin, R. H. (2003). Treatment of herpes zoster and post-herpetic neuralgia. *BMJ, 326*(7392), 748–750. doi:10.1136/bmj.326.7392.748

Knijnik, L. M., Dussán-Sarria, J. A., Rozisky, J. R., Torres, I. L., Brunoni, A. R., Fregni, F., & Caumo, W. (2016). Repetitive transcranial magnetic stimulation for fibromyalgia: Systematic review and meta-analysis. *Pain Pract, 16*(3), 294–304. doi:10.1111/papr.12276

Mailis, A., & Taenzer, P. (2012). Evidence-based guideline for neuropathic pain interventional treatments: Spinal cord stimulation, intravenous infusions, epidural injections and nerve blocks. *Pain Res Manag, 17*(3), 150–158.

Malik, R. A. (2014). Which test for diagnosing early human diabetic neuropathy? *Diabetes, 63*(7), 2206–2208. doi:10.2337/db14-0492

Mashayekh, A., Christo, P. J., Yousem, D. M., & Pillai, J. J. (2011). CT-guided injection of the anterior and middle scalene muscles: technique and complications. *AJNR Am J Neuroradiol, 32*(3), 495–500. doi:10.3174/ajnr.A2319

Max, M. B., Lynch, S. A., Muir, J., Shoaf, S. E., Smoller, B., & Dubner, R. (1992a). Effects of desipramine, amitriptyline, and fluoxetine on pain in diabetic neuropathy. *N Engl J Med, 326*(19), 1250–1256. doi:10.1056/NEJM199205073261904

McCabe, C. S., Haigh, R. C., Ring, E. F., Halligan, P. W., Wall, P. D., & Blake, D. R. (2003). A controlled pilot study of the utility of mirror visual feedback in the treatment of complex regional pain syndrome (type 1). *Rheumatology (Oxford), 42*(1), 97–101.

McGreevy, K., & Williams, K. A. (2012). Contemporary insights into painful diabetic neuropathy and treatment with spinal cord stimulation. *Curr Pain Headache Rep, 16*(1), 43–49. doi:10.1007/s11916-011-0230-2

McGuire, K. B., Stojanovic-Radic, J., Strober, L., Chiaravalloti, N., & DeLuca, J. (2015). Development and effectiveness of a psychoeducational wellness program for people with multiple sclerosis: Description and outcomes. *Int J MS Care, 17*(1), 1–8. doi:10.7224/1537-2073.2013-045

McNicol, E. D., Midbari, A., & Eisenberg, E. (2013). Opioids for neuropathic pain. *Cochrane Database Syst Rev*(8), CD006146. doi:10.1002/14651858.CD006146.pub2

Mittal, S. O., Safarpour, D., & Jabbari, B. (2016). Botulinum toxin treatment of neuropathic pain. *Semin Neurol, 36*(1), 73–83. doi:10.1055/s-0036-1571953

Nalamachu, S., & Morley-Forster, P. (2012). Diagnosing and managing post-herpetic neuralgia. *Drugs Aging, 29*(11), 863–869. doi:10.1007/s40266-012-0014-3

Oxman, M. N., Levin, M. J., Johnson, G. R., Schmader, K. E., Straus, S. E., Gelb, L. D., . . . Group, Shingles Prevention Study. (2005). A vaccine to prevent herpes zoster and postherpetic neuralgia in older adults. *N Engl J Med, 352*(22), 2271–2284. doi:10.1056/NEJMoa051016

Petropoulos, I. N., Alam, U., Fadavi, H., Marshall, A., Asghar, O., Dabbah, M. A., . . . Malik, R. A. (2014). Rapid automated diagnosis of diabetic peripheral neuropathy with in vivo corneal confocal microscopy. *Invest Ophthalmol Vis Sci, 55*(4), 2071–2078. doi:10.1167/iovs.13-13787

Raja, S. N., Haythornthwaite, J. A., Pappagallo, M., Clark, M. R., Travison, T. G., Sabeen, S., . . . Max, M. B. (2002). Opioids versus antidepressants in postherpetic neuralgia: a randomized, placebo-controlled trial. *Neurology, 59*(7), 1015–1021.

Rochlin, D. H., Gilson, M. M., Likes, K. C., Graf, E., Ford, N., Christo, P. J., & Freischlag, J. A. (2013). Quality-of-life scores in neurogenic thoracic outlet syndrome patients undergoing first rib resection and scalenectomy. *J Vasc Surg, 57*(2), 436–443. doi:10.1016/j.jvs.2012.08.112

Shibuya, N., Humphers, J. M., Agarwal, M. R., & Jupiter, D. C. (2013). Efficacy and safety of high-dose vitamin C on complex regional pain syndrome in extremity trauma and surgery—Systematic review and meta-analysis. *J Foot Ankle Surg, 52*(1), 62–66. doi:10.1053/j.jfas.2012.08.003

Smith, H. S., Harris, R., & Clauw, D. (2011). Fibromyalgia: an afferent processing disorder leading to a complex pain generalized syndrome. *Pain Physician, 14*(2), E217–245.

Stampacchia, G., Gerini, A., & Mazzoleni, S. (2016). Effects of severe spasticity treatment with intrathecal Baclofen in multiple sclerosis patients: Long term follow-up. *NeuroRehabilitation, 38*(4), 385–393. doi:10.3233/NRE-161329

Tsuda, M., Inoue, K., & Salter, M. W. (2005). Neuropathic pain and spinal microglia: a big problem from molecules in "small" glia. *Trends Neurosci, 28*(2), 101–107. doi:10.1016/j.tins.2004.12.002

van Rijn, M. A., Marinus, J., Putter, H., Bosselaar, S. R., Moseley, G. L., & van Hilten, J. J. (2011). Spreading of complex regional pain syndrome: not a random process. *J Neural Transm (Vienna), 118*(9), 1301–1309. doi:10.1007/s00702-011-0601-1

Whiting, P. F., Wolff, R. F., Deshpande, S., Di Nisio, M., Duffy, S., Hernandez, A. V., . . . Kleijnen, J. (2015). Cannabinoids for Medical Use: A Systematic Review and Meta-analysis. *JAMA, 313*(24), 2456–2473. doi:10.1001/jama.2015.6358

Zakrzewska, J. M., & Linskey, M. E. (2014). Trigeminal neuralgia. *BMJ, 348*, g474.

## Chapter 5

Aasvang, E. K., Møhl, B., Bay-Nielsen, M., & Kehlet, H. (2006). Pain related sexual dysfunction after inguinal herniorrhaphy. *Pain, 122*(3), 258–263. doi:10.1016/j.pain.2006.01.035

Buffenoir, K., Rioult, B., Hamel, O., Labat, J. J., Riant, T., & Robert, R. (2015). Spinal cord stimulation of the conus medullaris for refractory pudendal neuralgia: A prospective study of 27 consecutive cases. *Neurourol Urodyn, 34*(2), 177–182. doi:10.1002/nau.22525

Christo P. J, & Hobelmann G. (2009). Pelvic pain. In Smith HS ed. *Current therapy in pain*. Philadelphia, PA: Saunders.

Harlow, B. L., & Stewart, E. G. (2005). Adult-onset vulvodynia in relation to childhood violence victimization. *Am J Epidemiol, 161*(9), 871-880. doi:10.1093/aje/kwi108

Hunter, C., Davé, N., Diwan, S., & Deer, T. (2013). Neuromodulation of pelvic visceral pain: review of the literature and case series of potential novel targets for treatment. *Pain Pract, 13*(1), 3–17. doi:10.1111/j.1533-2500.2012.00558.x

Latthe, P., Latthe, M., Say, L., Gülmezoglu, M., & Khan, K. S. (2006). WHO systematic review of prevalence of chronic pelvic pain: A neglected reproductive health morbidity. *BMC Public Health*, 6, 177. doi:10.1186/1471-2458-6-177

Latthe, P., Mignini, L., Gray, R., Hills, R., & Khan, K. (2006). Factors predisposing women to chronic pelvic pain: Systematic review. *BMJ, 332*(7544), 749–755. doi:10.1136/bmj.38748.697465.55

Laumann, E. O., Paik, A., & Rosen, R. C. (1999). Sexual dysfunction in the United States: Prevalence and predictors. *JAMA, 281*(6), 537–544.

Luzzi, G., & Law, L. (2005). A guide to sexual pain in men. *Practitioner, 249*(1667), 73, 75, 77 passim.

Manchikanti, L., Singh, V., Pampati, V., Falco, F. J., & Hirsch, J. A. (2015). Comparison of the efficacy of caudal, interlaminar, and transforaminal epidural injections in managing lumbar disc herniation: Is one method superior to the other? *Korean J Pain, 28*(1), 11–21. doi:10.3344/kjp.2015.28.1.11

Pitts, M., Ferris, J., Smith, A., Shelley, J., & Richters, J. (2008). Prevalence and correlates of three types of pelvic pain in a nationally representative sample of Australian men. *J Sex Med, 5*(5), 1223–1229. doi:10.1111/j.1743-6109.2007.00784.x

Popeney, C., Ansell, V., & Renney, K. (2007). Pudendal entrapment as an etiology of chronic perineal pain: Diagnosis and treatment. *Neurourol Urodyn, 26*(6), 820–827. doi:10.1002/nau.20421

Rosen, R., Altwein, J., Boyle, P., Kirby, R. S., Lukacs, B., Meuleman, E., . . . Giuliano, F. (2003). Lower urinary tract symptoms and male sexual dysfunction: The multinational survey of the aging male (MSAM-7). *Eur Urol, 44*(6), 637–649.

Rowland, D. C., Wright, D., Moir, L., FitzGerald, J. J., & Green, A. L. (2016). Successful treatment of pelvic girdle pain with dorsal root ganglion stimulation. *Br J Neurosurg, 30*(6), 685–686. doi:10.1080/02688697.2016.1208810

Sokal, P., Zieli?ski, P., & Harat, M. (2015). Sacral roots stimulation in chronic pelvic pain. *Neurol Neurochir Pol, 49*(5), 307–312. doi:10.1016/j.pjnns.2015.07.003

World Health Organization. Global and regional estimates of violence against women, 2013. http://www.who.int/reproductivehealth/publications/violence/9789241564625/en (accessed on May 11, 2016).

## Chapter 6

Akcan, E., Yiğit, R., & Atici, A. (2009). The effect of kangaroo care on pain in premature infants during invasive procedures. *Turk J Pediatr, 51*(1), 14–18.

Anand, K. J., Aranda, J. V., Berde, C. B., Buckman, S., Capparelli, E. V., Carlo, W., . . . Walco, G. A. (2006). Summary proceedings from the neonatal pain-control group. *Pediatrics, 117*(3 Pt 2), S9–S22. doi:10.1542/peds.2005-0620C

Carbajal, R., Rousset, A., Danan, C., Coquery, S., Nolent, P., Ducrocq, S., . . . Bréart, G. (2008). Epidemiology and treatment of painful procedures in neonates in intensive care units. *JAMA, 300*(1), 60–70. doi:10.1001/jama.300.1.60

Harrison, D., Larocque, C., Bueno, M., Stokes, Y., Turner, L., Hutton, B., & Stevens, B. (2017). Sweet Solutions to Reduce Procedural Pain in Neonates: A Meta-analysis. *Pediatrics, 139*(1). doi:10.1542/peds.2016-0955

Harrison, D., Yamada, J., & Stevens, B. (2010). Strategies for the prevention and management of neonatal and infant pain. *Curr Pain Headache Rep, 14*(2), 113–123. doi:10.1007/s11916-009-0091-0

Johnston, C. C., Filion, F., Campbell-Yeo, M., Goulet, C., Bell, L., McNaughton, K., . . . Walker, C. D. (2008). Kangaroo mother care diminishes pain from heel lance in very preterm neonates: a crossover trial. *BMC Pediatr, 8*, 13. doi:10.1186/1471-2431-8-13

Pillai Riddell, R. R., Racine, N. M., Turcotte, K., Uman, L. S., Horton, R. E., Din Osmun, L., . . . Gerwitz-Stern, A. (2011). Non-pharmacological management of infant and young child procedural pain. *Cochrane Database Syst Rev* (10), CD006275. doi:10.1002/14651858.CD006275.pub2

Prymula, R., Siegrist, C. A., Chlibek, R., Zemlickova, H., Vackova, M., Smetana, J., . . . Schuerman, L. (2009). Effect of prophylactic paracetamol administration at time of vaccination on febrile reactions and antibody responses in children: Two open-label, randomised controlled trials. *Lancet, 374*(9698), 1339–1350. doi:10.1016/S0140-6736(09)61208-3

Shah, P. S., Aliwalas, L. L., & Shah, V. S. (2006). Breastfeeding or breast milk for procedural pain in neonates. *The Cochrane Library.*

Wilson-Smith, E. M., & Morton, N. S. (2009). Survey of i.v. paracetamol (acetaminophen) use in neonates and infants under 1 year of age by UK anesthetists. *Paediatr Anaesth, 19*(4), 329–337. doi:10.1111/j.1460-9592.2009.02947.x

Yamada, J., Stinson, J., Lamba, J., Dickson, A., McGrath, P. J., & Stevens, B. (2008). A review of systematic reviews on pain interventions in hospitalized infants. Pain Res Manag, 13*(5), 413–420.*

## Chapter 7

Abernethy, B., Baker, J., & Côté, J. (2005). Transfer of pattern recall skills may contribute to the development of sport expertise. *Applied Cognitive Psychology, 19*(6), 705–718.

Caine, D., DiFiori, J., & Maffulli, N. (2006). Physeal injuries in children's and youth sports: Reasons for concern? *British journal of sports medicine, 40*(9), 749–760.

D'Arcy, Y. M. (2011). *Compact clinical guide to acute pain management: an evidence-based approach for nurses.* York: Springer Publishing Company.

DiFiori, J. P., Benjamin, H. J., Brenner, J. S., Gregory, A., Jayanthi, N., Landry, G. L., & Luke, A. (2014). Overuse injuries and burnout in youth sports: a position statement from the American Medical Society for Sports Medicine. *Br J Sports Med, 48*(4), 287–288. doi:10.1136/bjsports-2013-093299

DiFiori, J. P., Caine, D. J., & Malina, R. M. (2006). Wrist pain, distal radial physeal injury, and ulnar variance in the young gymnast. *Am J Sports Med, 34*(5), 840–849. doi:10.1177/0363546505284848

Galer, B. S., Rowbotham, M., Perander, J., Devers, A., & Friedman, E. (2000). Topical diclofenac patch relieves minor sports injury pain: Results of a multicenter controlled clinical trial. *J Pain Symptom Manage, 19*(4), 287–294.

Hauser, R. A., Lackner, J. B., Steilen-Matias, D., & Harris, D. K. (2016). A systematic review of dextrose prolotherapy for chronic musculoskeletal pain. *Clin Med Insights Arthritis Musculoskelet Disord, 9,* 139–159. doi:10.4137/CMAMD.S39160

How much physical activity do children need? Centers for Disease Control and Prevention 2008. www.cdc.gov/physicalactivity/everyone /guidelines/children.html (accessed on July 28, 2009).

Jayanthi, N., Pinkham, C., Dugas, L., Patrick, B., & Labella, C. (2013). Sports specialization in young athletes: Evidence-based recommendations. *Sports Health, 5*(3), 251–257. doi:10.1177/1941738112464626

Luke, A., Lazaro, R. M., Bergeron, M. F., Keyser, L., Benjamin, H., Brenner, J., . . . Smith, A. (2011). Sports-related injuries in youth athletes: is overscheduling a risk factor? *Clin J Sport Med, 21*(4), 307–314. doi:10.1097/JSM.0b013e3182218f71

McCarberg, B., & D'Arcy, Y. (2013). Options in topical therapies in the management of patients with acute pain. *Postgrad Med, 125*(4 Suppl 1), 19–24. doi:10.1080/00325481.2013.1110567011

Schwellnus, M., Soligard, T., Alonso, J. M., Bahr, R., Clarsen, B., Dijkstra, H. P., . . . Engebretsen, L. (2016a). How much is too much? (Part 2) International Olympic Committee consensus statement on load in sport and risk of illness. *Br J Sports Med, 50*(17), 1043–1052. doi:10.1136/bjsports-2016-096572

Strong, W. B., Malina, R. M., Blimkie, C. J., Daniels, S. R., Dishman, R. K., Gutin, B., . . . Trudeau, F. (2005). Evidence based physical activity for school-age youth. *J Pediatr, 146*(6), 732–737. doi:10.1016/j.jpeds.2005.01.055

Wall, E. J. (1997). Growth plate overuse syndrome of The ankle in athletes 1703. *Medicine & Science in Sports & Exercise, 29*(5), 299.

Winsley, R., & Matos, N. (2011a). Overtraining and elite young athletes. *Med Sport Sci, 56,* 97–105. doi:10.1159/000320636

## Chapter 8

Akbar, A., Yiangou, Y., Facer, P., Walters, J. R., Anand, P., & Ghosh, S. (2008). Increased capsaicin receptor TRPV1-expressing sensory fibres in irritable bowel syndrome and their correlation with abdominal pain. *Gut, 57*(7), 923–929. doi:10.1136/gut.2007.138982

Arnold, J., Barcena de Arellano, M. L., Rüster, C., Vercellino, G. F., Chiantera, V., Schneider, A., & Mechsner, S. (2012). Imbalance between sympathetic and sensory innervation in peritoneal endometriosis. *Brain Behav Immun, 26*(1), 132–141. doi:10.1016/j.bbi.2011.08.004

Asmus, S. E., Parsons, S., & Landis, S. C. (2000). Developmental changes in the transmitter properties of sympathetic neurons that innervate the periosteum. *J Neurosci, 20*(4), 1495–1504.

Bjurholm, A. (1991). Neuroendocrine peptides in bone. *Int Orthop, 15*(4), 325–329.

Chapurlat, R. D., Gensburger, D., Jimenez-Andrade, J. M., Ghilardi, J. R., Kelly, M., & Mantyh, P. (2012). Pathophysiology and medical treatment of pain in fibrous dysplasia of bone. *Orphanet J Rare Dis, 7* Suppl 1, S3. doi:10.1186/1750-1172-7-S1-S3

Feinberg, S. D. (2000). Prescribing analgesics. How to improve function and avoid toxicity when treating chronic pain. *Geriatrics, 55*(11), 44, 49–50, 53 passim.

Health Quality Ontario. (2016). Vertebral augmentation involving vertebroplasty or kyphoplasty for cancer-related vertebral compression fractures: A systematic review. *Ontario health technology assessment series, 16*(11), 1.

Jimenez-Andrade, J. M., & Mantyh, P. W. (2012). Sensory and sympathetic nerve fibers undergo sprouting and neuroma formation in the painful arthritic joint of geriatric mice. *Arthritis Res Ther, 14*(3), R101. doi:10.1186/ar3826

Jimenez-Andrade, J. M., Mantyh, W. G., Bloom, A. P., Freeman, K. T., Ghilardi, J. R., Kuskowski, M. A., & Mantyh, P. W. (2012). The effect of aging on the density of the sensory nerve fiber innervation of bone and acute skeletal pain. *Neurobiol Aging, 33*(5), 921–932. doi:10.1016/j.neurobiolaging.2010.08.008

Jimenez-Andrade, J. M., Mantyh, W. G., Bloom, A. P., Xu, H., Ferng, A. S., Dussor, G., . . . Mantyh, P. W. (2010). A phenotypically restricted set of primary afferent nerve fibers innervate the bone versus skin: Therapeutic opportunity for treating skeletal pain. *Bone, 46*(2), 306–313. doi:10.1016/j.bone.2009.09.013

Lane, N. E., Schnitzer, T. J., Birbara, C. A., Mokhtarani, M., Shelton, D. L., Smith, M. D., & Brown, M. T. (2010). Tanezumab for the treatment of pain from osteoarthritis of the knee. *N Engl J Med, 363*(16), 1521–1531. doi:10.1056/NEJMoa0901510

Mantyh, W. G., Jimenez-Andrade, J. M., Stake, J. I., Bloom, A. P., Kaczmarska, M. J., Taylor, R. N., . . . Mantyh, P. W. (2010). Blockade of nerve sprouting and neuroma formation markedly attenuates the development of late stage cancer pain. *Neuroscience, 171*(2), 588–598. doi:10.1016/j.neuroscience.2010.08.056

McMahon, S. B., Bennett, D. L. H., & Bevan, S. (2006). Inflammatory mediators and modulators of pain. *Wall and Melzack's textbook of Pain, 5,* 49–72.

Pezet, S., & McMahon, S. B. (2006). Neurotrophins: Mediators and modulators of pain. *Annu Rev Neurosci, 29,* 507–538. doi:10.1146/annurev.neuro.29.051605.112929

Schaible, H. G., Richter, F., Ebersberger, A., Boettger, M. K., Vanegas, H., Natura, G., . . . Segond von Banchet, G. (2009). Joint pain. *Exp Brain Res, 196*(1), 153–162. doi:10.1007/s00221-009-1782-9

Vitté, C., Fleisch, H., & Guenther, H. L. (1996). Bisphosphonates induce osteoblasts to secrete an inhibitor of osteoclast-mediated resorption. *Endocrinology, 137*(6), 2324–2333. doi:10.1210/endo.137.6.8641182

## Chapter 9

Dammers, J. W., Roos, Y., Veering, M. M., & Vermeulen, M. (2006). Injection with methylprednisolone in patients with the carpal tunnel syndrome: A randomised double blind trial testing three different doses. *J Neurol, 253*(5), 574–577. doi:10.1007/s00415-005-0062-2

Dempsey, P. G., & Filiaggi, A. J. (2006). Cross-sectional investigation of task demands and musculoskeletal discomfort among restaurant wait staff. *Ergonomics, 49*(1), 93–106. doi:10.1080/00140130500415225

Gellman, H., Gelberman, R. H., Tan, A. M., & Botte, M. J. (1986). Carpal tunnel syndrome. An evaluation of the provocative diagnostic tests. *J Bone Joint Surg Am, 68*(5), 735–737.

Hamamoto Filho, P. T., Leite, F. V., Ruiz, T., & Resende, L. A. (2009). A systematic review of anti-inflammatories for mild to moderate carpal tunnel syndrome. *J Clin Neuromuscul Dis, 11*(1), 22–30. doi:10.1097/CND.0b013e3181ac8364

Hirata, H. (2007). [Carpal tunnel syndrome & cubital tunnel syndrome]. *Rinsho Shinkeigaku, 47*(11), 761–765.

Kao, S. Y. (2003). Carpal tunnel syndrome as an occupational disease. *J Am Board Fam Pract, 16*(6), 533–542.

Laperrière, E., Ngomo, S., Thibault, M. C., & Messing, K. (2006). Indicators for choosing an optimal mix of major working postures. *Appl Ergon, 37*(3), 349–357. doi:10.1016/j.apergo.2005.06.014

Management of carpal tunnel syndrome. *Drug Ther Bull.* 2009;47(8):86–89.

Marshall, S., Tardif, G., & Ashworth, N. (2007). Local corticosteroid injection for carpal tunnel syndrome. *Cochrane Database Syst Rev* (2), CD001554. doi:10.1002/14651858.CD001554.pub2

Pomerance, J., Zurakowski, D., & Fine, I. (2009). The cost-effectiveness of nonsurgical versus surgical treatment for carpal tunnel syndrome. *J Hand Surg Am, 34*(7), 1193–1200. doi:10.1016/j.jhsa.2009.04.034

Silverstein, B. A., Fine, L. J., & Armstrong, T. J. (1987). Occupational factors and carpal tunnel syndrome. *Am J Ind Med, 11*(3), 343–358.

Swedler, D. I., Verma, S. K., Huang, Y. H., Lombardi, D. A., Chang, W. R., Brennan, M., & Courtney, T. K. (2015). A structural equation modelling approach examining the pathways between safety climate, behaviour performance and workplace slipping. *Occup Environ Med, 72*(7), 476–481. doi:10.1136/oemed-2014-102496

Wills, A. C., Davis, K. G., & Kotowski, S. E. (2013, September). Quantification of the physical demands for servers in restaurants. In *Proceedings of the Human Factors and Ergonomics Society Annual Meeting* (Vol. 57, No. 1, pp. 981–984). Los Angeles, CA: Sage Publications.

Witt, J. C., Hentz, J. G., & Stevens, J. C. (2004). Carpal tunnel syndrome with normal nerve conduction studies. *Muscle Nerve, 29*(4), 515–522. doi:10.1002/mus.20019

## Chapter 10

Andreae, M. H., & Andreae, D. A. (2013). Regional anaesthesia to prevent chronic pain after surgery: A Cochrane systematic review and meta-analysis. *Br J Anaesth, 111*(5), 711–720. doi:10.1093/bja/aet213

Barrington, M. J., & Kluger, R. (2013). Ultrasound guidance reduces the risk of local anesthetic systemic toxicity following peripheral nerve blockade. *Reg Anesth Pain Med, 38*(4), 289–299. doi:10.1097/AAP.0b013e318292669b

Fletcher, D., Fermanian, C., Mardaye, A., Aegerter, P., & (SFAR), Pain and Regional Anesthesia Committee of the French Anesthesia and Intensive Care Society. (2008). A patient-based national survey on postoperative pain management in France reveals significant achievements and persistent challenges. *Pain, 137*(2), 441–451. doi:10.1016/j.pain.2008.02.026

Gerbershagen, H. J., Aduckathil, S., van Wijck, A. J., Peelen, L. M., Kalkman, C. J., & Meissner, W. (2013). Pain intensity on the first day after surgery: a prospective cohort study comparing 179 surgical procedures. *Anesthesiology, 118*(4), 934–944. doi:10.1097/ALN.0b013e31828866b3

Gerbershagen, H. J., Pogatzki-Zahn, E., Aduckathil, S., Peelen, L. M., Kappen, T. H., van Wijck, A. J., . . . Meissner, W. (2014). Procedure-specific risk factor analysis for the development of severe postoperative pain. *Anesthesiology, 120*(5), 1237–1245. doi:10.1097/ALN.0000000000000108

Kalkman, C. J., Visser, K., Moen, J., Bonsel, G. J., Grobbee, D. E., & Moons, K. G. (2003). Preoperative prediction of severe postoperative pain. *Pain, 105*(3), 415–423.

Katz, J., & Seltzer, Z. (2009). Transition from acute to chronic postsurgical pain: Risk factors and protective factors. *Expert Rev Neurother, 9*(5), 723–744. doi:10.1586/ern.09.20

Kehlet, H., Jensen, T. S., & Woolf, C. J. (2006a). Persistent postsurgical pain: Risk factors and prevention. *Lancet, 367*(9522), 1618–1625. doi:10.1016/S0140-6736(06)68700-X

Kehlet, H., Jensen, T. S., & Woolf, C. J. (2006b). Persistent postsurgical pain: rRsk factors and prevention. *Lancet, 367*(9522), 1618–1625. doi:10.1016/S0140-6736(06)68700-X

Ladha, K. S., Patorno, E., Huybrechts, K. F., Liu, J., Rathmell, J. P., & Bateman, B. T. (2016). Variations in the use of perioperative multimodal analgesic therapy. *Anesthesiology, 124*(4), 837–845. doi:10.1097/ALN.0000000000001034

Macrae, W. A. (2008). Chronic post-surgical pain: 10 years on. *Br J Anaesth, 101*(1), 77–86. doi:10.1093/bja/aen099

Maier, C., Nestler, N., Richter, H., Hardinghaus, W., Pogatzki-Zahn, E., Zenz, M., & Osterbrink, J. (2010). The quality of pain management in German hospitals. *Dtsch Arztebl Int, 107*(36), 607–614. doi:10.3238/arztebl.2010.0607

Manchikanti, L., Cash, K. A., Pampati, V., Wargo, B. W., & Malla, Y. (2013). A randomized, double-blind, active control trial of fluoroscopic cervical interlaminar epidural injections in chronic pain of cervical disc herniation: results of a 2-year follow-up. *Pain Physician, 16*(5), 465–478.

Perkins, F. M., & Kehlet, H. (2000). Chronic pain as an outcome of surgery. A review of predictive factors. *Anesthesiology, 93*(4), 1123–1133.

Weiser, T. G., Regenbogen, S. E., Thompson, K. D., Haynes, A. B., Lipsitz, S. R., Berry, W. R., & Gawande, A. A. (2008). An estimation of the global volume of surgery: A modelling strategy based on available data. *Lancet, 372*(9633), 139–144. doi:10.1016/S0140-6736(08)60878-8

## Chapter 11

Aouizerat, B. E., Miaskowski, C. A., Gay, C., Portillo, C. J., Coggins, T., Davis, H., . . . Lee, K. A. (2010). Risk factors and symptoms associated with pain in HIV-infected adults. *J Assoc Nurses AIDS Care, 21*(2), 125–133. doi:10.1016/j.jana.2009.10.003

Ballas, S. K., Gupta, K., & Adams-Graves, P. (2012). Sickle cell pain: A critical reappraisal. *Blood, 120*(18), 3647–3656. doi:10.1182/blood-2012-04-383430

Batheja, S., Nields, J. A., Landa, A., & Fallon, B. A. (2013). Post-treatment Lyme syndrome and central sensitization. *J Neuropsychiatry Clin Neurosci, 25*(3), 176–186. doi:10.1176/appi.neuropsych.12090223

Bockenstedt, L. K., Mao, J., Hodzic, E., Barthold, S. W., & Fish, D. (2002). Detection of attenuated, noninfectious spirochetes in Borrelia burgdorferi-infected mice after antibiotic treatment. *J Infect Dis, 186*(10), 1430–1437. doi:10.1086/345284

Brandow, A. M., Farley, R. A., & Panepinto, J. A. (2014). Neuropathic pain in patients with sickle cell disease. *Pediatr Blood Cancer, 61*(3), 512–517. doi:10.1002/pbc.24838

Cairns, V., & Godwin, J. (2005). Post-Lyme Borreliosis syndrome: A meta-analysis of reported symptoms. *Int J Epidemiol, 34*(6), 1340–1345. doi:10.1093/ije/dyi129

Charache, S., Dover, G. J., Moyer, M. A., & Moore, J. W. (1987). Hydroxyurea-induced augmentation of fetal hemoglobin production in patients with sickle cell anemia. *Blood, 69*(1), 109–116.

Charache, S., Terrin, M. L., Moore, R. D., Dover, G. J., Barton, F. B., Eckert, S. V., . . . Bonds, D. R. (1995). Effect of hydroxyurea on the frequency of painful crises in sickle cell anemia. Investigators of the Multicenter Study of Hydroxyurea in Sickle Cell Anemia. *N Engl J Med, 332*(20), 1317–1322. doi:10.1056/NEJM199505183322001

Christensen, P. B., Wermuth, L., Hinge, H. H., & Bømers, K. (1990). Clinical course and long-term prognosis of acute transverse myelopathy. *Acta Neurol Scand, 81*(5), 431–435.

Defresne, P., Hollenberg, H., Husson, B., Tabarki, B., Landrieu, P., Huault, G., . . . Sébire, G. (2003). Acute transverse myelitis in children: Clinical course and prognostic factors. *J Child Neurol, 18*(6), 401–406. doi:10.1177/08830738030180060601

Dotevall, L., Eliasson, T., Hagberg, L., & Mannheimer, C. (2003). Pain as presenting symptom in Lyme neuroborreliosis. *Eur J Pain, 7*(3), 235–239. doi:10.1016/S1090-3801(02)00121-0

Elander, J., Lusher, J., Bevan, D., Telfer, P., & Burton, B. (2004). Understanding the causes of problematic pain management in sickle cell disease: evidence that pseudoaddiction plays a more important role than genuine analgesic dependence. *J Pain Symptom Manage, 27*(2), 156–169. doi:10.1016/j.jpainsymman.2003.12.001

Embers, M. E., Barthold, S. W., Borda, J. T., Bowers, L., Doyle, L., Hodzic, E., . . . Philipp, M. T. (2012). Persistence of Borrelia burgdorferi in rhesus macaques following antibiotic treatment of disseminated infection. *PLoS One, 7*(1), e29914. doi:10.1371/journal.pone.0029914

Fallon, B. A., Keilp, J. G., Corbera, K. M., Petkova, E., Britton, C. B., Dwyer, E., . . . Sackeim, H. A. (2008). A randomized, placebo-controlled trial of repeated IV antibiotic therapy for Lyme encephalopathy. *Neurology, 70*(13), 992–1003. doi:10.1212/01.WNL.0000284604.61160.2d

Hsieh, M. M., Kang, E. M., Fitzhugh, C. D., Link, M. B., Bolan, C. D., Kurlander, R., . . . Tisdale, J. F. (2009). Allogeneic hematopoietic stem-cell transplantation for sickle cell disease. *N Engl J Med, 361*(24), 2309–2317. doi:10.1056/NEJMoa0904971

Jeffery, D. R., Mandler, R. N., & Davis, L. E. (1993). Transverse myelitis: Retrospective analysis of 33 cases, with differentiation of cases associated with multiple sclerosis and parainfectious events. *Arch Neurol, 50*(5), 532–535.

Kuehn, B. M. (2013). CDC estimates 300,000 U.S. cases of Lyme disease annually. *Jama, 310*(11).

The management of sickle cell disease. national institutes of health national heart lung and blood institute division of blood diseases and resources. NIH publication 04-2117, revised 2004.

Maree, J. E., Dreyer Wright, S. C., & Makua, M. R. (2013). The management of HIV- and AIDS-related pain in a primary health clinic in Tshwane, South Africa. *Pain Manag Nurs, 14*(2), 94–101. doi:10.1016/j.pmn.2010.10.037

Marques, A. R. (2010). Lyme disease: A review. *Curr Allergy Asthma Rep, 10*(1), 13–20. doi:10.1007/s11882-009-0077-3

Merlin, J. S., Cen, L., Praestgaard, A., Turner, M., Obando, A., Alpert, C., . . . Frank, I. (2012). Pain and physical and psychological symptoms in ambulatory HIV patients in the current treatment era. *J Pain Symptom Manage, 43*(3), 638–645. doi:10.1016/j.jpainsymman.2011.04.019

Miaskowski, C., Penko, J. M., Guzman, D., Mattson, J. E., Bangsberg, D. R., & Kushel, M. B. (2011). Occurrence and characteristics of chronic pain in a community-based cohort of indigent adults living with HIV infection. *J Pain, 12*(9), 1004–1016. doi:10.1016/j.jpain.2011.04.002

Pachner, A. R., & Steiner, I. (2007). Lyme neuroborreliosis: Infection, immunity, and inflammation. *Lancet Neurol, 6*(6), 544–552. doi:10.1016/S1474-4422(07)70128-X

Platt, O. S., Thorington, B. D., Brambilla, D. J., Milner, P. F., Rosse, W. F., Vichinsky, E., & Kinney, T. R. (1991). Pain in sickle cell disease. Rates and risk factors. *N Engl J Med, 325*(1), 11–16. doi:10.1056/NEJM199107043250103

Rupprecht, T. A., Koedel, U., Fingerle, V., & Pfister, H. W. (2008). The pathogenesis of lyme neuroborreliosis: From infection to inflammation. *Mol Med, 14*(3-4), 205–212. doi:10.2119/2007-00091.Rupprecht

Steere, A. C., Gross, D., Meyer, A. L., & Huber, B. T. (2001). Autoimmune mechanisms in antibiotic treatment-resistant Lyme arthritis. *J Autoimmun, 16*(3), 263–268. doi:10.1006/jaut.2000.0495

Steinberg, M. H., Barton, F., Castro, O., Pegelow, C. H., Ballas, S. K., Kutlar, A., . . . Terrin, M. (2003). Effect of hydroxyurea on mortality and morbidity in adult sickle cell anemia: Risks and benefits up to 9 years of treatment. *JAMA, 289*(13), 1645–1651. doi:10.1001/jama.289.13.1645

U.S. Centers for Disease Control and Prevention. Sickle cell disease: Data and statistics. http://www.cdc.gov/ncbddd/sicklecell/data.html (accessed on March 8, 2014).

Wormser, G. P., Dattwyler, R. J., Shapiro, E. D., Halperin, J. J., Steere, A. C., Klempner, M. S., . . . Nadelman, R. B. (2006). The clinical assessment, treatment, and prevention of Lyme disease, human granulocytic anaplasmosis, and babesiosis: Clinical practice guidelines by the Infectious Diseases Society of America. *Clin Infect Dis, 43*(9), 1089–1134. doi:10.1086/508667

Yawn, B. P., Buchanan, G. R., Afenyi-Annan, A. N., Ballas, S. K., Hassell, K. L., James, A. H., . . . John-Sowah, J. (2014). Management of sickle cell disease: Summary of the 2014 evidence-based report by expert panel members. *JAMA, 312*(10), 1033–1048. doi:10.1001/jama.2014.10517

## Chapter 12

Abrams, D. I., Couey, P., Shade, S. B., Kelly, M. E., & Benowitz, N. L. (2011). Cannabinoid-opioid interaction in chronic pain. *Clin Pharmacol Ther, 90*(6), 844–851. doi:10.1038/clpt.2011.188

Araki, K., Kobayashi, M., Ogata, T., & Takuma, K. (1994). Colorectal carcinoma metastatic to skeletal muscle. *Hepatogastroenterology, 41*(5), 405–408.

Bloomfield, D. J. (1998). Should bisphosphonates be part of the standard therapy of patients with multiple myeloma or bone metastases from other cancers? An evidence-based review. *J Clin Oncol, 16*(3), 1218–1225. doi:10.1200/JCO.1998.16.3.1218

Bottros, M. M., & Christo, P. J. (2014). Current perspectives on intrathecal drug delivery. *J Pain Res, 7*, 615–626. doi:10.2147/JPR.S37591

Cancer pain relief: With a guide to opioid availability. (1996). World Health Organization.

Carter, G. T., Flanagan, A. M., Earleywine, M., Abrams, D. I., Aggarwal, S. K., & Grinspoon, L. (2011). Cannabis in palliative medicine: Improving care and reducing opioid-related morbidity. *Am J Hosp Palliat Care, 28*(5), 297–303. doi:10.1177/1049909111402318

Christo, P. J., & Mazloomdoost, D. (2008a). Cancer pain and analgesia. *Ann N Y Acad Sci, 1138*, 278–298. doi:10.1196/annals.1414.033

Christo, P. J., & Mazloomdoost, D. (2008b). Interventional pain treatments for cancer pain. *Ann N Y Acad Sci, 1138*, 299–328. doi:10.1196/annals.1414.034

Cleeland, C. S., Gonin, R., Hatfield, A. K., Edmonson, J. H., Blum, R. H., Stewart, J. A., & Pandya, K. J. (1994). Pain and its treatment in outpatients with metastatic cancer. *N Engl J Med, 330*(9), 592–596. doi:10.1056/NEJM199403033300902

Davies, A. N. (2014). Breakthrough cancer pain. *Curr Pain Headache Rep, 18*(6), 420. doi:10.1007/s11916-014-0420-9

Edwards, M. J. (2005). Opioids and benzodiazepines appear paradoxically to delay inevitable death after ventilator withdrawal. *J Palliat Care, 21*(4), 299–302.

ESMO. 2007. Management of cancer pain: ESMO clinical recommendations. *Annals of Oncology, 18*(suppl 2), ii92–ii94.

Ferrandina, G., Salutari, V., Testa, A., Zannoni, G. F., Petrillo, M., & Scambia, G. (2006). Recurrence in skeletal muscle from squamous cell carcinoma of the uterine cervix: A case report and review of the literature. *BMC Cancer, 6*, 169. doi:10.1186/1471-2407-6-169

Ferreira, K. A. S. L., Kimura, M., & Teixeira, M. J. (2006). The WHO analgesic ladder for cancer pain control, twenty years of use: How much pain relief does one get from using it? *Supportive care in cancer, 14*(11), 1086–1093.

Fishman, B. (1990). The treatment of suffering in patients with cancer pain-cognitive-behavioral approaches. In K. M. Foley, J. J. Bonica, & V. Ventafridda (Eds.). Second International Congress on Cancer Pain. Advances in pain research and therapy, vol 16. (301–316). NY: Raven Press.

Health Quality Ontario. (2016). Vertebral augmentation involving vertebroplasty or kyphoplasty for cancer-related vertebral compression fractures: A systematic review. *Ontario health technology assessment series, 16*(11), 1.

Kahan, A., Uebelhart, D., De Vathaire, F., Delmas, P. D., & Reginster, J. Y. (2009). Long-term effects of chondroitins 4 and 6 sulfate on knee osteoarthritis: The study on osteoarthritis progression prevention, a two-year, randomized, double-blind, placebo-controlled trial. *Arthritis Rheum, 60*(2), 524–533. doi:10.1002/art.24255

Keefe, F. J., Abernethy, A. P., & C Campbell, L. (2005a). Psychological approaches to understanding and treating disease-related pain. *Annu Rev Psychol, 56*, 601–630. doi:10.1146/annurev.psych.56.091103.070302

Keefe, F. J., Abernethy, A. P., & C Campbell, L. (2005b). Psychological approaches to understanding and treating disease-related pain. *Annu Rev Psychol, 56*, 601–630. doi:10.1146/annurev.psych.56.091103.070302

Keefe, F. J., Abernethy, A. P., & C Campbell, L. (2005c). Psychological approaches to understanding and treating disease-related pain. *Annu Rev Psychol, 56*, 601–630. doi:10.1146/annurev.psych.56.091103.070302

Kutner, J. S., Smith, M. C., Corbin, L., Hemphill, L., Benton, K., Mellis, B. K., . . . Fairclough, D. L. (2008a). Massage therapy versus simple touch to improve pain and mood in patients with advanced cancer: a randomized trial. Ann Intern Med, 149(6), 369–379.

Kutner, J. S., Smith, M. C., Corbin, L., Hemphill, L., Benton, K., Mellis, B. K., . . . Fairclough, D. L. (2008b). Massage therapy versus simple touch to improve pain and mood in patients with advanced cancer: A randomized trial. *Ann Intern Med, 149*(6), 369–379.

Lillemoe, K. D., Cameron, J. L., Kaufman, H. S., Yeo, C. J., Pitt, H. A., & Sauter, P. K. (1993). Chemical splanchnicectomy in patients with unresectable pancreatic cancer. A prospective randomized trial. *Ann Surg, 217*(5), 447–455; discussion 456–447.

Linton S. L. & Melin, L. Applied relaxation in the management of chronic pain. *Behav Psychother* 1983; 11-337-50.

Lynch, M. E. (2001). Antidepressants as analgesics: a review of randomized controlled trials. *J Psychiatry Neurosci, 26*(1), 30–36.

Macaluso, C., Weinberg, D., & Foley, K. M. (1988). Opioid abuse and misuse in a cancer pain population. *Journal of Pain and Symptom Management, 3*, S24.

Max, M. B., Payne R., Edwards W. T., et al. (1999). *Principles of analgesic use in the treatment of acute pain and cancer pain,* (4th ed.). Glenview, IL: American Pain Society.

Morita, T., Tsunoda, J., Inoue, S., & Chihara, S. (2001a). Effects of high dose opioids and sedatives on survival in terminally ill cancer patients. *J Pain Symptom Manage,* 21(4), 282–289.

Passik, S. D., Kirsh, K. L., McDonald, M. V., Ahn, S., Russak, S. M., Martin, L., . . . Portenoy, R. K. (2000). A pilot survey of aberrant drug-taking attitudes and behaviors in samples of cancer and AIDS patients. *J Pain Symptom Manage, 19*(4), 274–286.

Shah, R., Baqai-Stern, A., & Gulati, A. (2015). Managing intrathecal drug delivery (ITDD) in cancer patients. *Curr Pain Headache Rep, 19*(6), 20. doi:10.1007/s11916-015-0488-x

Sridhar, K. S., Rao, R. K., & Kunhardt, B. (1987). Skeletal muscle metastases from lung cancer. *Cancer, 59*(8), 1530–1534.

Sykes, N., & Thorns, A. (2003a). The use of opioids and sedatives at the end of life. *Lancet Oncol, 4*(5), 312–318.

Van den Beuken-van Everdingen, M. H. J., De Rijke, J. M., Kessels, A. G., Schouten, H. C., Van Kleef, M., & Patijn, J. (2007). Prevalence of pain in patients with cancer: A systematic review of the past 40 years. *Annals of Oncology, 18*(9), 1437–1449.

Ward, S. E., Goldberg, N., Miller-McCauley, V., Mueller, C., Nolan, A., Pawlik-Plank, D., . . . Weissman, D. E. (1993). Patient-related barriers to management of cancer pain. *Pain, 52*(3), 319–324.

Williams, M.R. (1984). The place of surgery in terminal care. In C. Saunders (Ed.), *The management of terminal disease* (148–153). London: Edward Arnold.

## Chapter 13

Agha, A., Phillips, J., O'Kelly, P., Tormey, W., & Thompson, C. J. (2005). The natural history of post-traumatic hypopituitarism: Implications for assessment and treatment. *Am J Med,* 118(12), 1416. doi:10.1016/j.amjmed.2005.02.042

Alexander, L., Mannion, R. O., Weingarten, B., Fanelli, R. J., & Stiles, G. L. (2014). Development and impact of prescription opioid abuse deterrent formulation technologies. *Drug Alcohol Depend,* 138, 1–6. doi:10.1016/j.drugalcdep.2014.02.006

Baptist Memorial Hospital, Memphis. (1977, August 16). Postmortem No. A77–160.

Baugh, C. M., Stamm, J. M., Riley, D. O., Gavett, B. E., Shenton, M. E., Lin, A., . . . & Stern, R. A. (2012). Chronic traumatic encephalopathy: Neurodegeneration following repetitive concussive and subconcussive brain trauma. *Brain Imaging Behav,* 6(2), 244–254. doi:10.1007/s11682-012-9164-5

Campbell P.N., Doniach D., Hudson R.V., & Roitt I. M. (1956). Auto-antibodies in Hashimoto's disease (lymphadenoid goitre). *Lancet,* 271(6947): 820–821

Caturegli, P., Newschaffer, C., Olivi, A., Pomper, M. G., Burger, P. C., & Rose, N. R. (2005). Autoimmune hypophysitis. *Endocr Rev,* 26(5), 599–614. doi:10.1210/er.2004-0011

Dallek, R. (2002). The medical ordeals of JFK. *Atlantic Monthly,* 290(5), 49–61.

Davies, A. L., Hayes, K. C., & Dekaban, G. A. (2007). Clinical correlates of elevated serum concentrations of cytokines and autoantibodies in patients with spinal cord injury. *Arch Phys Med Rehabil,* 88(11), 1384–1393. doi:10.1016/j.apmr.2007.08.004

Helmick, K., Baugh, L., Lattimore, T., & Goldman, S. (2012). Traumatic brain injury: Next steps, research needed, and priority focus areas. *Mil Med,* 177(8 Suppl), 86–92.

Henry, D. E., Chiodo, A. E., & Yang, W. (2011). Central nervous system reorganization in a variety of chronic pain states: a review. *PM R,* 3(12), 1116–1125. doi:10.1016/j.pmrj.2011.05.018

Holmquist, G. L. (2009). Opioid metabolism and effects of cytochrome P450. *Pain Medicine,* 10(s1), S20–S29.

Kelman J. President Kennedy's health secrets. PBS Newshour. http://www.pbs.org/newshour/bbhealth/july-dec02/jfk_11-18.html (accessed August 3, 2012).

Laker, S. R. (2011). Epidemiology of concussion and mild traumatic brain injury. *PM R,* 3(10 Suppl 2), S354–358. doi:10.1016/j.pmrj.2011.07.017

Lopalco, G., Cantarini, L., Vitale, A., Iannone, F., Anelli, M. G., Andreozzi, L., . . . & Rigante, D. (2015). Interleukin-1 as a common denominator from autoinflammatory to autoimmune disorders: premises, perils, and perspectives. *Mediators Inflamm,* 2015, 194864. doi:10.1155/2015/194864

Lucas, S. (2011). Headache management in concussion and mild traumatic brain injury. *PM R,* 3(10 Suppl 2), S406–412. doi:10.1016/j.pmrj.2011.07.016

Lundberg, G. D. (1992). Closing the case in JAMA on the John F. Kennedy autopsy. *JAMA,* 268(13), 1736–1738.

Mandel, L. R. (2009). Endocrine and autoimmune aspects of the health history of John F. Kennedy. *Ann Intern Med,* 151(5), 350–354.

McKee, A. C., Stern, R. A., Nowinski, C. J., Stein, T. D., Alvarez, V. E., Daneshvar, D. H., . . . & Cantu, R. C. (2013). The spectrum of disease in chronic traumatic encephalopathy. *Brain,* 136(Pt 1), 43–64. doi:10.1093/brain/aws307

Milligan, E. D., & Watkins, L. R. (2009). Pathological and protective roles of glia in chronic pain. *Nat Rev Neurosci,* 10(1), 23-36. doi:10.1038/nrn2533

O'Leary C., Walsh C.H., Wieneke P., O'Regan, P., Buckley, B., O'Halloran, D. J., . . . Cronin, C. C. (2002). Coeliac disease and autoimmune Addison's disease: a clinical pitfall. *QJM,* 95(2), 79–82.

Ren, K., & Torres, R. (2009). Role of interleukin-1beta during pain and inflammation. *Brain Res Rev,* 60(1), 57–64. doi:10.1016/j.brainresrev.2008.12.020

Saag, K. G. (2003). Glucocorticoid-induced osteoporosis. *Endocrinology and metabolism clinics of North America, 32*(1), 135–157.

Sherman, K. B., Goldberg, M., & Bell, K. R. (2006). Traumatic brain injury and pain. *Phys Med Rehabil Clin N Am, 17*(2), 473–490, viii. doi:10.1016/j.pmr.2005.11.007

Signoretti, S., Lazzarino, G., Tavazzi, B., & Vagnozzi, R. (2011). The pathophysiology of concussion. *PM R, 3*(10 Suppl 2), S359–368. doi:10.1016/j.pmrj.2011.07.018

Tennant, F. (2011). Genetic screening for defects in opioid metabolism: Historical characteristics and blood levels. *Pract Pain Manag, 11*, 1–2.

Travell, J. G. (1968). *Office Hours: Day and night: The autobiography of Janet Travell, MD.* Cleveland: World Publishing Company.

Travell, J., & Travell, W. (1946). Therapy of lowback pain by manipulation and of referred pain in the lower extremity by procaine infiltration. *Arch Phys Med Rehabil, 27*, 537–547.

Wass, J. A. H., White, K. G., & Elliott, A. (2006). Osteoporosis, osteopaenia, and osteoarthritis in autoimmune hypoadrenalism.

Zhang, J. M., & An, J. (2007). Cytokines, inflammation, and pain. *Int Anesthesiol Clin, 45*(2), 27–37. doi:10.1097/AIA.0b013e318034194e

## Chapter 14

Abrams, D. I., Jay, C. A., Shade, S. B., Vizoso, H., Reda, H., Press, S., . . . & Petersen, K. L. (2007). Cannabis in painful HIV-associated sensory neuropathy: A randomized placebo-controlled trial. *Neurology, 68*(7), 515–521. doi:10.1212/01.wnl.0000253187.66183.9c

Angst, M. S., & Clark, J. D. (2006). Opioid-induced hyperalgesia: A qualitative systematic review. *Anesthesiology, 104*(3), 570–587.

Backonja, M. M. (2002). Use of anticonvulsants for treatment of neuropathic pain. *Neurology, 59*(5 Suppl 2), S14–17.

Ballantyne, J. C., & Mao, J. (2003). Opioid therapy for chronic pain. *N Engl J Med, 349*(20), 1943–1953. doi:10.1056/NEJMra025411

Broussard, C. S., Rasmussen, S. A., Reefhuis, J., Friedman, J. M., Jann, M. W., Riehle-Colarusso, T., & Honein, M. A. (2011). National birth defects prevention study. Maternal treatment with opioid analgesics and risk for birth defects. *Am J Obstet Gynecol, 204*(4), 314.e311–311. doi:10.1016/j.ajog.2010.12.039

Budney, A. J., Roffman, R., Stephens, R. S., & Walker, D. (2007). Marijuana dependence and its treatment. *Addict Sci Clin Pract, 4*(1), 4–16.

Butler, S. F., Cassidy, T. A., Chilcoat, H., Black, R. A., Landau, C., Budman, S. H., & Coplan, P. M. (2013). Abuse rates and routes of administration of reformulated extended-release oxycodone: initial findings from a sentinel surveillance sample of individuals assessed for substance abuse treatment. *J Pain, 14*(4), 351–358. doi:10.1016/j.jpain.2012.08.008

Center for Disease Control and Prevention. (2015). Wide-ranging online data for epidemiologic research (WONDER). Multiple-cause-of-death file, 2000–2014. Retrieved from http://www.cdc.gov/nchs/data/healthpolicy/AADR_US_2000-2014.pdf

Chang, G., Chen, L., & Mao, J. (2007). Opioid tolerance and hyperalgesia. *Med Clin North Am, 91*(2), 199–211. doi:10.1016/j.mcna.2006.10.003

Cicero, T. J., & Ellis, M. S. (2015). Abuse-deterrent formulations and the prescription opioid abuse epidemic in the United States: Lessons learned from OxyContin. *JAMA Psychiatry, 72*(5), 424–430. doi:10.1001/jamapsychiatry.2014.3043

Cicero, T. J., Ellis, M. S., & Surratt, H. L. (2012). Effect of abuse-deterrent formulation of OxyContin. *N Engl J Med, 367*(2), 187–189. doi:10.1056/NEJMc1204141

Coplan, P. M., Chilcoat, H. D., Butler, S. F., Sellers, E. M., Kadakia, A., Harikrishnan, V., . . . & Dart, R. C. (2016). The effect of an abuse-deterrent opioid formulation (OxyContin) on opioid abuse-related outcomes in the postmarketing setting. *Clin Pharmacol Ther, 100*(3), 275–286. doi:10.1002/cpt.390

Corey-Bloom, J., Wolfson, T., Gamst, A., Jin, S., Marcotte, T. D., Bentley, H., & Gouaux, B. (2012). Smoked cannabis for spasticity in multiple sclerosis: a randomized, placebo-controlled trial. *CMAJ, 184*(10), 1143–1150. doi:10.1503/cmaj.110837

du Plessis, S. S., Agarwal, A., & Syriac, A. (2015). Marijuana, phytocannabinoids, the endocannabinoid system, and male fertility. *J Assist Reprod Genet, 32*(11), 1575–1588. doi:10.1007/s10815-015-0553-8

Dworkin, R. H., O'Connor, A. B., Backonja, M., Farrar, J. T., Finnerup, N. B., Jensen, T. S., . . . & Wallace, M. S. (2007). Pharmacologic management of neuropathic pain: evidence-based recommendations. *Pain, 132*(3), 237–251. doi:10.1016/j.pain.2007.08.033

Fishbain, D. A., Cole, B., Lewis, J., Rosomoff, H. L., & Rosomoff, R. S. (2008a). What percentage of chronic nonmalignant pain patients exposed to chronic opioid analgesic therapy develop abuse/addiction and/or aberrant drug-related behaviors? A structured evidence-based review. *Pain Med, 9*(4), 444–459. doi:10.1111/j.1526-4637.2007.00370.x

Friedewald, V. E., Bennett, J. S., Christo, J. P., Pool, J. L., Scheiman, J. M., Simon, L. S., . . . & Roberts, W. C. (2010). AJC Editor's consensus: Selective and nonselective nonsteroidal anti-inflammatory drugs and cardiovascular risk. *Am J Cardiol, 106*(6), 873–884. doi:10.1016/j.amjcard.2010.04.006

Grant, I., Atkinson, J. H., Gouaux, B., & Wilsey, B. (2012). Medical marijuana: clearing away the smoke. *Open Neurol J, 6*, 18–25. doi:10.2174/1874205X01206010018

Hasin, D. S., Kerridge, B. T., Saha, T. D., Huang, B., Pickering, R., Smith, S. M., . . . & Grant, B. F. (2016). Prevalence and correlates of DSM-5 cannabis use disorder, 2012-2013: Findings from the National Epidemiologic Survey on Alcohol and Related Conditions-III. *Am J Psychiatry, 173*(6), 588–599. doi:10.1176/appi.ajp.2015.15070907

Hill, K. P. (2015). Medical marijuana for treatment of chronic pain and other medical and psychiatric problems: A clinical review. *JAMA, 313*(24), 2474–2483. doi:10.1001/jama.2015.6199

Kellogg, A., Rose, C. H., Harms, R. H., & Watson, W. J. (2011). Current trends in narcotic use in pregnancy and neonatal outcomes. *Am J Obstet Gynecol, 204*(3), 259.e251–254. doi:10.1016/j.ajog.2010.12.050

Lynch, M. E., & Ware, M. A. (2015). Cannabinoids for the treatment of chronic non-cancer pain: An updated systematic review of random-ized controlled trials. *J Neuroimmune Pharmacol, 10*(2), 293–301. doi:10.1007/s11481-015-9600-6

Majithia, N., Smith, T. J., Coyne, P. J., Abdi, S., Pachman, D. R., Lachance, D., . . . & Loprinzi, C. L. (2016). Scrambler therapy for the management of chronic pain. *Support Care Cancer, 24*(6), 2807–2814. doi:10.1007/s00520-016-3177-3

Manchikanti, L., Kaye, A. M., Knezevic, N. N., McAnally, H., Slavin, K., Trescot, A. M., . . . & Hirsch, J. A. (2017). Responsible, safe, and effective prescription of opioids for chronic non-cancer pain: American Society of Interventional Pain Physicians (ASIPP) guidelines. *Pain Physician, 20*(2S), S3–S92.

Miller, M., Stürmer, T., Azrael, D., Levin, R., & Solomon, D. H. (2011). Opioid analgesics and the risk of fractures in older adults with arthritis. *J Am Geriatr Soc, 59*(3), 430–438. doi:10.1111/j.1532-5415.2011.03318.x

Noble, M., Treadwell, J. R., Tregear, S. J., Coates, V. H., Wiffen, P. J., Akafomo, C., & Schoelles, K. M. (2010). Long-term opioid management for chronic noncancer pain. *Cochrane Database Syst Rev, 1*(1).

Office of the President of the United States. (2011). Epidemic: Responding to America's prescription drug abuse crisis. Washington, DC: Office of National Drug Control Policy Executive. Retrieved from http://www.whitehouse.gov/sites/default/files/ondcp/policy-and-research/rx_abuse_plan.pdf

Pravetoni, M. (2016). Biologics to treat substance use disorders: Current status and new directions. *Hum Vaccin Immunother, 12*(12), 3005–3019. doi:10.1080/21645515.2016.1212785

See, S., & Ginzburg, R. (2008). Skeletal muscle relaxants. *Pharmacotherapy, 28*, 207–213.

Sindrup, S. H., Otto, M., Finnerup, N. B., & Jensen, T. S. (2005). Antidepressants in the treatment of neuropathic pain. *Basic Clin Pharmacol Toxicol, 96*(6), 399–409. doi:10.1111/j.1742-7843.2005.pto_96696601.x

Whiting, P. F., Wolff, R. F., Deshpande, S., Di Nisio, M., Duffy, S., Hernandez, A. V., . . . & Kleijnen, J. (2015). Cannabinoids for medical use: A systematic review and meta-analysis. *JAMA, 313*(24), 2456–2473. doi:10.1001/jama.2015.6358

Williams, B.S., & Christo, P.J. (2011). Antipyretic Analgesics: Nonsteroidals, acetaminophen and phenazone derivatives. In L. Manchikanti, P. J. Christo, A. Trescot A, & F. J. E. Falco (Eds.). *Foundations of pain medicine and interventional pain management: A comprehensive review.* Paducah, KY: American Society of Interventional Pain Physicians.

## Chapter 15

Berthoud, H. R., & Neuhuber. W. L. (2000). Functional and chemical anatomy of the afferent vagal system. *Auton Neurosci, 85*(1-3), 1–17. doi: 10.1016/S1566-0702(00)00215-0

Bottros, M. M., & Christo, P. J. (2014). Current perspectives on intrathecal drug delivery. *J Pain Res, 7,* 615–626. doi:10.2147/JPR.S37591

The British Pain Society. (2013, June 15). *Spinal cord stimulation for the management of pain: Recommendations for best clinical practice.* Retrieved from http://www.britishpainsociety.org/book_scs_main

Chakravarthy, K., Nava, A., Christo, P. J., & Williams, K. (2016). Review of recent advances in peripheral nerve stimulation (PNS). *Curr Pain Headache Rep, 20*(11), 60. doi:10.1007/s11916-016-0590-8

Chakravarthy, K., Chen, Y., He, C., & Christo, P. J. (2017). Stem cell therapy for chronic pain management: Review of uses, advances, and adverse effects. *Pain Physician, 20,* 293–305.

Cruccu, G., Garcia-Larrea, L., Hansson, P., Keindl, M., Lefaucheur, J. P., Paulus, W., . . . & Attal, N. (2016). EAN guidelines on central neurostimulation therapy in chronic pain conditions. *Eur J Neurol, 23*(10), 1489–1499. doi:10.1111/ene.13103

Deer, T. R., Krames, E., Mekhail, N., Pope, J., Leong, M., Stanton-Hicks, M., . . . & Golovac, S. (2014). The appropriate use of neurostimulation: new and evolving neurostimulation therapies and applicable treatment for chronic pain and selected disease states. Neuromodulation Appropriateness Consensus Committee. *Neuromodulation, 17*(6), 599–615; discussion 615. Neuromodulation Appropriateness Consensus Committee. doi:10.1111/ner.12204

Deer, T. R., Mekhail, N., Provenzano, D., Pope, J., Krames, E., Leong, M., . . . & Levy, R. M. (2014). The appropriate use of neurostimulation of the spinal cord and peripheral nervous system for the treatment of chronic pain and ischemic diseases. The Neuromodulation Appropriateness Consensus Committee. *Neuromodulation, 17*(6), 515–550; discussion 550. doi:10.1111/ner.12208

Deer, T. R., Prager, J., Levy, R., Rathmell, J., Buchser, E., Burton, A., . . . & Mekhail, N. (2012). Recommendations for the management of pain by intrathecal (intraspinal) drug delivery: Report of an interdisciplinary expert panel. Polyanalgesic Consensus Conference 2012. *Neuromodulation, 15*(5), 436–464; discussion 464-436. doi:10.1111/j.1525-1403.2012.00476.x

Dowell, D., Haegerich, T. M., & Chou, R. (2016). CDC guideline for prescribing opioids for chronic pain—United States, 2016. *Jama, 315*(15), 1624–1645.

Dubinsky, R. M., & Miyasaki, J. (2010). Assessment: Efficacy of transcutaneous electric nerve stimulation in the treatment of pain in neurologic disorders (an evidence-based review). Therapeutics and Technology Assessment Subcommittee of the American Academy of Neurology. *Neurology, 74*(2), 173–176. doi:10.1212/WNL.0b013e3181c918fc

Ellrich, J. (2011). Transcutaneous vagus nerve stimulation. *Eur Neurol Rev, 6*(4), 254–256.

Froholdt, A., Reikeraas, O., Holm, I., Keller, A., & Brox, J. I. (2012). No difference in 9-year outcome in CLBP patients randomized to lumbar fusion versus cognitive intervention and exercises. *Eur Spine J, 21*(12), 2531–2538. doi:10.1007/s00586-012-2382-0

Guan, Y. (2012). Spinal cord stimulation: neurophysiological and neurochemical mechanisms of action. *Curr Pain Headache Rep, 16*(3), 217–225. doi:10.1007/s11916-012-0260-4

Hayek, S. M., Deer, T. R., Pope, J. E., Panchal, S. J., & Patel, V. B. (2011). Intrathecal therapy for cancer and non-cancer pain. *Pain Physician, 14*(3), 219–248.

Kumar, K., Hunter, G., & Demeria, D. D. (2002). Treatment of chronic pain by using intrathecal drug therapy compared with conventional pain therapies: a cost-effectiveness analysis. *J Neurosurg, 97*(4), 803–810. doi:10.3171/jns.2002.97.4.0803

Kumar, K., Malik, S., & Demeria, D. (2002). Treatment of chronic pain with spinal cord stimulation versus alternative therapies: cost-effectiveness analysis. *Neurosurgery, 51*(1), 106–116.

Kumar, K., Rizvi, S., & Bishop, S. (2013). Cost effectiveness of intrathecal drug therapy in management of chronic nonmalignant pain. *Clin J Pain, 29*(2), 138–145. doi:10.1097/AJP.0b013e31824b5fc9

Kumar, K., Rizvi, S., Nguyen, R., Abbas, M., Bishop, S., & Murthy, V. (2014). Impact of wait times on spinal cord stimulation therapy outcomes. *Pain Pract, 14*(8), 709–720. doi:10.1111/papr.12126

Lange, G. Janal, M. N. Maniker, A., Fitzgibbons, J. Fobler, M. Cook, D., & Natelson, B. H. (2011). Safety and efficacy of vagus nerve stimulation in fibromyalgia: A phase I/II proof of concept trial. *Pain Med, 12*(9), 1406–1413. doi:10.1111/j.1526-4637.2011.01203.x

Liem, L., Russo, M., Huygen, F. J., Van Buyten, J. P., Smet, I., Verrills, P., . . . & Kramer, J. (2013). A multicenter, prospective trial to assess the safety and performance of the spinal modulation dorsal root ganglion neurostimulator system in the treatment of chronic pain. *Neuromodulation, 16*(5), 471–482; discussion 482. doi:10.1111/ner.12072

Nnoaham, K. E., & Kumbang, J. (2008). Transcutaneous electrical nerve stimulation (TENS) for chronic pain. *Cochrane Database Syst Rev* (3), CD003222. doi:10.1002/14651858.CD003222.pub2

Pain management devices market by device type (neurostimulation, SCS, TENS, RF ablation, infusion pumps), application (cancer, neuropathy, musculoskeletal, migraine, facial), by mode of purchase (OTC, prescription-based)–Global Forecast to 2020.

Poitras, S., & Brosseau, L. (2008). Evidence-informed management of chronic low back pain with transcutaneous electrical nerve stimulation, interferential current, electrical muscle stimulation, ultrasound, and thermotherapy. *Spine J, 8*(1), 226–233. doi:10.1016/j.spinee.2007.10.022

Poree, L., Krames, E., Pope, J., Deer, T. R., Levy, R., & Schultz, L. (2013). Spinal cord stimulation as treatment for complex regional pain syndrome should be considered earlier than last resort therapy. *Neuromodulation, 16*(2), 125–141. doi:10.1111/ner.12035

Rizvi, S., & Kumar, K. (2015). History and present state of targeted intrathecal drug delivery. *Curr Pain Headache Rep, 19*(2), 474. doi:10.1007/s11916-014-0474-8

Simpson, E. L., Duenas, A., Holmes, M. W., Papaioannou, D., & Chilcott, J. (2009). Spinal cord stimulation for chronic pain of neuropathic or ischaemic origin: Systematic review and economic evaluation. *Health Technol Assess, 13*(17), iii, ix–x, 1–154. doi:10.3310/hta13170

Stadler, J. A., Ellens, D. J., & Rosenow, J. M. (2011). Deep brain stimulation and motor cortical stimulation for neuropathic pain. *Curr Pain Headache Rep, 15*(1), 8–13. doi:10.1007/s11916-010-0161-3

Sukul, V. V., & Slavin, K. V. (2014). Deep brain and motor cortex stimulation. *Curr Pain Headache Rep, 18*(7), 427. doi:10.1007/s11916-014-0427-2

Welberg, L. (2012). Techniques: Optogenetic control in monkey brains. *Nature Reviews Neuroscience, 13*(9).

## Chapter 16

Bashir, J., Panero, A. J., & Sherman, A. L. (2015). The emerging use of platelet-rich plasma in musculoskeletal medicine. *J Am Osteopath Assoc, 115*(1), 24–31. doi:10.7556/jaoa.2015.004

Chakravarthy, K., Chaudhry, H., Williams, K., & Christo, P. J. (2015). Review of the uses of vagal nerve stimulation in chronic pain management. *Curr Pain Headache Rep, 19*(12), 54. doi:10.1007/s11916-015-0528-6

Chiew, S. K., Ramasamy, T. S., & Amini, F. (2016). Effectiveness and relevant factors of platelet-rich plasma treatment in managing plantar fasciitis: A systematic review. *J Res Med Sci, 21*, 38. doi:10.4103/1735-1995.183988

Correa, D., & Lietman, S. A. (2017). Articular cartilage repair: Current needs, methods and research directions. *Semin Cell Dev Biol, 62*, 67–77. doi:10.1016/j.semcdb.2016.07.013

Cui, G. H., Wang, Y. Y., Li, C. J., Shi, C. H., & Wang, W. S. (2016). Efficacy of mesenchymal stem cells in treating patients with osteoarthritis of the knee: A meta-analysis. *Exp Ther Med, 12*(5), 3390–3400. doi:10.3892/etm.2016.3791

Engebretsen, L., Steffen, K., Alsousou, J., Anitua, E., Bachl, N., Devilee, R., . . . & Verrall, G. (2010). IOC consensus paper on the use of platelet-rich plasma in sports medicine. *Br J Sports Med, 44*(15), 1072–1081. doi:10.1136/bjsm.2010.079822

Fernandez-Moure, J. S., Van Eps, J. L., Cabrera, F. J., Barbosa, Z., Medrano Del Rosal, G., Weiner, B. K., . . . & Tasciotti, E. (2017). Platelet-rich plasma: A biomimetic approach to enhancement of surgical wound healing. *J Surg Res, 207*, 33–44. doi:10.1016/j.jss.2016.08.063

Fitzpatrick, J., Bulsara, M., & Zheng, M. H. (2016). Effectiveness of platelet-rich plasma in the treatment of tendinopathy: Response. *Am J Sports Med, 44*(10), NP55–NP56. doi:10.1177/0363546516669322

Franchi, S., Castelli, M., Amodeo, G., Niada, S., Ferrari, D., Vescovi, A., . . . & Sacerdote, P. (2014). Adult stem cell as new advanced therapy for experimental neuropathic pain treatment. *Biomed Res Int, 2014*, 470983. doi:10.1155/2014/470983

Franz, C. K., Singh, B., Martinez, J. A., Zochodne, D. W., Midha, R. (2012). Brief transvertebral electrical stiumulation of the spinal cord improves the specificity of femoral nerve. *Biomed Res Int, 2014*, 470983. doi:10.1155/2014/470983

Freitag, J., Bates, D., Boyd, R., Shah, K., Barnard, A., Huguenin, L., & Tenen, A. (2016). Mesenchymal stem cell therapy in the treatment of osteoarthritis: Reparative pathways, safety and efficacy—a review. *BMC Musculoskelet Disord, 17*, 230. doi:10.1186/s12891-016-1085-9

Hauser, R. A., Lackner, J. B., Steilen-Matias, D., & Harris, D. K. (2016). A systematic review of dextrose prolotherapy for chronic musculoskeletal pain. *Clin Med Insights Arthritis Musculoskelet Disord, 9*, 139–159. doi:10.4137/CMAMD.S39160

Kim, A., Shin, D. M., & Choo, M. S. (2016). Stem cell therapy for interstitial cystitis/bladder pain syndrome. *Curr Urol Rep, 17*(1), 1. doi:10.1007/s11934-015-0563-1

Knezevic, N. N., Candido, K. D., Desai, R., & Kaye, A. D. (2016). Is platelet-rich plasma a future therapy in pain management? *Med Clin North Am, 100*(1), 199–217. doi:10.1016/j.mcna.2015.08.014

Knoepfler, P. S. (2015). From bench to FDA to bedside: U.S. regulatory trends for new stem cell therapies. *Adv Drug Deliv Rev, 82-83*, 192–196. doi:10.1016/j.addr.2014.12.001

Knoepfler, P. S. (2017). The stem cell hard sell: Report from a clinic's patient recruitment seminar. *Stem Cells Transl Med, 6*(1), 14–16. doi:10.5966/sctm.2016-0208

Kuffler, D. P. (2015). Platelet-rich plasma promotes axon regeneration, wound healing, and pain reduction: Fact or fiction. *Mol Neurobiol, 52*(2), 990–1014. doi:10.1007/s12035-015-9251-x

Meheux, C. J., McCulloch, P. C., Lintner, D. M., Varner, K. E., & Harris, J. D. (2016). Efficacy of intra-articular platelet-rich plasma injections in knee osteoarthritis: A systematic review. *Arthroscopy, 32*(3), 495–505. doi:10.1016/j.arthro.2015.08.005

Melrose, J. (2016). Strategies in regenerative medicine for intervertebral disc repair using mesenchymal stem cells and bioscaffolds. *Regen Med, 11*(7), 705–724. doi:10.2217/rme-2016-0069

Moriguchi, Y., Alimi, M., Khair, T., Manolarakis, G., Berlin, C., Bonassar, L. J., & Härtl, R. (2016). Biological treatment approaches for degenerative disk disease: A literature review of in vivo animal and clinical data. *Global Spine J, 6*(5), 497–518. doi:10.1055/s-0036-1571955

Osborne, H., Anderson, L., Burt, P., Young, M., & Gerrard, D. (2016). Australasian College of Sports Physicians-position statement: The place of mesenchymal stem/stromal cell therapies in sport and exercise medicine. *Br J Sports Med, 50*(20), 1237–1244. doi:10.1136/bjsports-2015-095711

Rabago, D., Patterson, J. J., Mundt, M., Kijowski, R., Grettie, J., Segal, N. A., & Zgierska, A. (2013). Dextrose prolotherapy for knee osteoarthritis: A randomized controlled trial. *Ann Fam Med, 11*(3), 229–237. doi:10.1370/afm.1504

Reeves, K. D., Sit, R. W., & Rabago, D. P. (2016). Dextrose prolotherapy: A narrative review of basic science, Clinical research, and best treatment recommendations. *Phys Med Rehabil Clin N Am, 27*(4), 783–823. doi:10.1016/j.pmr.2016.06.001

Richardson, S. M., Kalamegam, G., Pushparaj, P. N., Matta, C., Memic, A., Khademhosseini, A., . . . & Mobasheri, A. (2016). Mesenchymal stem cells in regenerative medicine: Focus on articular cartilage and intervertebral disc regeneration. *Methods, 99*, 69–80. doi:10.1016/j.ymeth.2015.09.015

Sánchez, M., Anitua, E., Delgado, D., Sanchez, P., Prado, R., Orive, G., & Padilla, S. (2017). Platelet-rich plasma, a source of autologous growth factors and biomimetic scaffold for peripheral nerve regeneration. *Expert Opin Biol Ther, 17*(2), 197–212. doi:10.1080/14712598.2017.1259409

Turner, L. (2015). U.S. stem cell clinics, patient safety, and the FDA. *Trends Mol Med, 21*(5), 271–273. doi:10.1016/j.molmed.2015.02.008

Vickers, E. R., Karsten, E., Flood, J., & Lilischkis, R. (2014). A preliminary report on stem cell therapy for neuropathic pain in humans. *J Pain Res, 7*, 255–263. doi:10.2147/JPR.S63361

Wu, T., Song, H. X., Dong, Y., & Li, J. H. (2016). Cell-based therapies for lumbar discogenic low back pain: Systematic review and single arm meta-analysis. *Spine (Phila Pa 1976)* . doi:10.1097/BRS.0000000000001549

Yu, H., Fischer, G., Ebert, A. D., Wu, H. E., Bai, X., & Hogan, Q. H. (2015). Analgesia for neuropathic pain by dorsal root ganglion transplantation of genetically engineered mesenchymal stem cells: Initial results. *Mol Pain, 11*, 5. doi:10.1186/s12990-015-0002-9

Zeckser, J., Wolff, M., Tucker, J., & Goodwin, J. (2016). Multipotent mesenchymal stem cell treatment for discogenic low back pain and disc degeneration. *Stem Cells Int, 2016*, 3908389. doi:10.1155/2016/3908389

Zochodne, D. W. (2012). The challenges and beauty of peripheral nerve regrowth. 2011 Peripheral Nerve Society Meeting Presidential Lecture. *Journal of the Peripheral Nervous System 17*, 1–18.

Zochodne, D. W. (2012). Reversing neuropathic deficits. *Journal of the Peripheral Nervous System17*, supplement, 4–9.

## Chapter 17

Baena-Beato, P. A., Arroyo-Morales, M., Delgado-Fernández, M., Gatto-Cardia, M. C., & Artero, E. G. (2013). Effects of different frequencies (2–3 days/week) of aquatic therapy program in adults with chronic low back pain. A non-randomized comparison trial. *Pain Med, 14*(1), 145–158. doi:10.1111/pme.12022

Brady, S. R., Mamuaya, B. B., Cicuttini, F., Wluka, A. E., Wang, Y., Hussain, S. M., & Urquhart, D. M. (2015). Body composition is associated with multisite lower body musculoskeletal pain in a community-based study. *J Pain, 16*(8), 700–706. doi:10.1016/j.jpain.2015.04.006

Briggs, M. S., Givens, D. L., Schmitt, L. C., & Taylor, C. A. (2013). Relations of C-reactive protein and obesity to the prevalence and the odds of reporting low back pain. *Arch Phys Med Rehabil, 94*(4), 745–752. doi:10.1016/j.apmr.2012.11.026

Choi, J., Joseph, L., & Pilote, L. (2013). Obesity and C-reactive protein in various populations: A systematic review and meta-analysis. *Obes Rev, 14*(3), 232–244. doi:10.1111/obr.12003

Ford, E. S., Li, C., Pearson, W. S., Zhao, G., Strine, T. W., & Mokdad, A. H. (2008). Body mass index and headaches: Findings from a national sample of U.S. adults. *Cephalalgia, 28*(12), 1270–1276. doi:10.1111/j.1468-2982.2008.01671.x

Frilander, H., Solovieva, S., Mutanen, P., Pihlajamäki, H., Heliövaara, M., & Viikari-Juntura, E. (2015). Role of overweight and obesity in low back disorders among men: A longitudinal study with a life course approach. *BMJ Open, 5*(8), e007805. doi:10.1136/bmjopen-2015-007805

Geneen, L. J., Moore, R. A., Clarke, C., Martin, D., Colvin, L. A., & Smith, B. H. (2017). Physical activity and exercise for chronic pain in adults: An overview of Cochrane reviews. *Cochrane Database Syst Rev, 1,* CD011279. doi:10.1002/14651858.CD011279.pub2

Guh, D. P., Zhang, W., Bansback, N., Amarsi, Z., Birmingham, C. L., & Anis, A. H. (2009). The incidence of co-morbidities related to obesity and overweight: A systematic review and meta-analysis. *BMC Public Health, 9,* 88. doi:10.1186/1471-2458-9-88

Hagen, K. B., Jamtvedt, G., Hilde, G., & Winnem, M. F. (2005). The updated Cochrane review of bed rest for low back pain and sciatica. *Spine (Phila Pa 1976), 30*(5), 542–546.

Heffner, K. L., France, C. R., Trost, Z., Ng, H. M., & Pigeon, W. R. (2011). Chronic low back pain, sleep disturbance, and interleukin-6. *Clin J Pain, 27*(1), 35–41.

Hitt, H. C., McMillen, R. C., Thornton-Neaves, T., Koch, K., & Cosby, A. G. (2007). Comorbidity of obesity and pain in a general population: Results from the Southern Pain Prevalence Study. *J Pain, 8*(5), 430–436. doi:10.1016/j.jpain.2006.12.003

Janke, E. A., Collins, A., & Kozak, A. T. (2007). Overview of the relationship between pain and obesity: What do we know? Where do we go next? *J Rehabil Res Dev, 44*(2), 245–262.

Jentzsch, T., Geiger, J., Slankamenac, K., & Werner, C. M. (2015). Obesity measured by outer abdominal fat may cause facet joint arthritis at the lumbar spine. *J Back Musculoskelet Rehabil, 28*(1), 85–91. doi:10.3233/BMR-140495

Jinks, C., Jordan, K., & Croft, P. (2006). Disabling knee pain—another consequence of obesity: Results from a prospective cohort study. *BMC Public Health, 6,* 258. doi:10.1186/1471-2458-6-258

Kayo, A. H., Peccin, M. S., Sanches, C. M., & Trevisani, V. F. (2012). Effectiveness of physical activity in reducing pain in patients with fibromyalgia: A blinded randomized clinical trial. *Rheumatol Int, 32*(8), 2285–2292. doi:10.1007/s00296-011-1958-z

Koltyn, K. F. (2000). Analgesia following exercise: A review. *Sports Med, 29*(2), 85–98.

Li, S., & Micheletti, R. (2011). Role of diet in rheumatic disease. *Rheum Dis Clin North Am, 37*(1), 119–133. doi:10.1016/j.rdc.2010.11.006

Liddle, S. D., Baxter, G. D., & Gracey, J. H. (2004). Exercise and chronic low back pain: What works? *Pain, 107*(1–2), 176–190.

Messier, S. P., Loeser, R. F., Miller, G. D., Morgan, T. M., Rejeski, W. J., Sevick, M. A., . . . & Williamson, J. D. (2004). Exercise and dietary weight loss in overweight and obese older adults with knee osteoarthritis: The arthritis, diet, and activity promotion trial. *Arthritis Rheum, 50*(5), 1501–1510. doi:10.1002/art.20256

Murtezani, A., Hundozi, H., Orovcanec, N., Sllamniku, S., & Osmani, T. (2011). A comparison of high intensity aerobic exercise and passive modalities for the treatment of workers with chronic low back pain: A randomized, controlled trial. *Eur J Phys Rehabil Med, 47*(3), 359–366.

Paley, C. A., & Johnson, M. I. (2016). Physical activity to reduce systemic inflammation associated with chronic pain and obesity: A narrative review. *Clin J Pain, 32*(4), 365–370. doi:10.1097/AJP.0000000000000258

Pisters, M. F., Veenhof, C., Schellevis, F. G., Twisk, J. W., Dekker, J., & De Bakker, D. H. (2010). Exercise adherence improving long-term patient outcome in patients with osteoarthritis of the hip and/or knee. *Arthritis Care Res (Hoboken), 62*(8), 1087–1094. doi:10.1002/acr.20182

Roffey, D. M., Ashdown, L. C., Dornan, H. D., Creech, M. J., Dagenais, S., Dent, R. M., & Wai, E. K. (2011). Pilot evaluation of a multidisciplinary, medically supervised, nonsurgical weight loss program on the severity of low back pain in obese adults. *Spine J, 11*(3), 197–204. doi:10.1016/j.spinee.2011.01.031

Sullivan, A. B., Scheman, J., Venesy, D., & Davin, S. (2012). The role of exercise and types of exercise in the rehabilitation of chronic pain: Specific or nonspecific benefits. *Curr Pain Headache Rep, 16*(2), 153–161. doi:10.1007/s11916-012-0245-3

Vandenkerkhof, E. G., Macdonald, H. M., Jones, G. T., Power, C., & Macfarlane, G. J. (2011). Diet, lifestyle and chronic widespread pain: Results from the 1958 British birth cohort study. *Pain Res Manag, 16*(2), 87–92.

Vincent, H. K., Heywood, K., Connelly, J., & Hurley, R. W. (2012). Obesity and weight loss in the treatment and prevention of osteoarthritis. *PM R, 4*(5 Suppl), S59–67. doi:10.1016/j.pmrj.2012.01.005

Van Middwekoop M, Rubinstein SM, Verhagen AP, Ostelo RW, Koes BW, van Tulder MW. Exercise therapy for chronic nonspecific low back pain. *Arch physMed Rehabil.* Mar 2013;94(3), 536–542.

Waller, B., Lambeck, J., & Daly, D. (2009). Therapeutic aquatic exercise in the treatment of low back pain: A systematic review. *Clin Rehabil, 23*(1), 3–14. doi:10.1177/0269215508097856

Weil, A. Dr. Weil's anti-inflammatory diet. Retrieved from http://www .drweil.com/drw/u/ART02012/anti-inflammatory-diet

Zdziarski, L. A., Wasser, J. G., & Vincent, H. K. (2015). Chronic pain management in the obese patient: A focused review of key challenges and potential exercise solutions. *J Pain Res, 8,* 63–77. doi:10.2147/JPR.S55360

# Chapter 18

Bernal, M., Haro, J. M., Bernert, S., Brugha, T., de Graaf, R., Bruffaerts, R., . . . & ESEMED/MHEDEA Investigators. (2007). Risk factors for suicidality in Europe: Results from the ESEMED study. *J Affect Disord, 101*(1-3), 27–34. doi:10.1016/j.jad.2006.09.018

Bongers, P. M., Ijmker, S., van den Heuvel, S., & Blatter, B. M. (2006). Epidemiology of work related neck and upper limb problems: Psychosocial and personal risk factors (part I) and effective interventions from a bio behavioural perspective (part II). *J Occup Rehabil, 16*(3), 279–302. doi:10.1007/s10926-006-9044-1

Carskadon, M. A., & Dement, W. C. (2005). Normal human sleep: An overview. *Principles and practice of sleep medicine, 4,* 13–23.

Chapman, C. R., Tuckett, R. P., & Song, C. W. (2008). Pain and stress in a systems perspective: Reciprocal neural, endocrine, and immune interactions. *J Pain, 9*(2), 122–145. doi:10.1016/j.jpain.2007.09.006

Correa, D., Farney, R. J., Chung, F., Prasad, A., Lam, D., & Wong, J. (2015). Chronic opioid use and central sleep apnea: A review of the prevalence, mechanisms, and perioperative considerations. *Anesth Analg, 120*(6), 1273–1285. doi:10.1213/ANE.0000000000000672

Devins, G. M., Edworthy, S. M., Paul, L. C., Mandin, H., Seland, T. P., Klein, G., . . . Shapiro, C. M. (1993). Restless sleep, illness intrusiveness, and depressive symptoms in three chronic illness conditions: Rheumatoid arthritis, end-stage renal disease, and multiple sclerosis. *J Psychosom Res, 37*(2), 163–170.

Diatchenko, L., Slade, G. D., Nackley, A. G., Bhalang, K., Sigurdsson, A., Belfer, I., . . . & Maixner, W. (2005). Genetic basis for individual variations in pain perception and the development of a chronic pain condition. *Hum Mol Genet, 14*(1), 135–143. doi:10.1093/hmg/ddi013

Fishbain, D. A. (1999). Approaches to treatment decisions for psychiatric comorbidity in the management of the chronic pain patient. *Med Clin North Am, 83*(3), 737–760, vii.

Foley, D., Ancoli-Israel, S., Britz, P., & Walsh, J. (2004). Sleep disturbances and chronic disease in older adults: Results of the 2003 National Sleep Foundation Sleep in America survey. *J Psychosom Res, 56*(5), 497–502. doi:10.1016/j.jpsychores.2004.02.010

Keefe, F. J., Rumble, M. E., Scipio, C. D., Giordano, L. A., & Perri, L. M. (2004). Psychological aspects of persistent pain: Current state of the science. *J Pain, 5*(4), 195–211. doi:10.1016/j.jpain.2004.02.004

Kripke, D. F., Langer, R. D., & Kline, L. E. (2012). Hypnotics' association with mortality or cancer: A matched cohort study. *BMJ Open, 2*(1), e000850. doi:10.1136/bmjopen-2012-000850

McCain, G. A. Fibromyalgia and myofascial pain syndromes. (1994). In P. D. Wall & R. Melzack (Eds.), *Textbook of Pain* (3rd ed.) (475–493). London: Churchill Livingstone.

McDonald, D. D. (1999). Postoperative pain after hospital discharge. *Clin Nurs Res, 8*(4), 355–367. doi:10.1177/105477389900800405

Menefee, L. A., Cohen, M. J., Anderson, W. R., Doghramji, K., Frank, E. D., & Lee, H. (2000). Sleep disturbance and nonmalignant chronic pain: A comprehensive review of the literature. *Pain Med, 1*(2), 156–172. doi:10.1046/j.1526-4637.2000.00022.x

Miaskowski, C., & Lee, K. A. (1999). Pain, fatigue, and sleep disturbances in oncology outpatients receiving radiation therapy for bone metastasis: A pilot study. *J Pain Symptom Manage, 17*(5), 320–332.

Miranda, C., Selleri, S., Pierotti, M. A., & Greco, A. (2002). The M581V mutation, associated with a mild form of congenital insensitivity to pain with anhidrosis, causes partial inactivation of the NTRK1 receptor. *J Invest Dermatol, 119*(4), 978–979. doi:10.1046/j.1523-1747.2002.00140.x

Möller, H. J. (2003). Suicide, suicidality and suicide prevention in affective disorders. *Acta Psychiatr Scand Suppl* (418), 73–80.

Onen, S. H., Alloui, A., Gross, A., Eschallier, A., & Dubray, C. (2001). The effects of total sleep deprivation, selective sleep interruption and sleep recovery on pain tolerance thresholds in healthy subjects. *J Sleep Res, 10*(1), 35–42.

Onen, S. H., Onen, F., Courpron, P., & Dubray, C. (2005). How pain and analgesics disturb sleep. *Clin J Pain, 21*(5), 422–431.

Rasmussen, B. K. (1993). Migraine and tension-type headache in a general population: Precipitating factors, female hormones, sleep pattern and relation to lifestyle. *Pain, 53*(1), 65–72.

Raymond, I., Nielsen, T. A., Lavigne, G., Manzini, C., & Choinière, M. (2001). Quality of sleep and its daily relationship to pain intensity in hospitalized adult burn patients. *Pain, 92*(3), 381–388.

Selye, H. (1998). A syndrome produced by diverse nocuous agents. 1936. *J Neuropsychiatry Clin Neurosci, 10*(2), 230–231. doi:10.1176/jnp.10.2.230a

Smith, M. T., Edwards, R. R., McCann, U. D., & Haythornthwaite, J. A. (2007). The effects of sleep deprivation on pain inhibition and spontaneous pain in women. *Sleep, 30*(4), 494–505.

Stephenson, J. L., Christou, E. A., & Maluf, K. S. (2011). Discharge rate modulation of trapezius motor units differs for voluntary contractions and instructed muscle rest. *Exp Brain Res, 208*(2), 203–215. doi:10.1007/s00221-010-2471-4

Tang, N. K., & Crane, C. (2006). Suicidality in chronic pain: A review of the prevalence, risk factors and psychological links. *Psychol Med, 36*(5), 575–586. doi:10.1017/S0033291705006859

Tracey, K. J. (2002). The inflammatory reflex. *Nature, 420*(6917), 853–859.

Tsigos, C., & Chrousos, G. P. (2002). Hypothalamic-pituitary-adrenal axis, neuroendocrine factors and stress. *J Psychosom Res, 53*(4), 865–871.

Turk, D. C. (2002). A diathesis-stress model of chronic pain and disability following traumatic injury. *Pain Res Manag, 7*(1), 9–19.

Vaccarino, V., Shah, A. J., Rooks, C., Ibeanu, I., Nye, J. A., Pimple, P., . . . Raggi, P. (2014). Sex differences in mental stress-induced myocardial ischemia in young survivors of an acute myocardial infarction. *Psychosom Med, 76*(3), 171–180. doi:10.1097/PSY.0000000000000045

Vizi, E. S., & Elenkov, I. J. (2002). Nonsynaptic noradrenaline release in neuro-immune responses. *Acta Biol Hung, 53*(1-2), 229–244. doi:10.1556/ABiol.53.2002.1-2.21

## Chapter 19

Adachi, T., Fujino, H., Nakae, A., Mashimo, T., & Sasaki, J. (2014). A meta-analysis of hypnosis for chronic pain problems: A comparison between hypnosis, standard care, and other psychological interventions. *Int J Clin Exp Hypn, 62*(1), 1–28. doi:10.1080/00207144.2013.841471

Astin, J. A., Beckner, W., Soeken, K., Hochberg, M. C., & Berman, B. (2002). Psychological interventions for rheumatoid arthritis: A meta-analysis of randomized controlled trials. *Arthritis Rheum, 47*(3), 291–302. doi:10.1002/art.10416

Berry, M. E., Chapple, I. T., Ginsberg, J. P., Gleichauf, K. J., Meyer, J. A., & Nagpal, M. L. (2014). Non-pharmacological intervention for chronic pain in veterans: A pilot study of heart rate variability biofeedback. *Glob Adv Health Med, 3*(2), 28–33. doi:10.7453/gahmj.2013.075

Colón, Y., & Avnet, M. S. (2014). Medical hypnotherapy for pain management. *J Pain Palliat Care Pharmacother, 28*(2), 174–176. doi:10.3109/15360288.2014.911792

De Benedittis, G. (2015). Neural mechanisms of hypnosis and meditation. *J Physiol Paris, 109*(4-6), 152–164. doi:10.1016/j.jphysparis.2015.11.001

deCharms, R. C., Maeda, F., Glover, G. H., Ludlow, D., Pauly, J. M., Soneji, D., . . . & Mackey, S. C. (2005). Control over brain activation and pain learned by using real-time functional MRI. *Proc Natl Acad Sci USA, 102*(51), 18626–18631. doi:10.1073/pnas.0505210102

Ehde, D. M., Dillworth, T. M., & Turner, J. A. (2014). Cognitive-behavioral therapy for individuals with chronic pain: Efficacy, innovations, and directions for research. *Am Psychol, 69*(2), 153–166. doi:10.1037/a0035747

Elkins, G., Jensen, M. P., & Patterson, D. R. (2007). Hypnotherapy for the management of chronic pain. *Int J Clin Exp Hypn, 55*(3), 275–287. doi:10.1080/00207140701338621

Facco, E. (2016). Hypnosis and anesthesia: Back to the future. *Minerva Anestesiol, 82*(12), 1343–1356.

Glombiewski, J. A., Bernardy, K., & Häuser, W. (2013). Efficacy of EMG- and EEG-biofeedback in fibromyalgia syndrome: A meta-analysis and a systematic review of randomized controlled trials. *Evid Based Complement Alternat Med, 2013*, 962741. doi:10.1155/2013/962741

Gracely, R. H., Geisser, M. E., Giesecke, T., Grant, M. A., Petzke, F., Williams, D. A., & Clauw, D. J. (2004). Pain catastrophizing and neural responses to pain among persons with fibromyalgia. *Brain, 127*(Pt 4), 835–843. doi:10.1093/brain/awh098

Guillory, J., Chang, P., Henderson, C. R., Shengelia, R., Lama, S., Warmington, M., . . . & Reid, M. C. (2015). Piloting a text message-based social support intervention for patients with chronic pain: Establishing feasibility and preliminary efficacy. *Clin J Pain, 31*(6), 548–556. doi:10.1097/AJP.0000000000000193

Hassett, A. L., Radvanski, D. C., Vaschillo, E. G., Vaschillo, B., Sigal, L. H., Karavidas, M. K., . . . & Lehrer, P. M. (2007). A pilot study of the efficacy of heart rate variability (HRV) biofeedback in patients with fibromyalgia. *Appl Psychophysiol Biofeedback, 32*(1), 1–10. doi:10.1007/s10484-006-9028-0

Jensen, M. P., & Patterson, D. R. (2014). Hypnotic approaches for chronic pain management: Clinical implications of recent research findings. *Am Psychol, 69*(2), 167–177. doi:10.1037/a0035644

Jensen, M. P., & Turk, D. C. (2014). Contributions of psychology to the understanding and treatment of people with chronic pain: Why it matters to ALL psychologists. *Am Psychol, 69*(2), 105–118. doi:10.1037/a0035641

Kaiser, R. S., Mooreville, M., & Kannan, K. (2015). Psychological interventions for the management of chronic pain: A review of current evidence. *Curr Pain Headache Rep, 19*(9), 43. doi:10.1007/s11916-015-0517-9

MacKinnon, S., Gevirtz, R., McCraty, R., & Brown, M. (2013). Utilizing heartbeat evoked potentials to identify cardiac regulation of vagal afferents during emotion and resonant breathing. *Appl Psychophysiol Biofeedback, 38*(4), 241–255. doi:10.1007/s10484-013-9226-5

Nestoriuc, Y., & Martin, A. (2007). Efficacy of biofeedback for migraine: A meta-analysis. *Pain, 128*(1-2), 111–127. doi:10.1016/j.pain.2006.09.007

Nestoriuc, Y., Rief, W., & Martin, A. (2008). Meta-analysis of biofeedback for tension-type headache: Efficacy, specificity, and treatment moderators. *J Consult Clin Psychol, 76*(3), 379–396. doi:10.1037/0022-006X.76.3.379

Nevedal, D. C., Wang, C., Oberleitner, L., Schwartz, S., & Williams, A. M. (2013). Effects of an individually tailored web-based chronic pain management program on pain severity, psychological health, and functioning. *J Med Internet Res, 15*(9), e201. doi:10.2196/jmir.2296

Sielski, R., Rief, W., & Glombiewski, J. A. (2017). Efficacy of biofeedback in chronic back pain: A meta-analysis. *Int J Behav Med, 24*(1), 25–41. doi:10.1007/s12529-016-9572-9

Thomas, D. A., Maslin, B., Legler, A., Springer, E., Asgerally, A., & Vadivelu, N. (2016). Role of alternative therapies for chronic pain syndromes. *Curr Pain Headache Rep, 20*(5), 29. doi:10.1007/s11916-016-0562-z

## Chapter 20

Andersson, S., Sundberg, T., Johansson, E., & Falkenberg, T. (2012). Patients' experiences and perceptions of integrative care for back and neck pain. *Altern Ther Health Med, 18*(3), 25–32.

Barnes, P. M., & Nahin, R.L. (2015). Trends in the use of complementary health approaches among adults: United States, 2002–2012. Retrieved from http:/ www.cdc.gov/nchs/data/nhsr/nhsr079.pdf

Bruckenthal, P., Marino, M. A., & Snelling, L. (2016). Complementary and integrative therapies for persistent pain management in older adults: A review. *J Gerontol Nurs, 42*(12), 40–48. doi:10.3928/00989134-20161110-08

Chrubasik, S., Eisenberg, E., Balan, E., Weinberger, T., Luzzati, R., & Conradt, C. (2000). Treatment of low back pain exacerbations with willow bark extract: A randomized double-blind study. *Am J Med, 109*(1), 9–14.

Chrubasik, S., Junck, H., Breitschwerdt, H., Conradt, C., & Zappe, H. (1999). Effectiveness of harpagophytum extract WS 1531 in the treatment of exacerbation of low back pain: A randomized, placebo-controlled, double-blind study. *Eur J Anaesthesiol, 16*(2), 118–129.

Deare, J. C., Zheng, Z., Xue, C. C., Liu, J. P., Shang, J., Scott, S. W., & Littlejohn, G. (2013). Acupuncture for treating fibromyalgia. *Cochrane Database Syst Rev* (5), CD007070. doi:10.1002/14651858.CD007070.pub2

Dorsher, P. T., & McIntosh, P. M. (2011). Acupuncture's effects in treating the sequelae of acute and chronic spinal cord injuries: A review of allopathic and traditional Chinese medicine literature. *Evid Based Complement Alternat Med, 2011*, 428108. doi:10.1093/ecam/nep010

Gagnier, J. J., Oltean, H., van Tulder, M. W., Berman, B. M., Bombardier, C., & Robbins, C. B. (2016). Herbal medicine for low back pain: A Cochrane review. *Spine (Phila Pa 1976), 41*(2), 116–133. doi:10.1097/BRS.0000000000001310

Goldman, N., Chen, M., Fujita, T., Xu, Q., Peng, W., Liu, W., . . . & Nedergaard, M. (2010). Adenosine A1 receptors mediate local antinociceptive effects of acupuncture. *Nat Neurosci, 13*(7), 883–888. doi:10.1038/nn.2562

Guillory, J., Chang, P., Henderson, C. R., Shengelia, R., Lama, S., Warmington, M., . . . & Reid, M. C. (2015). Piloting a text message-based social support intervention for patients with chronic pain: Establishing feasibility and preliminary efficacy. *Clin J Pain, 31*(6), 548–556. doi:10.1097/AJP.0000000000000193

Gutgsell, K. J., Schluchter, M., Margevicius, S., DeGolia, P. A., McLaughlin, B., Harris, M., . . . & Wiencek, C. (2013). Music therapy reduces pain in palliative care patients: A randomized controlled trial. *J Pain Symptom Manage, 45*(5), 822–831. doi:10.1016/j.jpainsymman.2012.05.008

Hashempur, M. H., Sadrneshin, S., Mosavat, S. H., & Ashraf, A. (2016). Green tea (Camellia sinensis) for patients with knee osteoarthritis: A randomized open-label active-controlled clinical trial. *Clin Nutr.* doi:10.1016/j.clnu.2016.12.004

Jensen, M. P., & Turk, D. C. (2014). Contributions of psychology to the understanding and treatment of people with chronic pain: Why it matters to ALL psychologists. *Am Psychol, 69*(2), 105–118. doi:10.1037/a0035641

Lam, M., Galvin, R., & Curry, P. (2013). Effectiveness of acupuncture for nonspecific chronic low back pain: A systematic review and meta-analysis. *Spine (Phila Pa 1976), 38*(24), 2124–2138. doi:10.1097/01.brs.0000435025.65564.b7

Lee, C., Crawford, C., Wallerstedt, D., York, A., Duncan, A., Smith, J., . . . & Jonas, W. (2012). The effectiveness of acupuncture research across components of the trauma spectrum response (TSR): A systematic review of reviews. *Syst Rev, 1*, 46. doi:10.1186/2046-4053-1-46

Lee, J. H., Choi, T. Y., Lee, M. S., Lee, H., & Shin, B. C. (2013). Acupuncture for acute low back pain: A systematic review. *Clin J Pain, 29*(2), 172–185. doi:10.1097/AJP.0b013e31824909f9

Malone, M. A., & Gloyer, K. (2013). Complementary and alternative treatments in sports medicine. *Prim Care, 40*(4), 945–968, ix. doi:10.1016/j.pop.2013.08.010

Manyanga, T., Froese, M., Zarychanski, R., Abou-Setta, A., Friesen, C., Tennenhouse, M., & Shay, B. L. (2014). Pain management with acupuncture in osteoarthritis: A systematic review and meta-analysis. *BMC Complement Altern Med, 14*, 312. doi:10.1186/1472-6882-14-312

McAlindon, T. E., Jacques, P., Zhang, Y., Hannan, M. T., Aliabadi, P., Weissman, B., . . . & Felson, D. T. (1996). Do antioxidant micronutrients

protect against the development and progression of knee osteoarthritis? *Arthritis Rheum, 39*(4), 648–656.

Myers, C. D., White, B. A., & Heft, M. W. (2002). A review of complementary and alternative medicine use for treating chronic facial pain. *J Am Dent Assoc, 133*(9), 1189–1196; quiz 1259-1160.

Napadow, V., Liu, J., Li, M., Kettner, N., Ryan, A., Kwong, K. K., . . . & Audette, J. F. (2007). Somatosensory cortical plasticity in carpal tunnel syndrome treated by acupuncture. *Hum Brain Mapp, 28*(3), 159–171. doi:10.1002/hbm.20261

Napadow, V., Liu, J., Li, M., Kettner, N., Ryan, A., Kwong, K. K., . . . & Audette, J. F. (2007). Somatosensory cortical plasticity in carpal tunnel syndrome treated by acupuncture. *Hum Brain Mapp, 28*(3), 159–171. doi:10.1002/hbm.20261

The National Institute of Health Consensus Development Program (1997). Acupuncture. NIH Consensus Development Conference Statement November 3–5, 1997. Retrieved from http://consessus.nih.gov/1997/1997 Acupuncture 107html.htm

Nguyen, C. T., & Wang, M. B. (2013). Complementary and integrative treatments: Atypical facial pain. *Otolaryngol Clin North Am, 46*(3), 367–382. doi:10.1016/j.otc.2013.01.002

Oltean, H., Robbins, C., van Tulder, M. W., Berman, B. M., Bombardier, C., & Gagnier, J. J. (2014). Herbal medicine for low-back pain. *Cochrane Database Syst Rev* (12), CD004504. doi:10.1002/14651858.CD004504.pub4

Qaseem, A., Wilt, T. J., McLean, R. M., Forciea, M. A., & Clinical Guidelines Committee of the American College of Physicians. (2017). Noninvasive treatments for acute, subacute, and chronic low back pain: A clinical practice guideline from the American College of Physicians. *Ann Intern Med, 166*(7), 514–530. doi:10.7326/M16-2367

Sardella, A., Demarosi, F., Barbieri, C., & Lodi, G. (2009). An up-to-date view on persistent idiopathic facial pain. *Minerva Stomatol, 58*(6), 289–299.

Stuyt, E. B., & Voyles, C. A. (2016). The National Acupuncture Detoxification Association protocol, auricular acupuncture to support patients with substance abuse and behavioral health disorders: Current perspectives. *Subst Abuse Rehabil, 7*, 169–180. doi:10.2147/SAR.S99161

Thomas, D. A., Maslin, B., Legler, A., Springer, E., Asgerally, A., & Vadivelu, N. (2016). Role of alternative therapies for chronic pain syndromes. *Curr Pain Headache Rep, 20*(5), 29. doi:10.1007/s11916-016-0562-z

Vickers, A. J., Cronin, A. M., Maschino, A. C., Lewith, G., MacPherson, H., Foster, N. E., . . . & Acupuncture Trialists' Collaboration. (2012). Acupuncture for chronic pain: Individual patient data meta-analysis. *Arch Intern Med, 172*(19), 1444–1453. doi:10.1001/archinternmed.2012.3654

Wang, W., & Wu, S. X. (2014). Treating pain with acupuncture. *JAMA, 312*(13), 1365–1365.

Witt, C. M., Pach, D., Brinkhaus, B., Wruck, K., Tag, B., Mank, S., & Willich, S. N. (2009). Safety of acupuncture: Results of a prospective observational study with 229,230 patients and introduction of a medical information and consent form. *Forsch Komplementmed, 16*(2), 91–97. doi:10.1159/000209315

Xu, M., Yan, S., Yin, X., Li, X., Gao, S., Han, R., . . . & Lei, G. (2013). Acupuncture for chronic low back pain in long-term follow-up: A meta-analysis of 13 randomized controlled trials. *Am J Chin Med, 41*(1), 1–19. doi:10.1142/S0192415X13500018

Zhang, Y. (2014). American adult acupuncture use: Preliminary findings from NHIS 2012 data. *J Altern Complement Med, 20*(5), A109–A110.

## Chapter 21

Altier, N., & Stewart, J. (1999). The role of dopamine in the nucleus accumbens in analgesia. *Life Sci, 65*(22), 2269–2287.

Bernatzky, G., Presch, M., Anderson, M., & Panksepp, J. (2011). Emotional foundations of music as a non-pharmacological pain management tool in modern medicine. *Neurosci Biobehav Rev, 35*(9), 1989–1999. doi:10.1016/j.neubiorev.2011.06.005

Blood, A. J., & Zatorre, R. J. (2001). Intensely pleasurable responses to music correlate with activity in brain regions implicated in reward and emotion. *Proc Natl Acad Sci U S A, 98*(20), 11818–11823. doi:10.1073/pnas.191355898

Boehm, K., Büssing, A., & Ostermann, T. (2012). Aromatherapy as an adjuvant treatment in cancer care—a descriptive systematic review. *Afr J Tradit Complement Altern Med, 9*(4), 503–518.

Bradt, J., Dileo, C., Grocke, D., & Magill, L. (2011). Music interventions for improving psychological and physical outcomes in cancer patients. *Cochrane Database Syst Rev* (8), CD006911. doi:10.1002/14651858.CD006911.pub2

Buckle, J. (2002). Clinical aromatherapy and AIDS. *J Assoc Nurses AIDS Care, 13*(3), 81–99. doi:10.1177/10529002013003006

Busch, V., Magerl, W., Kern, U., Haas, J., Hajak, G., & Eichhammer, P. (2012). The effect of deep and slow breathing on pain perception, autonomic activity, and mood processing—an experimental study. *Pain Med, 13*(2), 215–228. doi:10.1111/j.1526-4637.2011.01243.x

Cepeda, M. S., Carr, D. B., Lau, J., & Alvarez, H. (2006). Music for pain relief. *Cochrane Database Syst Rev* (2), CD004843. doi:10.1002/14651858.CD004843.pub2

Chanda, M. L., & Levitin, D. J. (2013). The neurochemistry of music. *Trends Cogn Sci, 17*(4), 179–193. doi:10.1016/j.tics.2013.02.007

Dhany, A. L., Mitchell, T., & Foy, C. (2012). Aromatherapy and massage intrapartum service impact on use of analgesia and anesthesia in women in labor: A retrospective case note analysis. *J Altern Complement Med, 18*(10), 932–938. doi:10.1089/acm.2011.0254

Fancourt, D., Ockelford, A., & Belai, A. (2014). The psychoneuroimmunological effects of music: A systematic review and a new model. *Brain Behav Immun, 36*, 15–26. doi:10.1016/j.bbi.2013.10.014

Garza-Villarreal, E. A., Wilson, A. D., Vase, L., Brattico, E., Barrios, F. A., Jensen, T. S., . . . & Vuust, P. (2014). Music reduces pain and increases functional mobility in fibromyalgia. *Front Psychol, 5*, 90. doi:10.3389/fpsyg.2014.00090

Gedney, J. J., Glover, T. L., & Fillingim, R. B. (2004). Sensory and affective pain discrimination after inhalation of essential oils. *Psychosom Med, 66*(4), 599–606. doi:10.1097/01.psy.0000132875.01986.47

Guétin, S., Coudeyre, E., Picot, M. C., Ginies, P., Graber-Duvernay, B., Ratsimba, D., . . . & Hérisson, C. (2005). Effect of music therapy among hospitalized patients with chronic low back pain: A controlled, randomized trial. *Ann Readapt Med Phys, 48*(5), 217–224. doi:10.1016/j.annrmp.2005.02.003

Guétin, S., Giniès, P., Siou, D. K., Picot, M. C., Pommié, C., Guldner, E., . . . & Touchon, J. (2012). The effects of music intervention in the management of chronic pain: A single-blind, randomized, controlled trial. *Clin J Pain, 28*(4), 329–337. doi:10.1097/AJP.0b013e31822be973

Hole, J., Hirsch, M., Ball, E., & Meads, C. (2015). Music as an aid for postoperative recovery in adults: A systematic review and meta-analysis. *Lancet, 386*(10004), 1659–1671. doi:10.1016/S0140-6736(15)60169-6

Huang, S. T., Good, M., & Zauszniewski, J. A. (2010). The effectiveness of music in relieving pain in cancer patients: A randomized controlled trial. *Int J Nurs Stud, 47*(11), 1354–1362. doi:10.1016/j.ijnurstu.2010.03.008

Juslin, P. N., & Västfjäll, D. (2008). Emotional responses to music: The need to consider underlying mechanisms. *Behav Brain Sci, 31*(5), 559–575; discussion 575–621. doi:10.1017/S0140525X08005293

Kim, J. T., Wajda, M., Cuff, G., Serota, D., Schlame, M., Axelrod, D. M., . . . & Bekker, A. Y. (2006). Evaluation of aromatherapy in treating postoperative pain: Pilot study. *Pain Pract, 6*(4), 273–277. doi:10.1111/j.1533-2500.2006.00095.x

Korhan, E. A., Uyar, M., Eyigör, C., Hakverdio?lu Yönt, G., Çelik, S., & Khorshıd, L. (2014). The effects of music therapy on pain in patients with neuropathic pain. *Pain Manag Nurs, 15*(1), 306–314. doi:10.1016/j.pmn.2012.10.006

Koyanagi, S., Himukashi, S., Mukaida, K., Shichino, T., & Fukuda, K. (2008). Dopamine D2-like receptor in the nucleus accumbens is involved in the antinociceptive effect of nitrous oxide. *Anesth Analg, 106*(6), 1904–1909. doi:10.1213/ane.0b013e318172b15b

Lakhan, S. E., Sheafer, H., & Tepper, D. (2016). The effectiveness of aromatherapy in reducing pain: A systematic review and meta-analysis. *Pain Res Treat, 2016*, 8158693. doi:10.1155/2016/8158693

Masaoka, Y., Takayama, M., Yajima, H., Kawase, A., Takakura, N., & Homma, I. (2013). Analgesia is enhanced by providing information

regarding good outcomes associated with an odor: Placebo effects in aromatherapy? *Evid Based Complement Alternat Med, 2013*, 921802. doi:10.1155/2013/921802

McCaffrey, R., & Freeman, E. (2003). Effect of music on chronic osteo-arthritis pain in older people. *J Adv Nurs, 44*(5), 517–524.

Mitchell, L. A., & MacDonald, R. A. (2006). An experimental investigation of the effects of preferred and relaxing music listening on pain perception. *J Music Ther, 43*(4), 295–316.

Rouwette, T., Vanelderen, P., Roubos, E. W., Kozicz, T., & Vissers, K. (2012). The amygdala, a relay station for switching on and off pain. *Eur J Pain, 16*(6), 782–792. doi:10.1002/j.1532-2149.2011.00071.x

Salimpoor, V. N., van den Bosch, I., Kovacevic, N., McIntosh, A. R., Dagher, A., & Zatorre, R. J. (2013). Interactions between the nucleus accumbens and auditory cortices predict music reward value. *Science, 340*(6129), 216–219. doi:10.1126/science.1231059

Shin, B. C., & Lee, M. S. (2007). Effects of aromatherapy acupressure on hemiplegic shoulder pain and motor power in stroke patients: A pilot study. *J Altern Complement Med, 13*(2), 247–251. doi:10.1089/acm.2006.6189

Stefano, G. B., Zhu, W., Cadet, P., Salamon, E., & Mantione, K. J. (2004). Music alters constitutively expressed opiate and cytokine processes in listeners. *Med Sci Monit, 10*(6), MS18–27.

Sunitha Suresh, B. S., De Oliveira, G. S., & Suresh, S. (2015). The effect of audio therapy to treat postoperative pain in children undergoing major surgery: A randomized controlled trial. *Pediatr Surg Int, 31*(2), 197–201. doi:10.1007/s00383-014-3649-9

Valnet, J. (1980). *The practice of aromatherapy.* Saffron Walden, UK: C. W. Daniel.

## Chapter 22

Abe, K., Ichinomiya, R., Kanai, T., & Yamamoto, K. (2012). Effect of a Japanese energy healing method known as Johrei on viability and proliferation of cultured cancer cells in vitro. *J Altern Complement Med, 18*(3), 221–228. doi:10.1089/acm.2011.0467

Agdal, R., von B Hjelmborg, J., & Johannessen, H. (2011). Energy healing for cancer: A critical review. *Forsch Komplementmed, 18*(3), 146–154. doi:10.1159/000329316

Anderson, J. G., & Taylor, A. G. (2011). Effects of healing touch in clinical practice: A systematic review of randomized clinical trials. *J Holist Nurs, 29*(3), 221–228. doi:10.1177/0898010110393353

Anderson, J. G., & Taylor, A. G. (2012). Biofield therapies and cancer pain. *Clin J Oncol Nurs, 16*(1), 43–48. doi:10.1188/12.CJON.

Easter, A., & Watt, C. (2011). It's good to know: How treatment knowledge and belief affect the outcome of distant healing intentionality for arthritis sufferers. *J Psychosom Res, 71*(2), 86–89. doi:10.1016/j.jpsychores.2011.02.003

Eisenberg, D. M., Davis, R. B., Ettner, S. L., Appel, S., Wilkey, S., Van Rompay, M., & Kessler, R. C. (1998). Trends in alternative medicine use in the United States, 1990–1997: Results of a follow-up national survey. *JAMA, 280*(18), 1569–1575.

Ernst, E. (2003). Distant healing—an "update" of a systematic review. *Wien Klin Wochenschr, 115*(7–8), 241–245.

Fazzino, D. L., Griffin, M. T., McNulty, R. S., & Fitzpatrick, J. J. (2010). Energy healing and pain: A review of the literature. *Holist Nurs Pract, 24*(2), 79–88. doi:10.1097/HNP.0b013e3181d39718

Fernros, L., Furhoff, A. K., & Wändell, P. E. (2008). Improving quality of life using compound mind-body therapies: Evaluation of a course intervention with body movement and breath therapy, guided imagery, chakra experiencing and mindfulness meditation. *Qual Life Res, 17*(3), 367–376. doi:10.1007/s11136-008-9321-x

Foley, M. K., Anderson, J., Mallea, L., Morrison, K., & Downey, M. (2016). Effects of healing touch on postsurgical adult outpatients. *J Holist Nurs, 34*(3), 271–279. doi:10.1177/0898010115609486

Hammerschlag, R., Jain, S., Baldwin, A. L., Gronowicz, G., Lutgendorf, S. K., Oschman, J. L., & Yount, G. L. (2012). Biofield research: A roundtable discussion of scientific and methodological issues. *J Altern Complement Med, 18*(12), 1081–1086. doi:10.1089/acm.2012.1502

Havey, J., Vlasses, F. R., Vlasses, P. H., Ludwig-Beymer, P., & Hackbarth, D. (2014). The effect of animal-assisted therapy on pain medication use after joint replacement. *Anthrozoös, 27*(3), 361–369.

Henneghan, A. M., & Schnyer, R. N. (2015). Biofield therapies for symptom management in palliative and end-of-life care. *Am J Hosp Palliat Care, 32*(1), 90–100. doi:10.1177/1049909113509400

Hutchison, C. P., D'Alessio, B., Forward, J. B., & Newshan, G. (1999). Body-mind-spirit: Healing touch: An energetic approach. *AJN, 99*(4), 43–48.

Jain, S., & Mills, P. J. (2010). Biofield therapies: Helpful or full of hype? A best evidence synthesis. *Int J Behav Med, 17*(1), 1–16.

Jhaveri, A., Walsh, S. J., Wang, Y., McCarthy, M., & Gronowicz, G. (2008). Therapeutic touch affects DNA synthesis and mineralization of human osteoblasts in culture. *J Orthop Res, 26*(11), 1541–1546. doi:10.1002/jor.20688

Lamke, D., Catlin, A., & Mason-Chadd, M. (2014). "Not just a theory": The relationship between Jin Shin Jyutsu® self-care training for nurses and stress, physical health, emotional health, and caring efficacy. *J Holist Nurs, 32*(4), 278–289. doi:10.1177/0898010114531906

Lu, D. F., Hart, L. K., Lutgendorf, S. K., & Perkhounkova, Y. (2013). The effect of healing touch on the pain and mobility of persons with osteoarthritis: A feasibility study. *Geriatr Nurs, 34*(4), 314–322. doi:10.1016/j.gerinurse.2013.05.003

Marcus, D. A., Bernstein, C. D., Constantin, J. M., Kunkel, F. A., Breuer, P., & Hanlon, R. B. (2012). Animal-assisted therapy at an outpatient pain management clinic. *Pain Med, 13*(1), 45–57. doi:10.1111/j.1526-4637.2011.01294.x

McFadden, K. L., & Hernández, T. D. (2010). Cardiovascular benefits of acupressure (Jin Shin) following stroke. *Complement Ther Med, 18*(1), 42–48. doi:10.1016/j.ctim.2010.01.001

Miller, R. N. (1982). Study on the effectiveness of remote mental healing. *Med Hypotheses, 8*(5), 481–490.

Mulkins, A., Verhoef, M., Eng, J., Findlay, B., & Ramsum, D. (2003). Evaluation of the Tzu Chi Institute for Complementary and Alternative Medicine's Integrative Care Program. *J Altern Complement Med, 9*(4), 585–592. doi:10.1089/107555303322284893

Palmer, R. F., Katerndahl, D., & Morgan-Kidd, J. (2004). A randomized trial of the effects of remote intercessory prayer: Interactions with personal beliefs on problem-specific outcomes and functional status. *J Altern Complement Med, 10*(3), 438–448. doi:10.1089/1075553041323803

Rubik, B. (2002). The biofield hypothesis: Its biophysical basis and role in medicine. *J Altern Complement Med, 8*(6), 703–717. doi:10.1089/10755530260511711

Searls, K., & Fawcett, J. (2011). Effect of Jin Shin Jyutsu energy medicine treatments on women diagnosed with breast cancer. *J Holist Nurs, 29*(4), 270–278. doi:10.1177/0898010111412186

Sempell, P. (2000). Jin Shin Jyutsu and modern medicine: Integrating the ancient healing art of Jin Shin Jyutsu with the modern medicine of heart transplants. *Massage & Bodywork.*

So, P. S., Jiang, J. Y., & Qin, Y. (2008). Touch therapies for pain relief in adults. *The Cochrane Library.*

Targ, E. (1997). Evaluating distant healing: A research review. *Altern Ther Health Med, 3*(6), 74–78.

Tsubono, K., Thomlinson, P., & Shealy, C. N. (2009). The effects of distant healing performed by a spiritual healer on chronic pain: A randomized controlled trial. *Altern Ther Health Med, 15*(3), 30–34.

Wardell, D. W., & Weymouth, K. F. (2004). Review of studies of healing touch. *J Nurs Scholarsh, 36*(2), 147–154.

Welcher, B., & Kish, J. (2001). Reducing pain and anxiety through healing touch. *Healing Touch Newsletter, 1*(3), 19.

Yu, T., Tsai, H. L., & Hwang, M. L. (2003). Suppressing tumor progression of in vitro prostate cancer cells by emitted psychosomatic

power through Zen meditation. *Am J Chin Med, 31*(3), 499–507. doi:10.1142/S0192415X03001132

Zacharia R, Højgaard L, Zachariae, C, Vaeth M, Bang B, & Skov L. (2005). The effect of spiritual healing *in vitro* tumour cell proliferation and viability—an experimental study. *Br J Cancer, 93*, 538–543.

## Chapter 23

Buchanan, P. A., & Ulrich, B. D. (2001). The Feldenkrais Method: A dynamic approach to changing motor behavior. *Res Q Exerc Sport, 72*(4), 315–323. doi:10.1080/02701367.2001.10608968

Büssing, A., Khalsa, S. B., Michalsen, A., Sherman, K. J., & Telles, S. (2012). Yoga as a therapeutic intervention. *Evid Based Complement Alternat Med, 2012*, 174291. doi:10.1155/2012/174291

Büssing, A., Ostermann, T., Lüdtke, R., & Michalsen, A. (2012). Effects of yoga interventions on pain and pain-associated disability: A meta-analysis. *J Pain, 13*(1), 1–9. doi:10.1016/j.jpain.2011.10.001

Carson, J. W., Carson, K. M., Jones, K. D., Bennett, R. M., Wright, C. L., & Mist, S. D. (2010). A pilot randomized controlled trial of the Yoga of Awareness program in the management of fibromyalgia. *Pain, 151*(2), 530–539. doi:10.1016/j.pain.2010.08.020

Chou, R., Huffman, L. H., American Pain Society, & American College of Physicians. (2007). Nonpharmacologic therapies for acute and chronic low back pain: A review of the evidence for an American Pain Society/American College of Physicians clinical practice guideline. *Ann Intern Med, 147*(7), 492–504.

Connors, K. A., Galea, M. P., & Said, C. M. (2011). Feldenkrais method balance classes improve balance in older adults: A controlled trial. *Evid Based Complement Alternat Med, 2011*, 873672. doi:10.1093/ecam/nep055

Cramer, H., Krucoff, C., & Dobos, G. (2013). Adverse events associated with yoga: A systematic review of published case reports and case series. *PLoS One, 8*(10), e75515. doi:10.1371/journal.pone.0075515

Crow, E. M., Jeannot, E., & Trewhela, A. (2015). Effectiveness of Iyengar yoga in treating spinal (back and neck) pain: A systematic review. *Int J Yoga, 8*(1), 3–14. doi:10.4103/0973-6131.146046

The Feldenkrais method of somatic education. (2012, December). Retrieved from http://www.feldenkrais.com

Haaz, S., & Bartlett, S. J. (2011). Yoga for arthritis: A scoping review. *Rheum Dis Clin North Am, 37*(1), 33–46. doi:10.1016/j.rdc.2010.11.001

Ives, J. C., & Shelley, G. A. (1998). The Feldenkrais Method® in rehabilitation: A review. *Work, 11*(1), 75–90. doi:10.3233/WOR-1998-11109

Kendall, S. A., Ekselius, L., Gerdle, B., Sörén, B., & Bengtsson, A. (2001). Feldenkrais intervention in fibromyalgia patients: A pilot study. *J Musculoskelet Pain, 9*(4), 25–35.

Kirkwood, G., Rampes, H., Tuffrey, V., Richardson, J., & Pilkington, K. (2005). Yoga for anxiety: A systematic review of the research evidence. *Br J Sports Med, 39*(12), 884–891; discussion 891. doi:10.1136/bjsm.2005.018069

Kuttner, L., Chambers, C. T., Hardial, J., Israel, D. M., Jacobson, K., & Evans, K. (2006). A randomized trial of yoga for adolescents with irritable bowel syndrome. *Pain Res Manag, 11*(4), 217–223.

Langhorst, J., Häuser, W., Bernardy, K., Lucius, H., Settan, M., Winkelmann, A., . . . & Arbeitsgemeinschaft der Wissen-schaftlichen Medizinischen Fachgesellschaften. (2012). Comple-mentary and alternative therapies for fibromyalgia syndrome: Systematic review, meta-analysis and guideline. *Schmerz, 26*(3), 311–317. doi:10.1007/s00482-012-1178-9

Lundqvist, L. O., Zetterlund, C., & Richter, H. O. (2014). Effects of Feldenkrais method on chronic neck/scapular pain in people with visual impairment: A randomized controlled trial with one-year follow-up. *Arch Phys Med Rehabil, 95*(9), 1656–1661. doi:10.1016/j.apmr.2014.05.013

Ohman, A., Aström, L., & Malmgren-Olsson, E. B. (2011). Feldenkrais® therapy as group treatment for chronic pain—a qualitative evaluation. *J Bodyw Mov Ther, 15*(2), 153–161. doi:10.1016/j.jbmt.2010.03.003

Paolucci, T., Zangrando, F., Iosa, M., De Angelis, S., Marzoli, C., Piccinini, G., & Saraceni, V. M. (2017). Improved interoceptive awareness in chronic low back pain: A comparison of back school versus Feldenkrais method. *Disabil Rehabil, 39*(10), 994–1001. doi:10.1080/09638288.2016.1175035

Plastaras, C., Schran, S., Kim, N., Darr, D., & Chen, M. S. (2013). Manipulative therapy (Feldenkrais, massage, chiropractic manipulation) for neck pain. *Curr Rheumatol Rep, 15*(7), 339. doi:10.1007/s11926-013-0339-x

Posadzki, P., Ernst, E., Terry, R., & Lee, M. S. (2011). Is yoga effective for pain? A systematic review of randomized clinical trials. *Complement Ther Med, 19*(5), 281–287. doi:10.1016/j.ctim.2011.07.004

Pugh, J. D., & Williams, A. M. (2014). Feldenkrais method empowers adults with chronic back pain. *Holist Nurs Pract, 28*(3), 171–183. doi:10.1097/HNP.0000000000000026

Qaseem, A., Wilt, T. J., McLean, R. M., Forciea, M. A., & Clinical Guidelines Committee of the American College of Physicians. (2017). Noninvasive treatments for acute, subacute, and chronic low back pain: A clinical practice guideline from the American College of Physicians. *Ann Intern Med, 166*(7), 514–530. doi:10.7326/M16-2367

Raub, J. A. (2002). Psychophysiologic effects of Hatha Yoga on musculoskeletal and cardiopulmonary function: A literature review. *J Altern Complement Med, 8*(6), 797–812. doi:10.1089/10755530260511810

Reis, P. (2012). Cochrane review: Relaxation and yoga may decrease pain during labour and increase satisfaction with pain relief, but better quality evidence is needed. *Evid Based Nurs, 15*(4), 105–106. doi:10.1136/ebnurs-2012-100795

Rosen, L., French, A., Sullivan, G., & RYT-200. (2015). Complementary, holistic, and integrative medicine: Yoga. *Pediatr Rev, 36*(10), 468–474. doi:10.1542/pir.36-10-468

Ullmann, G., Williams, H. G., Hussey, J., Durstine, J. L., & McClenaghan, B. A. (2010). Effects of Feldenkrais exercises on balance, mobility, balance confidence, and gait performance in community-dwelling adults age 65 and older. *J Altern Complement Med, 16*(1), 97–105. doi:10.1089/acm.2008.0612

Webb, R., Cofré Lizama, L. E., & Galea, M. P. (2013). Moving with ease: Feldenkrais method classes for people with osteoarthritis. *Evid Based Complement Alternat Med, 2013*, 479142. doi:10.1155/2013/479142

Wieland, L. S., Skoetz, N., Pilkington, K., Vempati, R., D'Adamo, C. R., & Berman, B. M. (2017). Yoga treatment for chronic non-specific low back pain. *Cochrane Database Syst Rev, 1*, CD010671. doi:10.1002/14651858.CD010671.pub2

Wolsko, P. M., Eisenberg, D. M., Davis, R. B., Kessler, R., & Phillips, R. S. (2003). Patterns and perceptions of care for treatment of back and neck pain: Results of a national survey. *Spine (Phila Pa 1976), 28*(3), 292–297; discussion 298. doi:10.1097/01.BRS.0000042225.88095.7C

Wren, A. A., Wright, M. A., Carson, J. W., & Keefe, F. J. (2011). Yoga for persistent pain: New findings and directions for an ancient practice. *Pain, 152*(3), 477–480. doi:10.1016/j.pain.2010.11.017

# Index

# About the Author

Paul J Christo, MD, MBA is listed as a Top Doctor and among the top 1% for Pain Management by *U.S. News & World Report*. He hosts an award-winning, nationally syndicated SIRIUS XM radio talk show on overcoming pain called, *Aches and Gains*®. The show features distinguished celebrity guests such as Naomi Judd, Joe Montana, and Maya Angelou.

An Associate Professor in the Division of Pain Medicine at the Johns Hopkins University School of Medicine, Dr. Christo is an international lecturer and serves on numerous journal editorial boards. He has published more than 100 articles and book chapters related to pain. He was honored by the American Society of Pain Educators as Pain Educator of the Year for his transformational work on public education through the media.

His show, *Aches and Gains*® has earned the John and Emma Bonica Public Service Award from the American Pain Society which recognizes distinguished contributions to the field of pain medicine through public education, dissemination of information, and public service. Dr. Christo was selected as a Mayday Pain and Society Fellow, and named a "Hero" by The Pain Community, a patient advocacy association for his work on *Aches and Gains*®. A member of *Men's Health Magazine* medical advisory board, Dr. Christo proudly serves as their first pain specialist.

Dr. Christo is a board-certified pain specialist and anesthesiologist. He completed his fellowship in pain medicine at Johns Hopkins Medicine, residency in anesthesiology at Harvard Medical School, Massachusetts General Hospital, and internship at Johns Hopkins Medicine. He is a graduate of the University of Notre Dame and the University of Louisville School of Medicine. He also earned an MBA from the Johns Hopkins Carey Business School. Dr. Christo is widely consulted by the media for his expertise in pain diagnosis and treatment.